As HIV infection in childhood increases, concomitant with the spread in adult infection, so too is there rapid expansion in our knowledge of the complexities of paediatric infection. Clearly general paediatricians and other members of the multidisciplinary team of carers will increasingly be seeking guidance on management strategies to address a wide range of complex clinical problems.

This very practical and concise volume discusses the epidemiology, diagnosis, natural history and care of the HIV-infected child. As the book draws upon an international team of contributors, the considerable differences between European treatment strategies and those of North America can be contrasted and evaluated. This guide will be of particular interest to paediatricians, whether in a hospital, specialist unit or community-based setting. General practitioners, obstetricians, nurses, counsellors and epidemiologists should also benefit from this book.

HIV infection in children

HIV infection in children
A guide to practical management

Edited by

Jacqueline Y. Q. Mok
Department of Child Life & Health,
University of Edinburgh

and

Marie-Louise Newell
Institute of Child Health, London

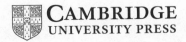
CAMBRIDGE
UNIVERSITY PRESS

Published by the Press Syndicate of the University of Cambridge
The Pitt Building, Trumpington Street, Cambridge CB2 1RP
40 West 20th Street, New York, NY 10011–4211, USA
10 Stamford Road, Oakleigh, Melbourne 3166, Australia

First published 1995

Printed in Great Britain at the University Press, Cambridge

A catalogue record for this book is available from the British Library

Library of Congress cataloguing in publication data available

ISBN 0 521 45421 2 hardback

Contents

Foreword

Paediatric HIV infection is associated with a wide range of complex clinical problems and knowledge is changing rapidly. Now, well into the second decade of the epidemic, it is timely to take stock of existing knowledge and expertise in a readily accessible form. Like many other chronic conditions, the management of paediatric HIV infection requires a coordinated approach, involving input from a range of disciplines.

Contributors to this book have been chosen because of their personal experience from working with children and families affected by HIV. This informed group of authors covers a diversity of subjects, ranging from the epidemiology of paediatric HIV infection, the diagnosis and immunology, clinical symptomatology and management, to the role of the nurse, the school and carers. Many of the contributors are active participants in the European Collaborative Study on children born to HIV-infected mothers.

The book brings together a range of areas relevant to paediatric HIV infection and will be of value to a wide readership. It should be of particular interest to paediatricians, whether they work in a specialist unit, a district hospital or as a community-based paediatrician. General practitioners, obstetricians, infectious disease specialists and other health care workers will also find the practical nature of the book useful. It should also appeal to epidemiologists in this field, as well as to anyone who may come into contact with HIV-infected people or their families. The editors are to be congratulated on their choice of authors and the readily accessible and up-to-date information provided in a concise and manageable form.

Professor Catherine Peckham

Contributors

A. Graham Bird

Churchill Hospital, Old Road, Headington, Oxford OX3 7LJ, UK

Stéphane Blanche

Unité d'Immuno-Hématologie, Département de Pédiatrie, Hôpital Necker-Enfants Malades, 149 rue de Sèvres, 75743 Paris, Cedex 15, France

Raymond P. Brettle

Regional Infectious Diseases Unit, City Hospital, Greenbank Drive, Edinburgh EH10 5SB, UK

M. Blake Caldwell

Department of Health and Human Services, Centers for Disease Control and Prevention (CDC), Atlanta, GA 30333, USA

Edward M. Connor

Medimmune, Inc., 35 West Watkins Mill Road, Gaithersburg, MD 20878, USA

Anita De Rossi

Istituto di Oncologia, Università di Padova, Via Gattamelata 64, 35128 Padua, Italy

Candy Duggan

The Hospitals for Sick Children, Great Ormond Street, London WC1N 3JH, UK

Carlo Giaquinto

Dipartimento di Pediatria, Università degli Studi di Padova, Via Giustiniani 3, 35100 Padua, Italy

Diana M. Gibb

Institute of Child Health, 30 Guilford Street, London WC1N 1EN, UK

Peta Hemmings

Orchard Project, Barnardos, Orchard House, Fenwick Terrace, Jesmond, Newcastle-upon-Tyne NE2 2JQ, UK

Naomi Honigsbaum — European Forum on HIV/AIDS Children and Families, National Children's Bureau, 8 Wakley Street, London EC1V 7QE, UK

Frank D. Johnstone — Simpson Memorial Maternity Pavilion, Lauriston Place, Edinburgh EH3 9EF, UK

Peter Jones — Haemophilia Centre, Royal Victoria Infirmary, Queen Victoria Road, Newcastle-upon-Tyne NE1 4LP, UK

Jack Levy — Paediatric Infectious Diseases Unit, 322 rue haute, Hôpital Universitaire Saint-Pierre, 1000 Brussels, Belgium

Mary Lou Lindegren — Department of Health and Human Services, Centers for Disease Control and Prevention (CDC), Atlanta, GA 30333, USA

Rebecca Lwin — The Hospitals for Sick Children, Great Ormond Street, London WC1N 3JH, UK

George D. McSherry — Department of Pediatrics, UMD-New Jersey Medical School, 185 South Orange Avenue, University Heights, Newark, NJ 07103, USA

Fiona Mitchell — Regional Infectious Diseases Unit, City Hospital, Greenbank Drive, Edinburgh EH10 5SB, UK

Jacqueline Y. Q. Mok — Regional Infectious Diseases Unit, City Hospital, Greenbank Drive, Edinburgh EH10 5SB, UK

Marie-Louise Newell — Institute of Child Health, 30 Guilford Street, London WC1N 1EN, UK

Margaret Oxtoby — Centers for Infectious Diseases, Centers for Disease Control and Prevention (CDC), Atlanta, GA 30333, USA

Pier-Angelo Tovo — Istituto Clinica Pediatrica, Corso Polonia 94, 10126 Turin, Italy

'A headteacher' and 'A parent' — c/o Jacqueline Mok, Regional Infectious Diseases Unit, City Hospital, Greenbank Drive, Edinburgh EH10 5SB, UK

Abbreviations

Ab	Antibody
ACTG	AIDS Clinical Trials Group
Ag	Antigen
AIDS	Acquired immune deficiency syndrome
ANRS	Agence Nationale de Recherches sur le SIDA
ARC	AIDS related complex
AZT	3'-Azido-3'-deoxythymidine (also known as ZDV)
BAL	Bronchoalveolar lavage
BHAP	Bis-heteroarylpiperazine
CD4	Also known as T helper cells, a subset of T lymphocytes
CD8	Also known as T suppressor cells, a subset of T lymphocytes
CDC	Centers for Disease Control and Prevention, Atlanta, Georgia
CMV	Cytomegalovirus
CNS	Central nervous system
CSF	Cerebrospinal fluid
CT	Computed tomography
CTL	Cytotoxic T lymphocyte
d4T	Stavudine
ddC	Dideoxycytidine, Zalcitabine
ddI	Dideoxyinosine, Didanosine
DNA	Deoxyribonucleic acid
dNTP	Deoxyribonucleotide triphosphate
dTTP	Deoxythymidine triphosphate
dUTP	Deoxyuracil triphosphate
EBV	Epstein–Barr virus
ECS	European Collaborative Study
ELISA	Enzyme-linked immunosorbent assay
ELISPOT	Enzyme-linked immunospot

FTT	Failure to thrive
gp 120	Glycoprotein 120 (HIV envelope protein)
gp 160	Glycoprotein 160 (HIV envelope protein)
Hib	*Haemophilus influenzae* type B
HIV	Human immunodeficiency virus
HIV-1	Human immunodeficiency virus type 1
HIVIG	HIV hyperimmune immunoglobulin
HLA	Human lymphocyte antigen
HSV	Herpes simplex virus
IC	Immunocomplexed
Ig	Immunoglobulin
IL	Interleukin
INSERM	Institut National de la Santé et de la Recherche Médicale
IV	Intravenous
IVAP	*In vitro* antibody production
IVDU/IDM	Intravenous drug user/injecting drug misuser
IVIG	Intravenous immunoglobulin
KS	Kaposi's sarcoma
LIP	Lymphoid interstitial pneumonitis
LTR	Long terminal repeats
MAC	*Mycobacterium avium* complex
MAI	*Mycobacterium avium intracellulare*
MHC	Major histocompatibility complex
MMR	Measles, mumps, rubella
NIAID	National Institute of Allergy and Infectious Diseases
NICHD	National Institute of Child Health and Development
NK	Natural killer
NVP	Nevirapine
OHL	Oral hairy leukoplakia
PBMC	Peripheral blood mononuclear cells
PCP	*Pneumocystis carinii* pneumonia
PCR	Polymerase chain reaction
PENTA	Paediatric European Network for Treatment of AIDS
PLH	Peribronchiolar lymphoid hyperplasia
PML	Progressive multifocal leucoencephalopathy
RNA	Ribonucleic acid
RSV	Respiratory syncytial virus
SIV	Simian immunodeficiency virus
STD	Sexually transmitted diseases
TB	Tuberculosis
3TC	3-Thiacytidine
TIBO	Tetrahydroimidazobenzodiazepinone

TMP-SMX	Trimethoprim-sulphamethoxazole
TNF	Tumour necrosis factor
UK	United Kingdom
USA	United States of America
VZV	Varicella zoster virus
WB	Western blot
WHO	World Health Organization
ZDV	Zidovudine (also known as AZT)
ZIg	Zoster immunoglobulin

1

Children and HIV infection

MARIE-LOUISE NEWELL

Introduction

Infection with the human immunodeficiency virus type 1 (HIV-1) has become a major public health problem in children as well as in adults. It is expected that by the year 2000 there will be 10 million HIV-infected children; most of these will be living in Africa, South and Southeast Asia and South America (Chin, 1990). However, it is also anticipated that there will be an increase in the numbers of infected children in Europe and the USA. By the end of 1993, more than 4500 children with acquired immunodeficiency syndrome (AIDS) had been reported from the USA and a similar number from Europe (World Health Organization/EC Collaborating Centre on AIDS, 1993).

Worldwide, heterosexual acquisition is the main route of infection for women and mother-to-child transmission is the main mode of acquisition of infection for children. With the increasing number of HIV-infected women of childbearing age there is a parallel increase in children with HIV infection. However, a proportion of children acquire infection through contaminated blood and blood products (Chapter 11) and the large number of children with AIDS from Romania highlights the need for continued vigilance in the use of needles and syringes. In countries where blood donations are not tested there remains a high risk of spread of HIV infection through this route. There is no evidence that HIV infection can be transmitted through any route other than blood, sexual contact or from mother to child (Fitzgibbon et al., 1993; Brownstein & Fricke, 1993).

Europe

By September 1993, a cumulative total of more than 103 000 cases of AIDS among adults and children had been reported from 44 European countries (World Health Organization/EC Collaborating Centre on AIDS,

Table 1.1. *AIDS in children less than 13 years of age by mode of acquisition (selected countries in Europe, September 1993)*

| | Mother's mode of acquisition in mother-to-child infection | | | | | | | | |
| | ivdu[a] | Hetero[b] | | Other | Haemo- philiac | Trans- fusion | Noso- comial | Other | Total |
		Endemic[c]	Other						
Romania	0	0	54	84	7	603	746	882	2376
Spain	270	0	99	77	54	14	0	11	525
France	138	136	70	35	27	66	0	5	477
Italy	206	0	107	33	15	7	0	6	377
UK	11	40	38	10	13	11	0	0	123
Germany	38	6	19	8	7	12	0	3	93
Belgium	2	2	51	6	3	8	0	4	76
Portugal	3	0	5	10	6	6	0	1	31
Total	709	194	477	302	153	745	748	1000	4331

From WHO (1993).
[a] History of intravenous drug use.
[b] Heterosexual contact; women from an HIV endemic area[c] or from another area.

1993). Most of the 15 000 women with AIDS were of childbearing age and the number of children reported from and within each country in Europe shows that the impact of the HIV epidemic varies across regions and populations. The majority of the 4300 children with AIDS were reported from Romania, Spain, France and Italy (Table 1.1). Excluding the reports from Romania, mother-to-child transmission accounted for about 80% of infection in children. This proportion is similar to that reported from the USA. About 40% of the mothers of the vertically infected children gave a history of intravenous drug use and a similar percentage had acquired infection through heterosexual contact. The relative proportions in each of these categories varied by country (Table 1.1).

HIV infection prevalence

AIDS surveillance is limited as an indicator of trends in HIV infection because of the long latent period between infection and serious symptoms, and because of under-reporting of AIDS (McCormick, 1991). To predict the spread of the epidemic, monitoring of HIV prevalence is essential. Increasingly the prevalence of HIV infection in a population is estimated through unlinked anonymous testing of blood taken for other purposes, although this may still result in a biased estimate as testing is limited to people who have blood taken.

Table 1.2. *Results of anonymous, unlinked antenatal or neonatal screening programmes*

Country or town	Year	Prevalence per 1000
Antenatal		
England	1990	1.14
London	1990	1.94
Paris	1990	4.14
Sweden	1986–91	0.10
Norway	1986–8	0.11
Neonatal		
Italy	1990	1.24
Paris	1990	2.75
Scotland	1990	0.29
Edinburgh	1990	2.46
Rome	1990	4.05

Since the main mode of acquisition of infection in children is vertical transmission from mother to child, the prevalence of HIV infection in the pregnant population is of particular relevance. In parallel with AIDS reports, there are marked differences in the seroprevalence of HIV infection among women of childbearing age between European countries, and between areas within one country. In Sweden (Lindgren *et al.*, 1993) and Norway (Jennum, 1988) the prevalence of HIV infection in the antenatal population was about 0.1 per 1000 women but it was 4 per 1000 in Paris (Couturier *et al.*, 1991) (Table 1.2). However, differences in the population tested make it difficult to compare results of various studies. For example, in Paris women were tested in early pregnancy, and the estimate includes women whose pregnancies were terminated. This group is known to have a higher HIV prevalence than women whose pregnancies continue to term. In England, women who had terminations are less likely to have been tested (PHLS Communicable Diseases Surveillance Centre, 1993). Continued surveillance will make it possible to look at changes over time.

HIV seroprevalence rates for women with live births are available for Italy, Southeast England and Scotland, based on unlinked anonymous testing of neonatal blood samples taken routinely from all newborns for metabolic screening (Holland *et al.*, 1994; Tappin *et al.*, 1991; Stegagno *et al.*, 1993). The estimated prevalence of HIV infection in newborns ranges from 0.3 per 1000 in Scotland in 1990 and Outer London in 1988 to 4 per 1000 in Rome 1990 (Table 1.2, Fig. 1.1). Trends over time are available only for London and Southeast England, and show a gradual increase (A.E. Ades, personal communication) (Fig. 1.1).

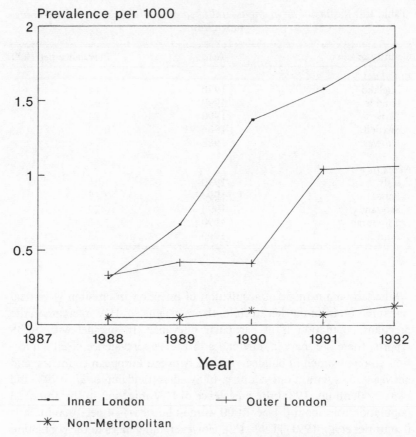

Fig. 1.1. HIV seroprevalence in neonates, Greater London 1988–92. From Ades *et al.* (1993 and personal communication).

Additional information on the extent and effect of the HIV epidemic comes from confidential surveillance schemes where HIV-seropositive pregnant women or HIV-seropositive children are reported to a central register. In the UK such a study has existed since 1989. Results of this surveillance programme can be compared with results from the unlinked anonymous neonatal screening programme in some regions to provide an estimate of the extent to which HIV infection is not recognised in pregnant women (Davison *et al.*, 1992; Ades *et al.*, 1993).

In Spain, the Spanish Paediatric Association carried out a survey in public hospitals of children born to HIV-positive mothers between 1981 and 1989 (Canosa *et al.*, 1991). A total of 1938 HIV-positive children were identified, with Madrid, Catalonia, Valencia, Basq and Andalucia reporting 85% of all cases; 93% of mothers were intravenous drug users.

In Italy the register of paediatric HIV infection and AIDS (Tovo *et al.*, 1992; Italian Register for HIV Infection in Children, 1994) has provided valuable information on children with infection, their presenting symptoms, the natural history of AIDS and survival. By June 1992, 2337 children had been reported, and for 1325 information was available from birth. In the UK, paediatricians report every month to a central register any child with HIV infection or born to an HIV-seropositive mother (Hall & Glickman, 1988). This paediatric surveillance is linked to the obstetric surveillance scheme to provide a comprehensive picture of vertically acquired infection in Britain (Davison *et al.*, 1992; Ades *et al.*, 1993). Additionally, in both the Italian and UK registers, follow-up information is obtained on the children reported.

In the UK, by October 1993, 660 children born to HIV-infected women had been reported: 235 were infected, 227 were not infected and for 198 HIV infection status was not yet determined (Ades *et al.*, 1993). Sixty per cent of these children were first identified by obstetricians reporting live births to infected women; the remaining two-fifths were first reported by paediatricians, generally after the child, a sibling or parent developed symptoms.

Mother-to-child transmission

Vertical transmission of HIV infection may occur before, during or after delivery, but because of the difficulty in diagnosis of infection in young infants (see Chapter 5) the relative importance of each of these routes is unknown. There is evidence that intrauterine infection occurs, although its contribution to vertical transmission cannot be quantified. Studies based on placentas and fetal tissues following pregnancy termination give conflicting results (Ehrnst *et al.*, 1991; Brossard *et al.*, 1993).

The importance of intrapartum acquisition of infection is debated. The exchange of blood between mother and child during labour and at the time of delivery, together with the detection of virus in cervical secretions, makes acquisition at this stage plausible, but it is difficult to confirm. Postnatal transmission of infection through breastfeeding can occur, both in children of women who were infected postnatally and in infants of women with established infection.

Diagnosis of infection in the infant

Early diagnosis of HIV infection and recognition of markers of disease progression in HIV-infected children are important if preventive and therapeutic interventions are to be implemented and evaluated. However, whereas in adults and older children the diagnosis of infection can be made on the basis of the detection of HIV antibodies, in infants born to HIV-antibody-positive women this method of diagnosis is hampered by the presence of passively acquired maternal antibody. Maternal immunoglobulin G (IgG) antibodies cross the placenta, and may persist in the child well into the second year of life. However, it is possible to exclude infection in a proportion of children at an earlier age, since half the uninfected children will have lost maternal antibody by age 10 months. Although an earlier diagnosis of HIV infection can be made using methods such as virus isolation or polymerase chain reaction (PCR), these techniques are costly, not widely available and currently performed only in specialised centres, mainly for research purposes (see Chapter 5). In experienced hands, using a multiplicity of clinical and laboratory information, a diagnosis of infection can usually be reached before the child is 6 months old. However, for most children, even in industrialised countries, diagnosis is still based on the persistence of antibodies beyond 15 or 18 months.

Vertical transmission rates

Estimates of the rates of vertical transmission vary widely (Newell & Peckham, 1993). Early studies are likely to have overestimated the risk of transmission as they were based on small selected groups with bias towards children or women with symptoms or mothers who already had an infected child. For example, Goedert and colleagues (Goedert *et al.*, 1991) showed that the rate of vertical transmission was 11% in children born to women known to be HIV infected at the time of delivery, whereas 65% of children identified after development of HIV-related symptoms or signs were infected.

The large majority of children born to HIV-infected women are not themselves infected. Published estimates of vertical transmission of HIV-1 from mother to child, based on studies where all children born to women known to be HIV infected at or before the time of delivery are enrolled and followed until their infection status is determined, range from 16% to 39% (Newell & Peckham, 1993; Table 1.3). In Europe the rate is 15–20%, in Africa 25–30% and in the USA 15–25% (Newell & Peckham, 1993).

In the French perinatal study (Rouzioux *et al.*, 1992) there were 47 infants born to mothers who were HIV-2 positive. None of the 25 who had been followed up to 18 months were infected (95% confidence interval 0–14%). Further evidence that the vertical transmission rate of HIV-2 is likely to be low comes from the Ivory Coast, where the results of specific immunoglobulin A (IgA) and PCR tests at 6 months of age suggest that

Table 1.3. *Estimates of mother-to-child transmission rates*

Study	Transmission rate (%)
European Collaborative Study (1992)	14
French Collaborative Study	18
Italian Multicentre Study (Gabiano *et al.*, 1992)	19
Swiss Perinatal Study (Kind *et al.*, 1992)	20
Ades *et al.* (1993) British Isles	14
Goedert *et al.* (1989) New York, NY	29
Hutto *et al.* (1991) Miami, FL	30
Nair *et al.* (1993) Baltimore, MD	23
Halsey *et al.* (1991) Haiti	25
St Louis (1994) Zaïre	26
Lepage *et al.* (1993) Rwanda	25
Sibailly *et al.* (1992) Ivory Coast	28

7 of 25 (28%; 95% confidence interval 12–49%) infants born to HIV-1 infected mothers are infected compared with 1 of 34 (3%; 95% confidence interval 0–15%) infants born to HIV-2 infected mothers (Sibailly *et al.*, 1992). It has been suggested that the lower rate of transmission of HIV-2 than of HIV-1 is due to differences in viral load (De Cock *et al.*, 1993).

Detailed review of the major HIV-1 vertical transmission studies suggest that the reported variation in transmission rates could be explained by differences in the distribution of possible risk factors, although differences in methodology could account for some of the variation (Newell & Peckham, 1993). Studies have used different definitions of infection, and the length of paediatric follow-up varies. Loss to follow-up can also have a substantial effect on the estimated transmission rate, as can the high infant mortality in developing countries where many children at-risk die before their infection status is known. Without sophisticated diagnostic facilities it is often not possible to attribute these deaths to HIV infection. To overcome this problem, comparisons have been made between children born to HIV-positive and HIV-negative mothers, and the excess infant mortality in the HIV-positive group used as an indication of HIV infection (Dabis *et al.*, 1993). This is not entirely satisfactory since children of infected mothers are likely to have a higher risk of dying, irrespective of their HIV infection status. Knowledge of risk factors associated with vertical transmission could explain the observed variation in transmission rates (Table 1.4).

Risk factors for vertical transmission

Maternal characteristics may influence vertical transmission rates (Newell & Peckham, 1993). Although it has been suggested that genetic

Table 1.4. *Risk factors for vertical transmission*

Maternal
Primary infection
Clinical status
HIV-related
Other
Immunological status
CD4 count
CD4 : CD8 ratio
Neutralising antibodies
Other
p24-antigenaemia
Delivery
Gestational age
Passage through birth canal
Mode of delivery
Procedures used
Length of labour
Breastfeeding
Mother infected postnatally
Mother with established infection at delivery

factors could relate to susceptibility to infection, no association with vertical transmission rates has been proven. A mother's clinical and immunological HIV-related status during pregnancy is likely to be related to viral load and infectivity (De Cock *et al.*, 1993). However, high plasma and cell virus loads do not always result in mother-to-child transmission (Puel *et al.*, 1992), although there is some evidence that a high level of maternal viraemia is associated with high risk of transmission. Not only virus load but also virus type, such as virulent fast-replicating HIV variants (either syncytium or non-syncytium inducing), could be associated with increased transmission (Puel *et al.*, 1992). It has been suggested that mucosal lesions resulting from another sexually transmitted disease could increase the HIV viral load in the genital tract and thus increase the risk of intrapartum infection (Nair *et al.*, 1993). Also, other viral or parasitic infections such as malaria may cause immunological impairment and lead to a greater HIV virus load in the mother. Both primary HIV infection during pregnancy (Johnson *et al.*, 1989) and later stage infection are likely to be associated with a period of viraemia and could pose an increased risk to the fetus (Hague *et al.*, 1993). In the Italian register, however, maternal seroconversion during pregnancy was not associated with increased transmission, and only 2 of 10 children born to seroconverting mothers were found to be infected (Tovo *et al.*, 1991). Primary infections in pregnancy are likely to occur in populations where the prevalence of HIV infection is high and heterosexual spread the major route of transmission.

Results from various prospective studies suggest that mothers with AIDS, or mothers who are p24-antigenaemic or who have a lower CD4 count or CD4 : CD8 ratio, are at increased risk of transmission of infection to their child (European Collaborative Study, 1992; Jackson *et al.*, 1993; Mayaux, 1993). In the Italian multicentre register transmission was associated with development of symptoms in the mother before delivery (Gabiano *et al.*, 1992). In Kinshasa, Zaïre, with an overall rate of transmission of 26% (69/261), transmission was associated with maternal p24-antigenaemia, and raised maternal CD8 counts (St Louis *et al.*, 1993). Low CD4 counts were associated with increased transmission only for women whose CD8 count did not indicate advanced disease. In Kigali, Rwanda, a CD4/CD8 ratio below 0.5 was the only maternal factor associated with an increased risk of mother-to-child transmission (Lepage *et al.*, 1993). In a study in Sweden, mothers of infected children were found to have been infected for longer and to be more likely to be symptomatic and/or to have low CD4 cell counts at follow-up than mothers of uninfected children (Lindgren *et al.*, 1991). However, in a study in the USA no association was found between transmission and pre-delivery levels of maternal CD4 cells, anti-p24 levels or neutralising antibodies (Goedert *et al.*, 1989).

It has been suggested that the presence of antibodies directed to certain viral antigens, such as gp120 or gp160, may confer some protection and reduce the likelihood of acquisition of HIV (Rossi *et al.*, 1989; Devash *et al.*, 1990). However, no consistent pattern has emerged (Parekh *et al.*, 1991) and further work is needed in different populations to explore the possible protective effect of different types of HIV antibodies (St Louis *et al.*, 1994). Differences in antibodies to HIV may reflect differences in maternal HIV burden and cannot be evaluated independently of virus load. The fact that HIV transmission can be discordant in twin offspring of HIV-infected mothers suggests that the protective effect of any maternal antibody, presumably shared by the twins, is incomplete at best.

Prematurity has been associated with an increased risk of infection in the infant (Goedert *et al.*, 1989; European Collaborative Study, 1992), although this has not been found in all studies (Gabiano *et al.*, 1992). Infants born before the transfer of adequate levels of maternal antibodies (which occurs late in pregnancy) could be more susceptible to transmission of infection during delivery. Chorioamnionitis has also been linked to increased transmission. In Zaïre, evidence of chorioamnionitis was found in the placentas of 21% of women with AIDS, but only rarely in the placentas of HIV-positive women without AIDS and seronegative controls (Ryder *et al.*, 1989). In an American study, transmission was associated with the presence of sexually transmitted diseases, birthweight less than 2500 g and possibly chorioamnionitits (Nair *et al.*, 1993), and in Kinshasa chorioamnionitis was associated with transmission but only in women who were not immunosuppressed (St Louis *et al.*, 1993). Chorioamnionitis could have a direct or indirect effect, either through increased transmission across the placenta or through its link with prematurity. Although there has been some evidence suggesting an association between the presence of syphilis and increased transmission (Nair *et al.*, 1993), other studies have not found this (Lepage *et al.*, 1993). However, definitions of chorioamnionitis vary and the diagnosis of syphilis or other sexually transmitted diseases can be difficult; further research in this area could contribute to the discussions about timing of mother-to-child transmission.

It has been suggested that delivery by elective caesarean section may reduce the rate of transmission by reducing exposure to contaminated blood or cervical secretions. A meta-analysis combining the results of six large prospective studies did find a marginally significant difference in the rate of transmission by mode of delivery (Villari *et al.*, 1993). This was confirmed by a joint analysis of data from 11 prospective studies including more than 3000 mother–child pairs (Dunn *et al.*, 1994). However, no distinction could be made between emergency and elective caesarean section deliveries, nor could potential confounding factors be taken into account. In the European Collaborative Study it was estimated that, if the rate of transmission following vaginal delivery was 18%, the risk following caesarean section would be about 10%. This would mean that about 12 caesarean section operations would need to be performed to prevent infection in one infant.

In the European prospective studies (European Collaborative Study, 1992; Mayaux, 1993; Kind *et al.*, 1992) transmission rates were not associated with maternal intravenous drug use, age, race or parity, or birthweight, nor with HIV-related manifestations not classified as AIDS.

Timing

There is increasing evidence to suggest that substantial transmission occurs around the time of delivery. The findings of the international registry of HIV-exposed twins showed that the first twin was more likely to be infected than the second and the authors concluded that a significant proportion of HIV transmission occurs during the birth period (Goedert *et al.*, 1991). The results from laboratory studies also lend support to the view that some infants acquire infection at birth (Ehrnst *et al.*, 1991;

Krivine *et al.*, 1992; De Rossi *et al.*, 1992). A significant proportion of children are negative at birth on HIV diagnostic tests such as PCR and specific IgA, but positive 3–6 months later (De Rossi *et al.*, 1993). Although this could be due to a relative insensitivity of the test at birth and the developing immune response of the neonate, it is also compatible with acquisition of infection immediately before or during delivery (Pollack *et al.*, 1993). In the European Collaborative Study perinatal findings were not associated with HIV infection in the infants, which could suggest that transmission occurs late in the pregnancy or at the time of delivery (European Collaborative Study, 1994). The lower rate of vertical transmission after a caesarean section delivery than after a vaginal delivery could also be indicative of transmission shortly before or during delivery.

Breastfeeding

Transmission of HIV through breastfeeding has been described in situations where the mother acquired the infection shortly after birth (either through contaminated blood or through heterosexual contact). The risk of infection from mother to child is high in mothers with a primary infection after birth (van de Perre *et al.*, 1991), when women are likely to be more viraemic than those with established infection. It has been estimated that the risk of transmission of infection through breastfeeding in women infected postnatally is about 29% (95% confidence interval 16–42%) (Dunn *et al.*, 1992).

It would be anticipated that children of mothers with established infection at the time of delivery would be at lower risk of infection from breastfeeding because they have maternal IgG antibodies which may have a protective role and their mothers, unless symptomatic, are probably less infectious. Valid estimates of the additional risk of transmission through breastfeeding can only be based on birth cohort studies of children born to mothers known to be already infected at the time of delivery, and which enroll both breast-fed and bottlefed infants. A recent analysis estimated that where the mother was infected prenatally the additional risk of transmission through breastfeeding, over and above transmission *in utero* or during delivery, was 14% (95% confidence interval 7–22%) (Dunn *et al.*, 1992). In both the French and the European prospective studies, breastfeeding doubled the risk of infection.

Van de Perre and colleagues (1993) present data to suggest that specific IgM in breastmilk could either be protective against postnatal transmission of HIV-1 or be an intermediate maternal factor reflecting low transmissibility. In their study, milk secretory IgA response was weak and frequently delayed as compared with many other viral infections. Seventy per cent of HIV-infected women in a Haitian study had HIV-DNA in their breastmilk in the first 4 days after delivery (Ruff *et al.*, 1994). Although the prevalence decreased over time, 12 months after delivery half the women still had HIV-DNA detectable in their breastmilk. This decreasing prevalence of HIV-DNA may reflect the normal decrease in breastmilk cells during lactation, and the association with transmission of infectious virus remains to be explored.

Newburg *et al.* (1992) have shown that a human milk factor inhibits binding of HIV to the CD4 receptor. However, the presence of this inhibitory factor was later found not to be associated with decreased transmission (Ruff *et al.*, 1993).

The World Health Organization has recently reiterated the guidelines regarding breastfeeding and HIV infection, stating that 'in settings where the main cause of death during infancy is not infectious diseases and the infant mortality rate is low, the usual advice to pregnant women known to be infected with HIV should be to use a safe alternative rather than breastfeed'. WHO further advises 'where infectious diseases and malnutrition are the main causes of infant deaths and the infant mortality rate is high, breastfeeding should be the usual advice to pregnant women, including those who are HIV-infected' (World Health Organization, 1992). However, similarly, HIV-negative women who are at-risk of becoming infected during the period of breastfeeding should also be advised to refrain from breastfeeding if safe alternatives are available.

Interventions to reduce mother-to-child transmission

Several approaches to reduce perinatal transmission have been suggested (Newell & Peckham, 1994). The proposed strategies include attempts to decrease the viral load of the infected pregnant woman, to prevent leaks across the placenta, to minimise the risk of transmission in the birth canal, to provide passive protection with HIV-antibody given to the pregnant woman and/or the newborn, and to enhance fetal/neonatal HIV-specific immunity (Borkowsky & Krasinski, 1992).

Unbiased estimates of the effect of caesarean section on the rate of vertical transmission can only be realised through randomised controlled trials. However, previous attempts at randomisation to mode of delivery in other contexts have not been successful. To avoid acquisition of infection during birth, cleansing of the birth canal with an antiseptic and/or virucidal agent to reduce transmission of infection has been proposed (Burman *et al.*, 1992). The agent used should have anti-HIV activity but no local or systemic toxicity and be simple to apply. Nonoxynol-9 is effective *in vitro*, but has resulted in an increase in genital ulcers and vaginitis when used for long periods (Kreiss *et al.*, 1992). Benzalkonium chloride is effective *in vitro*, well tolerated and inactivates other infectious agents that may favour HIV transmission (Wainberg *et al.*, 1990). Chlorhexidine is already widely used in obstetric practice in some countries. Another option is a combination of a non-nucleoside reverse transcriptase inhibitor and a virucidal antiseptic. Further research is needed to determine the most appropriate agent. However, if most transmission occurs via transplacental transfusion of maternal blood to the fetus or infant, cleansing of the birth canal will not be very effective in reducing vertical transmission.

Since there is some evidence that maternal viraemia is associated with risk of transmission, therapy aimed to reduce maternal viral load could have a role in reducing mother-to-child transmission (Pons *et al.*, 1991; Watts *et al.*, 1991; Sperling *et al.*, 1992). However, issues relating to the duration of the effect in reducing viral load, development of resistance and transmission of resistant virus, as well as safety, will need to be addressed.

Zidovudine (AZT) is already used during pregnancy for maternal indications. It has also been used specifically to reduce mother-to-child transmission (Ferrazin *et al.*, 1993) as it reduces viral replication thereby decreasing viral load, but this effect persists for only a limited time. Although it is known that the pharmacokinetics of AZT are not modified in pregnancy, few data are available on concentrations in fetal tissue (Watts *et al.*, 1991). No teratogenic effects have been detected after AZT use in pregnancy (Ferrazin *et al.*, 1993; McLeod & Hammer, 1992). In the USA a randomised, placebo-controlled trial was started in 1991 to evaluate the efficacy, safety and tolerance of AZT in HIV-infected pregnant women with CD4+ lymphocyte counts above 200 per mm^3, and their infants. AZT was given orally during the second and third trimesters of pregnancy to women who had previously not received antiretroviral drugs, and by infusion during labour. Infants were then treated with AZT or placebo for 6 weeks (Ukwu *et al.*, 1992). French groups participated in this study, which aimed to detect a reduction in vertical transmission rate from 30% to 20%. A first interim analysis in early 1994 showed a statistically significant difference in the rate of vertical transmission between the two groups (Choo, 1994). Of the 364 evaluable children, 53 were infected: 13 in the AZT arm and 40 in the placebo arm. It was estimated that the rate of vertical transmission was 8.3% in the treated group and 25.5% in the untreated group. On the basis of these results the investigators decided to halt enrolment and offer AZT to all women and infants already in the trial. The small numbers of infected children preclude multivariate analysis and no information is available on the effect of length of treatment. It is premature to issue general clinical guidelines based on these preliminary results. Further studies are required to identify the optimum method and timing of interventions.

Some newer antiretroviral drugs, such as non-nucleoside reverse transcriptase inhibitors (Pauwels *et al.*, 1993), are being evaluated as potential candidates to reduce transmission. Because of their rapid and marked initial effect on viral replication they may be suitable for use as an intervention to reduce vertical transmission. However, resistance develops quickly and these drugs cannot yet be used for treatment to delay progression of HIV disease (Koup *et al.*, 1993).

The humoral immune response is an important component of protective immunity against a number of infectious agents, possibly including HIV. Passive immunisation with HIV-specific immunoglobulin to prevent vertical transmission of HIV has therefore been proposed (Ukwu *et al.*, 1992). Problems still to be resolved include the selection of suitable donors, the standardisation of the preparation and the optimum timing of administering the immunisation. Phase I/II studies are under way in the USA and Uganda to address these issues (Cotton, 1993), and passive immunisation with human polyclonal antibodies should be seen as a step towards immunisation with monoclonal antibodies, either singly or in a cocktail. Monoclonal antibodies are being developed, and there is some evidence of an effect in laboratory conditions (Emini *et al.*, 1992).

Active immunisation is an attractive approach because it can potentially induce a long-lasting immunity. It may also induce fetal immunity (Englund & Glezen, 1991). Phase I trials with recombinant envelope vaccines based on the SF2 and MN strains, the prevalent strains in the USA, have started in pregnant women and newborns in the USA (P. Fast, personal communication 1993). Immunisation early in pregnancy should be avoided to decrease the risk of activation of the maternal immune system, inducing teratogenic effects or immunological tolerance in the infant. Further research is needed to establish whether vaccines developed in the USA are appropriate for other populations. Two phase I/II trials of active immunisation of infants and children are in progress in the USA, one aimed at prevention of infection acquired in the intrapartum period, the other of a therapeutic agent to prevent progression of disease. Data from these trials are anticipated in 1995.

Conclusion

The rate of vertical transmission of HIV infection is about 15–20% in Europe, 20–25% in the USA and 25–30% in Africa. Variation in the rates may be explained by the distribution of factors possibly associated with increased risk such as advanced clinical and immunological disease, delivery before 34 weeks gestation, and breastfeeding. There is some evidence to suggest that delivery by caesarean section would reduce transmission, but the data do not justify the routine use of caesarean section delivery for all HIV-infected women. Furthermore, morbidity and mortality associated with caesarean section in HIV-infected, immunocompromised women should be taken into account. Breastfeeding is a recognised route of acquisition of infection and it is estimated in Europe that breastfeeding doubles the risk of transmission of infection.

With increasing evidence to suggest that a substantial amount of infection occurs around the time of delivery, attention is now being given to interventions aimed at reducing vertical transmission. Suggested approaches include a safer alternative to breastfeeding, elective caesarean section delivery, and cleansing of the birth canal. Passive immunisation with hyperimmune immunoglobulin or with monoclonal antibodies has also been proposed, based on the assumption that neutralising antibodies confer protection. The role of antiretroviral therapy such as AZT in the prevention of vertical transmission of HIV is being investigated, as is the use of active immunisation. However, since there is no vaccine or cure for HIV infection, the most effective prevention of mother-to-child transmission is primary prevention of maternal infection.

References

Ades, A. E., Davison, C. F., Holland, F. J., *et al.* (1993). Vertically transmitted HIV infection in the British Isles. *British Medical Journal*, **306**, 1296–9.

Borkowsky, W. & Krasinski, K. (1992). Perinatal human immunodeficiency virus infection: ruminations on mechanisms of transmission and methods of intervention. *Pediatrics*, **90**, 133–6.

Brossard, Y., Bignozzi, C., Mandelbrot, L., *et al.* (1993). PCR prevalence of HIV in 99 fetal thymuses at mid-gestation [abstract PO-B05-1038]. Berlin: IXth International Conference on AIDS.

Brownstein A. & Fricke W. (1993). HIV transmission between two adolescent brothers with hemophilia. *Morbidity and Mortality Weekly Report*, **42**, 948–51.

Burman, L. G., Christensen, P., Christensen, K., *et al.* (1992). Prevention of excess neonatal morbidity associated with group B streptococci by vaginal chlorhexidine disinfection during labour. *Lancet*, **340**, 65–9.

Canosa, C. A., Delgado, A., Martin, F. G., Llorens, J., Omenaca, F., & Contreras, J. R. (1991). Asociacion Espanola de Pediatria. Madrid. Infeccion por el virus de la inmunodeficiencia humana. Encuesta multicentrica espanola. *Anales Espanoles de Pediatria*, **34**, 425–35.

Chin, J. (1990). Epidemiology. Current and future dimensions of the HIV/AIDS pandemic in women and children. *Lancet*, **336**, 221–4.

Choo, V. (1994). Maternal transmission of HIV. *Lancet*, **343**, 533.

Cotton, P. (1993). Delayed trial of HIV immune globulin to protect infants of infected mothers is likely to resume. *Journal of the American Medical Association*, **269**, 17.

Couturier, E., Brossard, Y., Larsen, C., *et al.* (1991). Prévalence de l'infection VIH chez les femmes enceintes de la région parisienne. Une enquête anonyme non correlée. *PREVAGEST Bulletin Epidemiologique Hebdomadaire*, **33**, 139.

Dabis, F., Msellati, P., Dunn, D., *et al.* (1993). Estimating the rate of mother-to-child transmission of HIV. Report of a workshop on methodological issues, Ghent (Belgium), 17–20 February 1992. *AIDS*, **7**, 1139–48.

Davison, C. F., Holland, F. J., Newell, M-L., Hudson, C. N., & Peckham, C. S. (1992). Screening for HIV infection in pregnancy. *AIDS Care*, **5**, 135–40.

De Cock, K. M., Adjorlolo, G., Ekpini, E., *et al.* (1993). Epidemiology and transmission of HIV-2: why there is no HIV-2 pandemic. *Journal of the American Medical Association*, **270**, 2083–6.

De Rossi, A., Ometto, L., Mammano, F., Zanotto, C., Giaquinto, C., & Chieco-Bianchi L. (1992). Vertical transmission of HIV 1: lack of detectable virus in peripheral blood cells of infected children at birth. *AIDS*, **6**, 117–20.

De Rossi, A., Ometto, L., Mammano, F., *et al.* (1993). Time course of antigenaemia and seroconversion in infants with vertically acquired HIV-1 infection. *AIDS*, **7**, 1528–9.

Devash, Y., Calvelli, T. A., Wood, D. G., Reagan, K. J., & Rubenstein, A. (1990). Vertical transmission of human immunodeficiency virus is correlated with the absence of high affinity/avidity maternal antibodies to the gp120 principal neutralising domain. *Proceedings of the National Academy of Sciences, USA*, **87**, 3445–9.

Dunn, D. T., Newell, M. L. Mayaux, M. J., *et al.* (1994). Mode of delivery and vertical transmission of HIV-1: a review of prospective studies. *Journal of Acquired Immune Deficiency Syndromes*, **7**, 1064–6.

Dunn, D. T., Newell, M. L., Ades, A. E., & Peckham, C. S. (1992). Risk of human immunodefiency virus type 1 transmission through breastfeeding. *Lancet*, **340**, 585–8.

Ehrnst, A., Lindgren, S., Dictor, M., *et al.* (1991). HIV in pregnant women and their offspring: evidence for late transmission. *Lancet*, **338**, 203–7.

Emini, E. A., Schleif, W. A., Nunberg, J. H., *et al.* (1992). Prevention of HIV-1 infection in chimpanzees by gp120 V3 domain-specific monoclonal antibody. *Nature*, **355**, 728–30.

Englund, J. A. & Glezen, W. P. (1991). Maternal immunization for the prevention of infection in early infancy. *Seminars in Pediatric Infectious Diseases*, **2**, 225–31.

European Collaborative Study (1992). Risk factors for mother-to-child transmission of HIV-1. *Lancet*, **339**, 1007–12.

European Collaborative Study (1994). Perinatal findings in children born to HIV-infected mothers. *British Journal of Obstetrics and Gynaecology*, **101**, 136–41.

Ferrazin, A., de Maria, A., Gotta, C., *et al.* (1993). Zidovudine therapy of HIV-1 infection during pregnancy: assessment of the effect on the newborns. *Journal of Acquired Immune Deficiency Syndrome*, **6**, 376–9.

Fitzgibbon, J. E., Gaur, S., Frenkel, L. D., Laraque, F., Edlin, B. R., & Dubin, D. T. (1993). Transmission from one child to another of human immunodeficiency virus type 1 with a zidovudine-resistance mutation. *New England Journal of Medicine*, **329**, 1835–41.

Gabiano, C., Tovo, P., de Martino, M., *et al.* (1992). Mother-to-child transmission of Human Immunodeficiency Virus Type 1: Risk of infection and correlates of transmission. *Pediatrics*, **90**, 369–74.

Goedert, J. J., Duliege, A.-M., Amos, C. I., *et al.* (1991). High risk of infection with human immunodeficiency virus type I for first-born, vaginally delivered twins. *Lancet*, **338**, 1471–5.

Goedert, J. J., Mendez, H., Drummond, J. E., *et al.* (1989). Mother-to-infant transmission of human immunodeficiency virus type 1: association with prematurity or low anti-gp120. *Lancet*, **ii**, 1351–4.

Hague, R. A., Mok, J. Y. Q., Johnstone, F. D., *et al.* (1993). Maternal factors in HIV transmission. *International Journal of STD & AIDS*, **4**, 142–6.

Hall, S. & Glickman, M. (1988). The British Paediatric Surveillance Unit. *Archives of Disease in Childhood*, **63**, 344–6.

Halsey, N. A., Boulos, R., Holt, E., Ruff, A., *et al.* (1991). Transmission of HIV-1 infection from mothers to infants in Haiti. *Journal of the American Medical Association*, **264**, 2088–92.

Hutto, C., Parks, W. P., Lai, S., *et al.* (1991). A hospital-based prospective study of perinatal infection with human immunodeficiency virus type 1. *Journal of Pediatrics*, **118**, 347–53.

Italian Register for HIV Infection in Children (1994). Features of children perinatally infected with HIV-1 surviving longer than 5 years. *Lancet*, **343**, 191–5.

Jackson, J. B., Kataaha, P., Hom D. L., *et al.* (1993). B(eta)2-microglobulin, HIV-1 p24 antibody and acid-dissociated HIV-1 p24 antigen levels: predictive markers for vertical transmission of HIV-1 in pregnant Ugandan women. *AIDS*, **7**, 1475–9.

Jennum, P. H. (1988). Anti-HIV screening of pregnant women in south-eastern Norway. *Norwegian Institute of Public Health Annals*, **11**, 54–8.

Johnson, J. P., Prasanna, N., Hines, S. E., *et al.* (1989). Natural history and serologic diagnosis of infants born to human immunodeficiency virus-infected women. *American Journal of Diseases of Children*, **143**, 1147–53.

Kind, C., Brandle, B., Wyler, C.-A., *et al.* (1992). Epidemiology of vertically transmitted HIV-1 infection in Switzerland: results of a nationwide prospective study. *European Journal of Pediatrics*, **151**, 442–8.

Koup, R. A., Brewster, F., Grob, P., & Sullivan, J. L. (1993). Nevirapine synergistically inhibits HIV-1 replication in combination with zidovudine, interferon or CD4 immunoadhesin. *AIDS*, **7**, 1181–4.

Kreiss, J., Ngugi, E., Holmes, K., *et al.* (1992). Efficacy of nonoxynol 9 contraceptive sponge use in preventing heterosexual acquisition of HIV in Nairobi prostitutes. *Journal of the American Medical Association*, **268**, 477–82.

Krivine, A., Firtion, G., Cao, L., Francoual, C., Henrion, R., & Lebon, P. (1992). HIV replication during the first few weeks of life. *Lancet*, **339**, 1187–9.

Lepage, P., Van de Perre, P., Msellati, P., *et al.* (1993). Mother-to-child transmission of HIV-1 and its determinants; a cohort study in Kigali, Rwanda. *Amercian Journal of Epidemiology*, **137**, 589–99.

Lindgren, S., Anzen, B., Bohlin, A., & Lidman, K. (1991). HIV and child-bearing:

clinical outcome and aspects of mother-to-infant transmission. *AIDS*, **5**, 1111–16.

Lindgren, S., Bohlin, A., Forsgren, M., *et al.* (1993). Screening for HIV-1 antibodies in pregnancy: results from the Swedish national programme. *British Medical Journal*, **307**, 1447–51.

Mayaux, M. J. (1993). Risk factors for mother-to-child transmission in the French national prospective study: a six years experience, vol. 1 [abstract WS-C10–11]. Berlini IXth International Conference on AIDS.

McCormick, A. (1991). Unrecognised HIV related deaths. *British Medical Journal*, **302**, 1365–7.

McLeod, G. X. & Hammer, S. M. (1992). Zidovudine: five years later. *Annals of Internal Medicine*, **117**, 487–501.

Nair, P., Alger, L., Hines, S., Seiden, S., Hebel, R., & Johnson, J. P. (1993). Maternal and neonatal characteristics associated with HIV infection in infants of seropositive women. *Journal of Acquired Immune Deficiency Syndromes*, **6**, 298–302.

Newburg, D. S., Viscidi, R. P., Ruff, A., & Yolken, R. H. (1992). A human milk factor inhibits binding of human immunodeficiency virus to CD4 receptor. *Pediatric Research*, **31**, 22–8.

Newell, M. L. & Peckham, C. S. (1993). Risk factors for vertical transmission of HIV-1 and early markers of HIV-1 infection in children. *AIDS*, **7**, S591–7.

Newell, M. L. & Peckham, C. S. (1994). Working towards a European strategy for intervention to reduce vertical transmission of HIV. *British Journal of Obstetrics and Gynaecology*, **101**, 192–196

Parekh, B. S., Shaffer, N., Pau, C-P., *et al.* (1991). Lack of correlation between maternal antibodies to V3 loop peptides of gp120 and perinatal HIV-1 transmission. *AIDS*, **5**, 1179–84.

Pauwels, R., Andries, K., Debyser, Z., *et al.* (1993). Potent and higly selective human immunodeficiency virus type 1 (HIV-1) inhibition by a series of alpha-anilinophenylacetamide derivatives targeted at HIV-1 reverse transcriptase. *Proceedings of the National Academy of Science, USA*, **90**, 1711–5.

PHLS Communicable Diseases Surveillance Centre (1993). Unlinked anonymous monitoring of HIV prevalence in England and Wales: 1990–92. *Communicable Disease Report*, **3**, R1–11.

Pollack, H., Zhan, M. X., Ilmet-Moore, T., Ajuang-Simbiri, K., Krasinski, K., & Borkowsky, W. (1993). Ontogeny of anti-human immunodeficiency virus (HIV) antibody production in HIV-1 infected infants. *Proceedings of the National Academy of Sciences, USA*, **90**, 2340–4.

Pons, J. C., Boubon, M. C., Taburet, A. M., *et al.* (1991). Fetoplacental passage of 2′,3′-dideoxyinosine. *Lancet*, **337**, 732.

Puel, J., Lheritier, D., Guyader, M., *et al.* (1992). Viral load and mother-to-infant HIV transmission. *Lancet*, **340**, 859.

Rossi, P., Moschese, V., Broliden, P. A., *et al.* (1989). Presence of maternal antibodies to human immunodeficiency virus 1 envelope glycoprotein gp120 epitopes correlates with the uninfected status of children born to seropositive mothers. *Proceedings of the National Academy of Sciences, USA*, **86**, 8055–8.

Rouzioux, C., Mayaux, M. J., Blanche, S., Burgard, M., & Griscelli, C. (1992). The materno-foetal transmission rates of HIV-1 and HIV-2 in France [abstract WeC 1063]. Amsterdam: Final Program and Oral Abstracts, VIII International Conference on AIDS.

Ruff, A. J., Coberly, J., Halsey, N. A., *et al.* (1994). Prevalence of HIV-1 DNA and p24 antigen in breastmilk and correlation with maternal factors. *Journal of Acquired Immune Deficiency Syndromes*, **7**, 68–73.

Ruff, A., Yolken, R., Desormeaux, J., *et al.* (1993). HIV-1 and HIV-1 inhibitory activity in breastmilk [abstract WS–CO2–3]. Berlin: IXth International Conference on AIDS.

Ryder, R. W., Nsa, W., Hassig, S. E., *et al.* (1989). Perinatal transmission of the human immunodeficiency virus type 1 to infants of seropositive women in Zaire. *New England Journal of Medicine*, **320**, 1637–42.

Scarlatti, G., Lombardi, V., Plebani, A., *et al.* (1991). Polymerase chain reaction, virus isolation and antigen assay in HIV-1-antibody-positive mothers and their children. *AIDS*, **5**, 1173–8.

Sibailly, S. T., Adjoriolo, G., Gayle, H., *et al.* (1992). Prospective study to compare HIV-1 and HIV-2 perinatal transmission in Abidjan, Cote D'Ivoire [abstract WeC 1065]. Amsterdam: Final Program and Oral Abstracts, VIII International Conference of AIDS.

Sperling, R. S., Stratton, P., O'Sullivan, M. J., *et al.* (1992). A survey of zidovudine use in pregnant women with human immunodeficiency virus infection. *New England Journal of Medicine*, **326**, 857–61.

St Louis, M. E., Kamenga, M., Brown, C., *et al.* (1993). Risk for perinatal HIV-1 transmission according to maternal immunologic, virologic, and placental factors. *Journal of the Amercian Medical Association*, **269**, 2853–9.

St Louis, M. E., Pau, C., Nsuami, M., *et al.* (1994). Lack of association between anti-V3 loop antibody and perinatal HIV-1 transmission in Kinshasa, Zaire, despite use of assays based on local HIV-1 strain. *Journal of Acquired Immune Deficiency Syndromes*, **7**, 63–7.

Stegagno, M., Ippolito, G., Costa, F., Aebischer, M. L., Guzzanti, E., Italian Collaborative Study Group of HIV Prevalence in Newborns (1993). Anti-HIV 1 antibodies prevalence in parturients through newborn testing: results of the Italian anonymous serosurvey. *European Journal of Epidemiology*, **9**, 430–5.

Tappin, D. M., Girdwood, R. W. A., Follett, E. A. C., Kennedy, R., Brown, A. J., & Cockburn, F. (1991). Prevalence of maternal HIV infection in Scotland based on unlinked anonymous testing of newborn babies. *Lancet*, **337**, 1565–7.

Tovo, P. A., de Martino, M., Gabiano, C., *et al.* (1992). Prognostic factors and survival in children with perinatal HIV-1 infection. *Lancet*, **339**, 1249–53.

Tovo, P. A., Palomba, E., Gabiano, C., Galli, L., & de Martino, M. (1991). Human immunodeficiency type 1 (HIV-1) seroconversion during pregnancy does not increase the risk of perinatal transmission. *British Journal of Obstetrics and Gynaecology*, **98**, 940–2.

Ukwu, H. N., Graham, B. S., Lambert, J. S., & Wright, P. F. (1992). Perinatal transmission of human immunodeficiency virus-1 infection and maternal immunization strategies for prevention. *Obstetrics and Gynecology*, **80**, 458–68.

van de Perre, P., Simonon, A., Hitimana, D., *et al.* (1993). Infective and anti-infective properties of breastmilk from HIV-1 infected women. *Lancet*, **341**, 914–18.

van de Perre, P., Simonon, A., Msellati, P., *et al.* (1991). Postnatal transmission of human immunodeficiency virus type 1 from mother to infant: a prospective cohort study in Kigali, Rwanda. *New England Journal of Medicine*, **325**, 593–8.

Villari, P., Spino C., Chalmers, T. C., Lau, J., & Sacks, H. S. (1993). Cesarean section to reduce perinatal transmission of Human Immunodeficiency Virus. *The Online Journal of Current Clinical Trials*, vol. 2.

Wainberg, M. A., Spira, B., Bleau, G., & Thomas, R. (1990). Inactivation of human immunodeficiency virus type 1 in tissue culture fluid and in genital secretions by the spermicide benzalkonium chloride. *Journal of Clinical Microbiology*, **28**, 156–8.

Watts, D. H., Brown, Z. A., Tartaglione, T., *et al*. (1991). Pharmacokinetic disposition of zidovudine during pregnancy. *Journal of Infectious Diseases*, **163**, 226–32.

World Health Organization, G. (1992). Consensus statement from the WHO/ UNICEF Consultation on HIV transmission and breastfeeding. *Weekly Epidemiological Record*, **67**, 177–9.

World Health Organization/EC Collaborating Centre on AIDS (1993). *AIDS Surveillance in Europe*. Paris: WHO, Quarterly Report no. 39.

Addenda

Further relevant references:

Holland, F. J., Ades, A. E., Davison, C. F., *et al*. (1994). Use of anonymous newborn serosurveys to evaluate antenatal HIV screening programmes. *Journal of Medical Screening*, **1**, 176–9.

The paper by Rouzioux *et al*. (1992) has been published as:

HIV Infection in Newborns French Collaborative Group (1994). Comparison of vertical HIV-2 and HIV-1 transmission in the French prospective cohort. *Pediatric Infectious Disease Journal*, **13**, 502–6.

The results of the American/French zidovudine trial (ACTG 076) have now been published as:

Connor, E. M., Sperling, R. S., Gelber, R., *et al*. (1994). Reduction of maternal– infant transmission of human immunodeficiency virus type 1 with zidovudine treatment. *New England Journal of Medicine*, **331**, 1173–80.

And for a discussion of the implications for antenatal screening:

Bayer, R. (1994). Ethical challenges posed by zidovudine treatment to reduce vertical transmission of HIV. *New England Journal of Medicine*, **331**, 1223–5.

Guidelines on the use of ZDV in pregnancy, specifically to reduce mother-to-child transmission, were issued in the USA after the reports of the 076 trial:

Centers for Disease Control (1994). Recommendations for the use of zidovudine to reduce perinatal transmission of HIV. *Morbidity and Mortality Weekly Report*, **43**, RR11: 1—20.

For the results of the ECS on mode of delivery see:

European Collaborative Study (1994). Caesarean section and risk of vertical transmission of HIV-1 infection. *Lancet*, **343**, 1464–7.

An international randomised trial has started to evaluate the effectiveness of an elective caesarean section in preventing perinatal transmission (for more information contact Dr Marie-Louise Newell at the Institute of Child Health in London, UK).

2

Paediatric HIV infection in the USA

MARY LOU LINDEGREN, M. BLAKE CALDWELL
and MARGARET OXTOBY

Introduction

HIV infection and AIDS was the seventh leading cause of death among children 1–4 years of age and the ninth leading cause of death among children 5–14 years of age in the USA in 1991 (National Center for Health Statistics, 1993). Since the first cases of AIDS were reported among adults in 1981 and among children in 1982 (Centers for Disease Control, 1982) in the USA, over 4900 children less than 13 years of age and over 40 000 adult and adolescent women had been reported with AIDS up to September 1993; these represented 1.4% and 12%, respectively, of all cases. Women have accounted for an increasing proportion of AIDS cases (14% in 1992) (Centers for Disease Control, 1993a). The majority of women (85%) reported with AIDS are in their childbearing years (15–44 years) (Ellerbrock et al., 1991; Fleming & Gwinn, 1994). From 1991 to 1992, while total cases increased by 3.5%, percentage increases were greater among women (9.8%) than among men (2.5%); among children aged <5 years (16.6%) compared with other age groups; and among persons infected via heterosexual (17.1%) and vertical (mother-to-child) transmission (13.4%) compared with other HIV-exposure categories (Centers for Disease Control, 1993a). Projections of AIDS cases suggest continued increases in the number of vertically infected children, persons infected through heterosexual transmission, and women diagnosed with AIDS (Centers for Disease Control, 1992b). The anonymous serosurvey of childbearing women (Gwinn et al., 1991) estimates that approximately 7000 infants were born to HIV-infected mothers each year in 1991 and 1992 (Davis et al., 1993). Among states conducting these surveys since 1989, the prevalence of HIV has remained relatively stable; however, trends varied regionally, with increases in the Southeast.

With the onset of the second decade of the epidemic, increasing numbers of HIV-infected women and children will need medical and social services in the coming years. Important advances have occurred in the

21

understanding of HIV infection in children and more recently in the prevention of vertical transmission of HIV through the administration of zidovudine to HIV-infected pregnant women (Connor *et al.*, 1994). Early identification of pregnant women and children with HIV infection is increasingly important for early intervention and prevention. This chapter will review the epidemiology of HIV infection in children in the USA by reviewing data collected through AIDS and HIV infection surveillance, and studies of HIV seroprevalence, vertical transmission, spectrum of disease and survival in the USA.

Epidemiology of paediatric HIV infection in the USA

Transmission of HIV to children has primarily occurred through vertical transmission during pregnancy, delivery or breastfeeding or through transfusion of HIV-infected blood or blood products (Curran *et al.*, 1988; Simonds & Chanock, 1993). In the USA the majority of all HIV infection in children is attributable to vertical transmission, following the implementation of heat treatment for clotting factors in 1984 (McDougal *et al.*, 1985) and the initiation of nationwide screening of blood and blood products for HIV in 1985.

Vertical transmission
AIDS surveillance methods

Since 1981, the Centers for Disease Control and Prevention (CDC) together with state and local health departments have conducted surveillance for AIDS, which is reportable in all states and territories in the USA. This surveillance system has been extremely useful in characterising cases, describing modes of transmission, following trends in severe HIV-related illness and death, developing HIV prevention strategies, allocating resources for prevention and treatment, and projecting the future impact of the disease. Initially, the AIDS surveillance case definition included only highly specific diseases associated with a severe deficiency in cell-mediated immunity. In 1985 and 1987, the AIDS case definition was revised to reflect increased use of the HIV-antibody test and greater understanding of the spectrum of HIV-related diseases. The 1987 definition included additional HIV-related conditions, and also some AIDS indicator diseases diagnosed presumptively (i.e. without laboratory confirmation) to be consistent with clinical practices (Centers for Disease Control, 1987b). Information on demographics, vital status, mode of transmission, laboratory evidence of HIV infection and the diagnosis of AIDS-defining conditions is collected on each AIDS case and transmitted to CDC without personal identifiers. Although overall completeness of AIDS case reporting has been estimated to be 85–90% (Buehler, *et al.*, 1992; Rosenblum *et al.*, 1992), limited data are available for children. AIDS case reports are updated to reflect mortality; however, additional clinical conditions that occur subsequent to the initial AIDS-defining illnesses are not systematically reported.

In 1993, CDC revised the classification system for HIV infection and the AIDS surveillance case definition for adolescents and adults (≥ 13 years of age) to include CD4 T-lymphocyte counts, which have consistently correlated with disease progression and immune dysfunction (Centers for Disease Control, 1992c). To monitor the number of persons with severe HIV-related immunosuppression and those at highest risk for severe HIV-related morbidity more accurately, the adolescent and adult AIDS surveillance case definition was expanded to include all HIV-infected persons with a CD4 cell count <200 cells/mm^3, a CD4 percentage of total lymphocytes of <14, or any of three clinical conditions: pulmonary tuberculosis, recurrent pneumonia and invasive cervical cancer. AIDS case definition (Centers for Disease Control, 1987b) and the paediatric classification system (Centers for Disease Control, 1987a) have been reconsidered (see Addenda, p. 51).

AIDS in women

In recent years, the number of new AIDS cases reported among homosexual/bisexual men in the USA appears to be levelling off (Centers for Disease Control, 1992b, 1993a; Thomas *et al.*, 1993); however, the number and proportions of cases are increasing in minority populations and among women. Trends in AIDS cases among adolescent and adult women and among children less than 13 years of age are shown in Figs. 2.1 and 2.2. Women account for an increasing number and proportion of AIDS cases reported in the USA (Ellerbrock *et al.*, 1991; Centers for Disease Control, 1993a), the majority of whom (85%) are of childbearing age. As of June 1993, 30 018 women diagnosed with AIDS by 1992 had been reported to CDC under the 1987 case definition. When examined by year of diagnosis and adjusted for reporting delays (Karon *et al.*, 1992), the number of cases diagnosed among women increased by 10% from 1991 to 1992 (Fig. 2.1). Minority women are disproportionately represented among women with AIDS: 53% are black, 21% are Hispanic, 25% are white, and <1% are Asian/Pacific Islander or American Indian/Alaska Native. Black and Hispanic women have had the highest cumulative incidence rates (Ellerbrock *et al.*, 1991). The proportion of cases diagnosed among black non-Hispanic women has increased from 51% in 1988 to

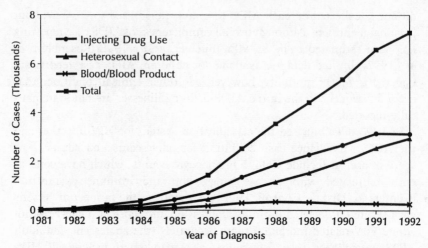

Fig. 2.1. Adult/adolescent female AIDS cases by mode of transmission and year of diagnosis up to December 1992, USA. (Reported up to the end of June 1993, adjusted for reporting delay, cases meeting 1987 case definition.)

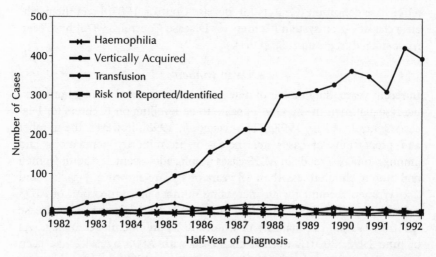

Fig. 2.2. Paediatric AIDS cases by mode of transmission and half-year of diagnosis up to the end of December 1992, USA. (Reported up to the end of June 1993, adjusted for reporting delay.)

55% in 1992. Although the majority of cases (49%) occurred in injecting drug users, an increasing proportion of cases in women are attributed to heterosexual contact (Fig. 2.1). Among cases with heterosexual transmission, most (58%) were attributed to sexual contact with an injecting drug user. In 1992, 41% of women diagnosed with AIDS acquired their

Table 2.1. *AIDS cases in children <13 years of age by mode of transmission (cumulative 1981–92 and 1992, by year of diagnosis, USA)*[a]

Transmission category	1981–92		1992	
Vertically acquired	4004	(87)	607	(94)
Injecting drug use (IDU)	1817	(40)	190	(29)
Sex with IDU	780	(17)	95	(15)
Other heterosexual contact	689	(15)	129	(20)
Transfusion/transplant	89	(2)	18	(3)
HIV infected, risk not specified	629	(14)	175	(27)
Haemophilia/coagulation disorder	198	(4)	12	(2)
Transfusion-acquired	318	(7)	15	(2)
Risk not reported/identified	64	(1)	15	(2)
Total	4584		649	

Values are number (percentage).
[a] Reported up to the end of June 1993.

infection through heterosexual contact – a 48% increase over the number diagnosed in 1990 with heterosexual contact. In 1992, 43% were infected through injecting drug use (Fig. 2.1). The greatest increases in heterosexually acquired AIDS were among women 20–29 years of age, among black women, and in the southern USA (Centers for Disease Control, 1993a). Patterns of transmission varied regionally, with injecting drug use the predominant mode in the northeast and heterosexual transmission more prominent among women in the rest of the country. As a result of the expansion of the 1993 AIDS case definition, the number of AIDS cases reported during 1993 compared with 1992 increased by 151% in women (6571 to 16 514) and 105% in men (42 445 to 86 986), largely due to the CD4 count criteria. The three additional clinical conditions accounted for 9% of AIDS cases reported during 1993 (Centers for Disease Control, 1994).

AIDS in children infected by vertical transmission

The increase in cases of AIDS among women is reflected in increases in AIDS in infants and children. By June 1993, 4004 vertically infected children had been diagnosed with AIDS up to December 1992 and reported to CDC. Virtually all (94%) paediatric AIDS cases diagnosed in 1992 acquired their infection vertically (Table 2.1). When examined by year of diagnosis and adjusted for reporting delay, from 1990 to 1992 there was an 18% increase in vertically acquired AIDS cases, despite an apparent decline in 1991 which occurred in certain geographic areas and may be the result of incomplete reporting or a delay in progression to AIDS due to medical intervention (Fig. 2.2). Like AIDS in women, the epidemic

Table 2.2. *AIDS cases diagnosed up to the end of 1992 in adult and adolescent women (≥13 years) and children (<13 years) by race/ethnicity and transmission category*[a]

Mode of transmission	White, non-Hispanic (%)	Black, non-Hispanic (%)	Hispanic (%)	Other[b] (%)	Total no.
Children (<13 years)					
Vertical	15	59	25	1	4 004
Haemophilia/coagulation disorder	68	13	17	2	198
Transfusion	51	23	24	2	318
No risk reported/identified	23	59	17	–	64
Women (≥13 years)					
Injecting drug use	21	58	20	<1	14 859
Heterosexual contact	23	53	23	1	10 927
Haemophilia/coagulation disorder	71	21	8	–	48
Transfusion	61	22	14	3	2 034
No risk reported/identified	25	53	20	2	2 150

[a] Reported up to the end of June 1993.
[b] Includes Asian/Pacific Islander/American Indian/Alaska Native.

continues to affect minority children disproportionately. Of vertically infected children with AIDS, 59% were black non-Hispanic, 25% Hispanic, 15% white non-Hispanic, and 1% were Asian/Pacific Islander or Indian/Native American (Table 2.2). The majority of children with AIDS were black non-Hispanic, increasing from 57% in 1988 to 62% of those diagnosed in 1992. Fifty per cent were male. Fifty-seven per cent had mothers who were either injecting drug users (40%) or were sex partners of injecting drug users (17%), suggesting prevention strategies should be targeted to this group. Thirty-two per cent of mothers of vertically infected children with AIDS were infected through heterosexual contact (Table 2.1). Recently, an increasing proportion of cases have been reported among children whose mothers acquired their HIV infection through heterosexual contact, specifically with an infected partner whose risk is not known or recognised and mothers whose risk is not known or reported. Of children reported with vertically acquired AIDS who were born in 1991, 40% had mothers who acquired their infection heterosexually and 31% had mothers who were injecting drug users.

Children with vertically acquired AIDS diagnosed up to and including 1992 have been reported from 46 states, the District of Columbia, Puerto Rico and the US Virgin Islands; 66% were from New York, Florida, New Jersey, California and Puerto Rico. The epidemic has been concentrated

Table 2.3. *Rates of AIDS among vertically infected children <13 years of age by metropolitan areas reporting the largest number of cases diagnosed in 1992, adjusted for reporting delay, USA*

Metropolitan area	No. of AIDS cases diagnosed in 1992	Rate per 100 000[a]
West Palm Beach, FL	32	24.9
Fort Lauderdale, FL	28	14.3
New York City, NY	172	11.8
Miami, FL	38	11.0
San Juan, PR	26	6.3
Baltimore, MD	25	5.7
Washington, DC	28	3.7
Philadelphia, PA	20	2.3
Chicago, IL	23	1.6
Los Angeles, CA	22	1.3

[a] Using 1990 census data.

in large urban areas on the east coast. Ten metropolitan areas accounted for 50% of vertically acquired AIDS cases diagnosed in 1992 (Table 2.3) Rates of vertically acquired AIDS greater than 10 per 100 000 population were reported in metropolitan areas in southern Florida and in New York City, NY. The metropolitan areas with the highest rates among women in 1992 were similar (Centers for Disease Control, 1993*a*). An increasing proportion of cases, however, have been reported from the south and from metropolitan areas with less than 500 000 population size. In 1992, 18% of diagnosed cases were in these less populated areas compared with 14% in 1988. Of cases diagnosed in 1992, 42% were from the South and 36% were from the Northeast compared with 28% and 52%, respectively, of cases diagnosed in 1988.

AIDS surveillance has continued to provide critical nationwide population-based information on trends in severe morbidity and mortality due to HIV infection in children. However, there are many HIV-infected children who have not met the AIDS case definition as well as children of indeterminate infection status in medical care who can not be classified on the basis of surveillance of end-stage disease alone. In addition, data from New York City suggest that many HIV-infected children may die without meeting the AIDS case definition (Lyon *et al.*, 1993).

Seroprevalence

Due to the incubation period between infection and onset of AIDS, seroprevalence data highlight the current epidemiology of HIV infection and complement AIDS surveillance data. Since 1988, CDC in collaboration with state and territorial health departments and the National Institute of

Child Health and Human Development has conducted a population-based anonymous serosurvey to measure the prevalence of HIV infection in women giving birth to live infants (Hoff *et al.*, 1988; Pappaionaou *et al.*, 1990a; Gwinn *et al.*, 1991). This serosurvey is conducted in 44 states, the District of Columbia, Puerto Rico and the US Virgin Islands (Fig. 2.3), using anonymous neonatal dried blood specimens. The 1991 and 1992 weighted national estimate of HIV prevalence in women bearing live infants was 1.7 per 1000 live births (Centers for Disease Control, 1993g). On the basis of this estimate, approximately 7000 children were born to HIV-seropositive women in 1992. Using a range of estimated rates of vertical transmission from 15% to 25%, approximately 1050–1750 infants with HIV infection were born in 1992 alone.

Seroprevalence rates varied regionally (Fig. 2.3). Births to HIV-seropositive women were detected in all but one participating area. Highest seroprevalence rates have been concentrated in urban metropolitan areas, primarily on the east coast (Wasser, *et al.*, 1993a). From 1987 to 1990, seroprevalence among women delivering live infants in New York City was 1.24%, with the highest rates (2.2%) among black women (Novick *et al.*, 1991). However, high rates of HIV infection were also found in non-urban areas of the USA, particularly the South (Wasser *et al.*, 1993a). High rates of syphilis have also been reported in non-urban areas of the Southeast, suggesting that heterosexual transmission has a substantial role in both epidemics (Rolfs & Nakashima, 1990). In 21 states with race data available in 1992, HIV seroprevalence among black childbearing women was 3–28 times higher than among white childbearing women (Centers for Disease Control, 1993g). These states accounted for approximately 75% of all HIV-infected childbearing women in the USA.

Among the 35 areas conducting the survey of childbearing women since 1989, HIV prevalence has remained relatively stable nationwide from 1989–90 (1.6 per 1000) to 1991–2 (1.7 per 1000) (Davis *et al.*, 1993). However, prevalence changed regionally. In the south, estimated births to HIV-positive women increased by 32% from 2283 in 1989 (1.7 per 1000) to 3011 (2.1 per 1000) in 1992. In the Northeast, prevalence decreased from 1989–90 (4.1 per 1000) to 1991–92 (3.6 per 1000) (Centers for Disease Control, 1993g). Although the anonymous survey of childbearing women has provided a critical population-based estimate of the number of children born to infected mothers, follow-up information on the infection status of these children or whether the child is in medical care is not available from the survey, nor is maternal risk, and demographic characteristics have been limited.

Data on HIV seroprevalence in women is also available from other anonymous unlinked surveys, conducted since 1988 in a variety of clinical

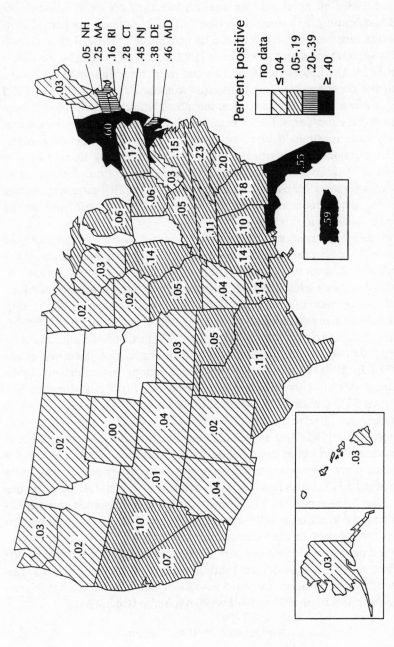

Fig. 2.3. HIV seroprevalence among childbearing women, USA, 1991 and 1992. (Results are for the last complete survey period that included births in 1992.)

settings (Pappaioanou *et al.*, 1990*b*; Centers for Disease Control, 1993*g*). Since 1985, all applicants for military service have been screened for human immunodeficiency virus type 1 (HIV-1) antibody as part of their routine medical examination (US Department of Defense, 1993). Of 546 977 women tested up to December 1992, 0.06% were positive for HIV-1 antibody. The highest rates were among women residing in states on the Atlantic coast and black non-Hispanic women. Data from 1987 to 1992 are available from routine screening of all students aged 16–21 years entering the Job Corps, a US federal training programme for socioeconomically and educationally disadvantaged youth. During this period, seroprevalence among female students increased significantly from 0.21% in 1988 to 0.42% in 1990 and remained fairly stable from 1990 to 1992 (Conway *et al.*, 1992). For female students, highest HIV rates were among blacks, increasing from 0.32% in 1988 to 0.66% in 1992, and among female students in the South.

In 1991–2, median seroprevalence among women attending 144 women's sentinel reproductive health clinics in 38 metropolitan areas in the US was 0.2% (range 0 to 3.3%) (Centers for Disease Control, 1993*g*). In 1988–9, median rates were higher among clinics offering prenatal services, with median rates of 0.6% (range 0 to 2.1%) in prenatal clinics, 0.8% (range 0 to 2.28%) in prenatal–family planning clinics, 0.15% (range 0 to 1.75%) in family planning clinics, 0.10% (range 0 to 1.9%) in abortion clinics and 0.2% (range 0.06–0.3%) in abortion–family planning clinics (Sweeney *et al.*, 1992). In 1991–2, median seroprevalence among heterosexually active women with no other acknowledged or recognised HIV risk attending 112 sentinel STD clinics in 46 metropolitan areas was 0.6% (range 0 to 8.5%) (Centers for Disease Control, 1993*g*). High median seroprevalence was found during 1991–2 among female injecting drug users attending 78 drug treatment centres in 35 metropolitan areas (median 6.3%; range 0 to 38.6%), particularly in areas on the Atlantic coast, and female injecting drug users attending STD clinics (median 4.5%; range 0 to 27.4%). High prevalence (median 5.1%; range 0 to 24.1%) was reported among women entering US correctional facilities in 1991–2, with rates either higher than or similar to rates among men in the same areas, most probably due to the high proportion of incarcerated women with a history of injecting drug use or prostitution, which is often associated with injecting drug use. The median rates among women with conditions not associated with HIV infection at 39 sentinel hospitals from 1991 to 1992 was 0.4% (range 0 to 5.2%).

Surveillance of HIV infection

Many states have added surveillance of HIV infection to surveillance of AIDS. By 1994, 25 states required reporting of HIV infection in women and 27 states required reporting of HIV infection in children (Centers for Disease Control, 1994c). Since 1992, CDC has funded active surveillance for HIV infection in these states. Children diagnosed with HIV infection as well as children who meet the 1987 paediatric AIDS case definition are reported through a standardised system in areas with HIV infection surveillance. Many of these areas also report all children with indeterminate infection status as they require continuing specialised health care, absorbing a significant proportion of clinical resources. States have implemented HIV infection surveillance to provide a minimum estimate of the number of infected persons in need of medical, social and prevention services, to monitor emerging trends in selected populations (i.e. adolescents) and to facilitate or document referrals to early treatment and prevention programmes (Centers for Disease Control, 1992d). Particularly in children, HIV infection surveillance can characterise incident infection, demonstrate the public health impact of the epidemic, provide referral for early medical intervention and prevention, help in planning for appropriate medical and social services and provide evaluation of the impact of public health recommendations (such as PCP prophylaxis guidelines, perinatal testing policies), use of zidovudine to reduce vertical HIV transmission and prevention programmes.

Data available from 22 states with HIV infection surveillance, which account for one-fifth of AIDS cases, found a higher proportion of adolescents with HIV infection compared with those reported with AIDS (3% HIV infection reports: <1% AIDS reports), women (17% : 10%) and black non-Hispanic (43% : 30%)(Fleming et al., 1993). However, the HIV data do not completely capture the population of HIV-infected persons, may be biased due to self-selection for HIV testing and over-representation of groups targeted by HIV screening programs, and currently are not implemented across the USA.

Characteristics of HIV exposed/infected children identified through paediatric HIV surveillance can be compared with estimates of the number of children born to infected mothers using the anonymous serosurvey of childbearing women to estimate the number of children who have not yet been identified. In Massachusetts, 223 newborn specimens tested HIV positive out of over 88 000 tested (2.5 per 1000 live births) during the 12 month survey period from November 1987 to October 1988 (Hsu et al., 1992). As of October 1991 when these children would have been 3–4 years of age, 78 (35%) of the 223 children born in this cohort had been medically evaluated for HIV infection and reported through statewide active paediatric HIV surveillance. Only 45% of the mothers of these 78 children were known to be HIV infected before the child's birth. The proportion of children born to HIV-infected mothers who were detected varied by geographic area. These data helped refine the areas for the targeting of physician education to improve early identification and treatment.

The Pediatric Spectrum of Disease (PSD) project is a special study conducted by CDC in seven sites in the USA. Children known to be infected or born to infected mothers are followed every 6 months by abstraction of the medical record. From 1989 to 1992, 1645 HIV-infected children who were born to HIV-infected mothers were enrolled in the project and were alive at the last clinical evaluation. Of these children, 42% had AIDS, 46% were symptomatic but did not have an AIDS defining condition and 12% were asymptomatic. In addition, 1012 children were of indeterminate HIV status (P-0), and 1053 had seroreverted and were considered uninfected. Thus, many children are in medical care and in need of resources who are HIV infected or being evaluated for HIV infection but who have not yet met the AIDS case definition. This project has provided important information on the spectrum of HIV disease in children. Although the project is population based in three of seven sites, the rural epidemic is not represented and the data may not be representative of all HIV-infected children.

Vertical transmission

A number of studies are continuing in the USA, as in Europe and other countries (see Chapter 1) to determine rates, timing and risk factors for transmission from mother to infant. Rates of vertical transmission of HIV infection from mother to infant have been reported in a variety of prospective studies and have ranged from 15% to 30% in studies in the USA (Goedert et al., 1989; Hutto et al., 1991; Mayers et al., 1991; Nair et al., 1993; Matheson et al., 1993; William-Herman et al., 1993; Bryson et al., 1993; Allen et al., 1993; Pitt et al., 1993a), from 14% to 33% in Europe (Italian Multicentre Study, 1988; Blanche et al., 1989; Lindgren et al., 1991; European Collaborative Study, 1992; Gabiano et al., 1992; Ades et al., 1993; Tibaldi et al., 1993), 25% in Haiti (Halsey et al., 1990) and somewhat higher (25–39%) in Africa (Hira et al., 1989; Ryder et al., 1989; Lepage et al., 1993; St Louis et al., 1993) (see Chapter 1). Differences in methodology (i.e. definitions of HIV infection, laboratory assessment), loss to follow-up and infant mortality have made comparisons between studies difficult (Dabis et al., 1993). These varying transmission rates may reflect different maternal clinical and immunological stage of disease as well as differences in the incidence of cofactors (e.g. chorioaminionitis) or postpartum transmission through breastfeeding (Dunn et al., 1992). In the USA and other countries where safe infant formula is available, breastfeeding is not recommended for women who are known to be HIV positive (Centers for Disease Control, 1985b). Three published prospective US studies conducted in Miami, Florida, Brooklyn, New York, and Baltimore, Maryland, report transmission rates of 23–30% (Goedert *et al.*, 1989; Hutto *et al.*, 1991; Nair *et al.*, 1993). Recent data from the New York City Perinatal HIV Transmission Collaborative Study estimated a transmission rate of 25% based on follow-up of almost 200 children (Matheson *et al.*, 1993). Other recent data on transmission rates have been reported from prospective studies in Los Angeles (28%; 22/74) (Bryson *et al.*, 1993), New York City (22.8%) (Allen *et al.*, 1993) and San Francisco (15.1%; 8/53) (William-Herman *et al.*, 1993). Several continuing multicentre prospective studies have studied correlates of transmission of HIV from mother to infant in the USA. These include the Perinatal AIDS Collaborative Transmission Studies (PACTS) coordinated at five sites by the Centers for Disease Control and Prevention, the Women and Infants Transmission Study (WITS) coordinated by the National Institutes of Health (NIH), the Ariel Project coordinated by the Pediatric AIDS Foundation to investigate maternal virological and immunological correlates of transmission, and the Pediatric Pulmonary and Cardiovascular Complication of Vertically Transmitted HIV Infection Study (P2C2) coordinated by the National Heart Lung Blood Institute, NIH, to determine the natural history of heart and lung disease in vertically infected children.

Determining the timing and risk factors for perinatal transmission of HIV infection is critical for designing appropriate intervention, prevention and maternal counselling strategies (Pizzo & Butler, 1991; Bryson *et al.*, 1992; Mofenson, *et al.*, 1992). Studies have evaluated the role of maternal, viral and immunological factors, placental factors and obstetric factors that may affect vertical transmission (see Chapter 1). Studies conducted in the USA have complemented studies in Europe and in Africa to highlight the multifactorial nature of vertical transmission. Higher transmission rates have been associated with advanced maternal clinical disease and low maternal CD4 lymphocyte count in US studies (Mayers *et al.*, 1991; Thomas *et al.*, 1992) as in studies in Europe and Africa (Ryder *et al.*, 1989; European Collaborative Study, 1992; Tibaldi *et al.*, 1993; St Louis *et al.*, 1993). Recent data from the WITS study suggest a decreased risk of transmission among mothers with high CD4% (>30) and with both high CD4% and maternal HIV cultures which were not consistently positive near the time of delivery (Pitt *et al.*, 1993*b*). The level of p24 antigenaemia has also been associated with transmission in studies in Europe and Africa (European Collaborative Study, 1992; Tibaldi *et al.*, 1993; St Louis *et al.*, 1993). Elevated maternal CD8 lymphocyte counts were associated with an increased risk of transmission in a study in Zaïre, which may be related to early maternal HIV infection with subsequent higher plasma viraemia (St Louis *et al.*, 1993). Data from the PACTS study suggest no increased risk of transmission to subsequent siblings born to infected mothers (Perinatal AIDS Collaborative Transmission Studies Group, 1992).

Placental factors and concurrent infections of the genital tract may also play a role in transmission and several studies suggest a higher transmission risk with chorioamnionitis (Ryder *et al.*, 1989; Nair *et al.*, 1993; St Louis *et al.*, 1993), seroevidence of syphilis (Allen *et al.*, 1993) or possibly other maternal sexually transmitted diseases during pregnancy (Nair *et al.*, 1993; Thomas *et al.*, 1992). As in the European Collaborative Study, studies in the USA have reported an association between preterm delivery (Goedert *et al.*, 1989) or low birthweight (Nair *et al.*, 1993) and vertical transmission. Several prospective studies conducted in the USA have evaluated the role of caesarean section in reducing HIV transmission (Hutto *et al.*, 1991; Nair *et al.*, 1993; William-Herman *et al.*, 1993; Allen *et al.*, 1993; Goedert *et al.*, 1993). A recent meta-analysis (Villari *et al.*, 1993) of six cohort studies, including three USA studies (Goedert *et al.*, 1991; Hutto *et al.*, 1991; Nair *et al.*, 1993), suggests a potentially protective effect of caesarean section on reduction of vertical transmission (odds ratio 0.65, 95% confidence interval 0.43 to 0.99), although limitations of these studies must be considered. Conflicting results have been reported concerning the role of other intrapartum factors such as invasive fetal monitoring (William-Herman *et al.*, 1993; Allen *et al.*, 1993). Further study is needed to clarify the contribution of mode of delivery and obstetric factors to the risk of vertical transmission (Tovo, 1993).

Several studies have reported that maternal antibodies to the envelope protein gp120, maternal antibodies to specific epitopes of the gp120 hypervariable V3 region or the avidity of maternal antibodies to gp120 principal neutralising domain were associated with a lower rate of vertical transmission (Goedert *et al.*, 1989; Rossi *et al.*, 1989; Devash *et al.*, 1990). However, other studies have not been able to confirm these findings (Parekh *et al.*, 1991). The role of maternal neutralising antibodies, maternal viral characteristics, maternal viral load and genetic factors is not clear and needs further study (Report of a consensus workshop, 1992).

Family and social impact of HIV infection

HIV affects the whole family (see Chapters 14 and 17). HIV-infected and uninfected children left motherless by the death of HIV-infected mothers will require increasing resources in the future. In 1991, HIV infection was the fifth leading cause of death in women 25–44 years of age in the USA, accounting for 6% of all deaths, and the seventh leading cause of death among women 15–24 years of age (National Center for Health Statistics, 1993; Centers for Disease Control, 1993e). Among women 25–44 years of age, HIV infection was the leading cause of death in nine cities in 1990 (Jersey City, Newark and Paterson, New Jersey; New Haven and Stamford, Connecticut; Baltimore, Maryland; New York City, New York; Fort Lauderdale and Miami, Florida), and in Newark, New Jersey, accounted for 43% of all deaths (Selik *et al.*, 1993*a*). By December 1991, it was estimated that in the USA there were at least 14 500 uninfected orphans of women with AIDS reported to have died who will require long-term care by relatives, foster parents or social service agencies, and that 93 000–112 000 uninfected children will have been born to infected women in the next decade, many of whom will also become orphans (Caldwell *et al.*, 1992*a*). Another study projected similar estimates (Michaels & Levine, 1992). However, due to conservative assumptions both estimates of future orphans most probably underestimate the number of motherless youth (Nicholas & Abrams, 1992). In addition, children born to HIV-infected mothers often do not live with biological parents due to maternal drug use (Caldwell *et al.*, 1992*b*). These children also often live in poverty and have other health and social service needs as well as being at high risk for HIV infection through sexual and drug use activities themselves (Nicholas & Abrams, 1992). The emotional impact on the family affected by HIV can also be profound. Public health resources are needed now and particularly in the future for all affected family members.

Transmission through receipt of blood, blood products or blood-containing tissue (see Chapter 11)

Since the implementation of heat treatment for clotting factors in 1984 and nationwide screening of blood and blood products in 1985 in conjunction with self-deferral of donations from individuals at high risk for HIV, incident cases of HIV infection attributed to these transmission routes have been virtually eliminated in the USA (Fig. 2.2). Overall, 7% (318/4584) of paediatric AIDS cases diagnosed by the end of 1992 and reported up to June 1993 acquired HIV infection from transfusion of blood or blood products (Table 2.1), with the number of cases diagnosed continuing to decline since 1988 (Fig. 2.2). The number of diagnosed cases among children less than 5 years of age peaked in 1985 (Selik, *et al.*, 1993*b*). The risk of transmission after transfusion of HIV-infected blood is over 89% and is proportional to the prevalence of HIV among donors as well as the number of transfusions received (Petersen, *et al.*, 1993). Most children with transfusion-acquired AIDS were transfused during infancy because of perinatal problems; therefore, the demographics of these cases reflect characteristics of children with increased perinatal morbidity (Jones *et al.*, 1992*a*). Two-thirds of AIDS cases associated with transfusion have been reported among males. Although the majority of children (51%) were white, a disproportionate number of black non-Hispanic (23%) and Hispanic (24%) children have been affected. Among children with transfusion-associated AIDS, the median age of AIDS diagnosis was 5 years and 11% were diagnosed at 12 months of age or younger. Cases have been reported from 36 states, Washington, DC, and Puerto Rico.

The risk of HIV transmission from transfusion of screened blood products has been estimated to be less than 1 in 150 000 (Petersen *et al.*, 1993) in the USA due to the possibility of transfusion during the period of time after infection and before seroconversion. There have also been rare reports of transmission from seronegative organ and tissue donors during this window period (Simonds *et al.*, 1992). As of September 1993, only two children and 19 adolescents/adults have developed AIDS following receipt of blood screened negative for HIV-antibody at the time of donation, where the donor later seroconverted.

By the end of 1992, haemophilia and other clotting disorders accounted for 4% (198/4584) of children diagnosed with AIDS, with the number of cases declining since 1989. Nearly all cases (96%) were in males, which reflects the genetic transmission of haemoglobinopathies. The racial distribution was 68% white non-Hispanic, 13% black non-Hispanic, 17% Hispanic, and 2% Asian, Pacific Islander, Indian or Native American. The median age at AIDS diagnosis was 10 years and only 2% of cases were diagnosed at 12 months of age or younger. Cases have been reported from 36 states and Puerto Rico. Sexual transmission of HIV infection to sex partners of male haemophiliacs and subsequent transmission to children has accounted for 20 children with vertically acquired HIV infection and represents 0.4% of all paediatric cases. Since 1987, the National Hemophilia Foundation, the Food and Drug Administration, and the Centers for Disease Control and Prevention have conducted a study, the Seroconversion Surveillance Project, to monitor the risk of transmission through clotting factor concentrates. Of 9496 patients from 131 haemophilia treatment centres in the USA, 46% have been reported seropositive. No seroconversions have been detected in patients who received only heat-treated concentrates made only from plasma tested for HIV-antibody (Fricke *et al.*, 1992).

Other modes of transmission

Sexual transmission of HIV infection to children through sexual abuse has been reported, although rarely (Gutman *et al.*, 1991; Gellert *et al.*, 1993; Hanson *et al.*, 1994). CDC is now systematically collecting information on sexual transmission of HIV infection in children less than 13 years of age reported with AIDS and in children reported with HIV infection from states with confidential HIV surveillance. Because the incidence of reported sexual abuse has increased in the USA (Krugman, 1986), the number of cases of paediatric AIDS identified or recognised as exposed through sexual transmission may increase. Screening policies for HIV-antibody among children who have been sexually abused have varied, and have included policies such as selective testing based on prevalence of HIV infection in the community and risk factors of the perpetrator (Gellert, *et al.*, 1990; American Academy of Pediatrics, 1991; Centers for Disease Control, 1993*d*). Standardised guidelines for HIV screening of abused children may assist in identifying more children who may have acquired HIV infection through sexual transmission.

As of September 1993, of over 4900 children reported to CDC with AIDS only 1% have no reported or identified risk. State and local health departments, with technical assistance from CDC, perform standardised follow-up investigations of these AIDS cases. Most AIDS cases initially reported with no risk are subsequently reclassified into known transmission modes (Lifson *et al.*, 1987; Castro *et al.*, 1988; Hammett *et al.*, 1993), usually vertical transmission for children. The majority of cases remaining without reported risk have incomplete information about the birth mother (Hammett, *et al.*, 1993). None of the investigations of these cases have documented transmission by other than recognised modes.

Concern has been raised about the possibility of transmission of HIV in settings such as households, day-care facilities and schools. A recent review paper (Simonds & Chanock, 1993) summarised studies of HIV infection prevalence among persons sharing households with HIV-infected persons. In 17 studies, ten conducted in the USA and seven in Europe, of 1167 household contacts, including more than 300 children, of infected persons with no other risks for HIV infection who were followed for 1700 person-years none were infected (95% confidence interval for rate of infection 0 to 0.18 per 100 person-years) (Simonds & Chanock, 1993; Simonds & Rogers, 1993). Several of these studies found no transmission despite considerable close personal contact among household members that may have resulted in exposure to blood or other body fluids (Lawrence *et al.*, 1985; Rogers *et al.*, 1990; Friedland *et al.*, 1990). There have been rare reports (Grint & McEvoy, 1985; Koenig *et al.*, 1986; Centers for Disease Control, 1986, 1992*a*) suggesting HIV transmission may have occurred during health care practices in the home through percutaneous or cutaneous exposure to blood or contaminated needles. These cases highlight the need for careful attention to proper infection control practices in any setting where exposure to blood is possible (Centers for Disease Control, 1987*c*, 1988). There have been rare reports of transmission of HIV in households between siblings where opportunities for skin or mucous membrane exposure to HIV-infected blood were present. A brief case report (Wahn *et al.*, 1986) suggested transmission of HIV-1 infection occurred between two siblings through biting, although there was no break in the child's skin. A recent report suggested transmission of HIV occurred between two young household members through presumed but undocumented contact of skin or mucous membranes to infected blood (Fitzgibbon *et al.*, 1993; Simonds & Rogers, 1993) and another report documented HIV transmission from an older brother with haemophilia and HIV infection to his younger adolescent brother with haemophilia, most likely through blood exposure (Centers for Disease Control, 1993*b*). However, because transmission of HIV is rare in settings such as homes, schools and day-care centres, and recommendations have been made to prevent exposure in these settings (American Public Health Association & American Academy of Pediatrics, 1992: Centers for Disease Control, 1985*a*), HIV-infected children should not be excluded because of their HIV infection alone. Nevertheless, to prevent these rare occurrences, precautions to prevent exposure to blood, as described in previously published guidelines (Centers for Disease Control, 1987*c*, 1988; American Public Health Association & American Academy of Pediatrics, 1992), should be taken in all settings, including the home (see Chapter 9).

Clinical spectrum of disease and survival

Since the first report of AIDS in children born to infected mothers in 1982, a great deal has been learnt about the spectrum of paediatric HIV disease. In the USA, AIDS surveillance is critical in providing information on severe morbidity and mortality of children meeting the AIDS surveillance case definition. Further information comes from prospective clinical studies such as those conducted by the AIDS Clinical Trials Groups; however, only a small proportion of the infected children are followed in these studies. A more thorough and broad-based description of HIV-related illness in children has been provided through several studies of children in Europe and the USA.

Information about the prevalence of AIDS-defining conditions in children less than 13 years of age diagnosed with AIDS by December 1992 and reported up to June 1993 is presented in Table 2.4. *Pneumocystis carinii* pneumonia (PCP) is the most common AIDS-defining condition in children (37%) regardless of mode of transmission. These reports are likely to represent minimum estimates of opportunistic infections due to incomplete reporting of subsequent opportunistic infections in AIDS surveillance.

Table 2.4. *AIDS indicator diseases most commonly reported for children >13 years of age, diagnosed up to December 1992 and reported up to June 1993, by mode of transmission, USA*

AIDS indicator disease	Vertical (%) (n = 4004)	Haemo-philia (%) (n = 198)	Transfu-sion (%) (n = 318)	Total[a] (%) (n = 4584)
Pneumocystis carinii pneumonia	37	32	31	37
Lymphoid interstitial pneumonitis	25	6	21	24
Recurrent bacterial infections	19	16	27	19
Candida oesophagitis	14	21	16	14
Wasting syndrome	14	20	17	14
HIV encephalopathy	13	13	13	12
Cytomegalovirus disease	8	3	6	8
Mycobacterium avium complex	4	10	12	5
Candidiasis of lung	4	4	3	4
Chronic herpes simplex	3	7	3	4
Cryptosporidiosis	3	8	4	3
Cryptococcosis, extrapulmonary	1	6	3	1

[a] Includes 64 cases with no risk reported/identified.

A recent study described the epidemiology of PCP in children reported with vertically acquired HIV infection. Fifty-three per cent of 1374 cases of PCP occurred in children 3–6 months of age (Simonds *et al.*, 1993). Median survival after diagnosis of PCP in 278 children with follow-up information was 19 months. An estimated minimum risk of developing PCP in the first year of life for HIV-infected children born to HIV-infected mothers in 1989 was 7–20%. However, of children reported with PCP, 44% had not been evaluated for HIV infection prior to the month before PCP diagnosis, including 63% of children less than 6 months of age at PCP diagnosis. Despite guidelines for PCP prophylaxis published in 1991 in the USA (Centers for Disease Control, 1991) and data suggesting that an increasing proportion of children in medical care are on prophylaxis (Caldwell *et al.*, 1992c), PCP is still the most common opportunistic infection in children with AIDS. CDC is currently evaluating the impact of the guidelines on the incidence of PCP and the effectiveness of the current guidelines (Simonds *et al.*, 1994).

Recent analysis of characteristics of children reported with *Mycobacterium avium* complex (MAC) suggest that this opportunistic infection occurs late in the course of HIV disease. Median CD4 counts of children within 6 months of their diagnosis of non-tuberculous mycobacterial infection was 17 cells/mm^3, and median survival from date of diagnosis was 5 months, regardless of mode of HIV transmission (Horsburgh, *et al.* 1993). Although data from AIDS surveillance suggest that a larger proportion of children with transfusion-associated HIV infection or haemophilia have been reported with MAC than those with vertically acquired HIV infection, this is most probably due to a larger proportion of children with transfusion-associated AIDS who have very low CD4 counts due to a longer duration of HIV infection. Another study also found that the risk of developing disseminated MAC in children was associated with increasing age and low CD4 cell count (Rutstein *et al.*, 1993). Recently published recommendations for prophylaxis and treatment for disseminated MAC infection for adults and adolescents suggest prophylaxis should be considered for HIV-infected children (Centers for Disease Control, 1993*c*). Recent guidelines for the medical management of HIV infection in children suggest that selected high-risk children (>2 years old with less than 150 CD4 lymphocytes/mm3) should receive Rifabutin prophylaxis (Working Group on Antiretroviral Therapy, 1993).

Deaths have been reported for 54% of children with AIDS. Mortality data related to HIV infection from the National Center for Health Statistics indicate that, in 1991, HIV infection accounted for 1% of all deaths in children 1–4 years of age and 0.3% of all deaths in children 5–14 years of age (National Center for Health Statistics, 1993). The impact of HIV/ AIDS on childhood mortality has been greatest in children aged 1–4 years, in the northeast and in black and Hispanic children (Chu *et al.*, 1991). In New York City, AIDS was the second leading cause of death among children aged 1–14 years in 1990 (Thomas *et al.*, 1993).

One of the goals of the PSD project is to describe the spectrum of morbidity among children known to be HIV infected or born to infected mothers. From 1989 to 1992, more than 4000 children had been enrolled. The prevalence of the many and varied non-specific signs and symptoms among infected children must be interpreted within the context of normal childhood illnesses among uninfected children from similar populations. Table 2.5 shows the prevalence of selected non-specific signs and symptoms among children eventually determined to be infected compared with those who seroreverted and were presumed uninfected. Chronic/persistent otitis media was more common in infected children (50%) but was recorded for 1 in 4 of the children who seroreverted. Other signs, such as lymphadenopathy and failure to achieve new developmental milestones, were recorded for nearly 10% of uninfected children but were far more common among infected children. Still other signs, such as thrombocytopenia, parotid enlargement and cardiomyopathy, were seen almost exclusively among infected children.

By age 15 months, more than 90% of children have at least mild symptoms attributable to HIV (Tovo *et al.*, 1992). Table 2.6 lists the prevalence of selected non-specific signs and symptoms comparing symptomatic ver-

Table 2.5. *Prevalence of selected non-specific signs and symptoms among children who are HIV infected (all modes of transmission) versus seroreverters*

Signs and symptoms	Infected (%) (*n*=2123)	Seroreverted (%) (*n*=1112)
Persistent otitis	50	27
Failure to thrive	34	8
Weight loss (>10% of baseline)	7	<1
Chronic diarrhoea (>2 months)	18	3
Recurrent diarrhoea	9	2
Fever (>2 months)	33	6
Lymphadenopathy	63	10
Hepatomegaly	54	9
Splenomegaly	42	3
Anaemia	36	8
Thrombocytopenia	15	<1
Nephropathy	4	<1
Herpes stomatitis	3	0
Herpes bronchitis/pneumonitis	<1	0
Disseminated herpes	3	0
Disseminated varicella	3	<1
Parotid enlargement	10	<1
Pulmonary tuberculosis	2	<1
Lower respiratory infection[a]	24	8
Failure to progress[b]	29	10
Motor failure[c]	11	2
Impaired brain growth	8	2
Cardiomyopathy	10	<1

Data from the Pediatric Spectrum of Disease Project, 1989–92.
[a] Lower respiratory infection of undetermined aetiology.
[b] Failure to achieve new developmental milestones.
[c] Failure of motor function.

tically infected children who have not yet met the AIDS case definition with those who have. Children with AIDS have a greater prevalence of all the listed conditions except lymphadenopathy ($p = 0.02$). Fever lasting more than 2 months, failure to thrive, weight loss (>10% of baseline weight), chronic diarrhoea, failure of motor function; and cardiomyopathy were among the conditions occurring twice as often in children with AIDS. Nephropathy occurred almost exclusively in children with AIDS (Table 2.6).

However, it appeared that the signs and symptoms alone did not predict the outcome in these children. Early in the paediatric epidemic, the French collaborative group described a bimodal distribution of clinical and

Table 2.6 *Prevalence of selected non-specific signs and symptoms among vertically infected symptomatic children*[a]

	(n=757) Not AIDS[a]		(n=683) AIDS	
Fever (>2 months)	208	(27)	340	(50)
Failure to thrive	180	(24)	363	(53)
Weight loss (>10%)	27	(4)	83	(12)
Chronic diarrhoea(>2 months)	99	(13)	183	(27)
Recurrent diarrhoea	54	(7)	91	(13)
Lymphadenopathy	540	(71)	448	(66)
Hepatomegaly	448	(59)	490	(72)
Splenomegaly	344	(45)	383	(56)
Parotid enlargement	66	(9)	89	(13)
Failure to progress[b]	186	(25)	323	(47)
Motor failure[c]	50	(7)	144	(21)
Impaired brain growth	35	(5)	103	(15)
Oral/pharyngeal candida	282	(37)	424	(62)
Herpes stomatitis	13	(2)	33	(5)
Herpes bronchitis/pneumonitis	1	(<1)	2	(<1)
Disseminated herpes	29	(4)	22	(3)
Disseminated varicella	17	(2)	26	(4)
Pulmonary tuberculosis	12	(2)	17	(2)
Persistent otitis	397	(52)	405	(59)
Lower respiratory infection[c]	164	(22)	219	(32)
Cardiomyopathy	36	(5)	132	(19)
Nephropathy	4	(<1)	47	(7)
Anaemia	259	(34)	349	(51)
Thrombocytopenia	97	(13)	132	(19)

[Values are number (percentage).
[a] Data from the Pediatric Spectrum of Disease Project, 1989–92.
[b] Failure to achieve new developmental milestones.
[c] Failure of motor function.
[d] Lower respiratory infection of undetermined aetiology.

biological symptoms (Blanche *et al.*, 1990). It was shown that onset of severe symptoms in the first 2 years of life was highly correlated with shortened survival (Duliege *et al.*, 1992). Using mathematical modelling, Auger *et al.* (1988), Costagliola *et al.* (1990), and then Commenges *et al.* (1992), demonstrated a bimodal distribution of the AIDS incubation period. More recently, similar techniques were used to show a bimodal distribution of survival, using data from the PSD Project and from national AIDS surveillance. The model estimated that 24–30% of perinatally infected children were short-term survivors and had an accelerated disease course with a median survival of 5 months if diagnosed with PCP and 19 months if not (R. Byers, Division of HIV/AIDS, CDC, Personal communication December 1993). The remaining 70–76% of children had a relative constant and low rate of death with a median survival greater than 8 years among those not diagnosed with PCP. Further work is necessarily to identify methods to predict survival prospectively in the clinical setting.

Tuberculosis has become increasingly common among HIV-infected persons, and cases of tuberculosis are being reported in children (Jones *et al.*, 1992*b*). Diagnosis in children is often difficult due to anergy and obtaining clinical specimens for culture. In addition, uninfected children of HIV-infected adults with tuberculosis are also at-risk. Prompt identification and treatment of contacts along with appropriate therapy will be essential to reduce the spread of tuberculosis.

Prevention of HIV infection

In order to prevent HIV infection in children, effective strategies must be developed to prevent infection in women by reducing risk behaviors such as needle-sharing drug use and high risk sexual behaviour. Recent studies provide evidence that latex condoms are highly effective in protecting against HIV infection when used properly (Centers for Disease Control, 1993*f*). However, many sexually active women do not use condoms on a consistent basis. In addition, recent data suggest that many women do not seek HIV testing early in the course of their disease. Data collected from interviews of persons diagnosed with AIDS between 1990 to 1992 through a Supplement to the HIV/AIDS surveillance project in the USA found that most women were tested for HIV because they were sick rather than aware of their risk for HIV infection. Thus, many were getting tested only 2 months before their AIDS diagnosis (Wortley, *et al.*, 1993). Public health programme and health care providers need to assess HIV risk and routinely provide HIV counselling and testing to those at-risk. Seroprevalence data from the survey of childbearing women have been evaluated as a means of selecting specific geographic areas where routine HIV testing of pregnant women would identify the most HIV positive women and their infants for early intervention and evaluation (Wasser *et al.*, 1993*b*). Strategies to prevent vertical transmission of HIV infection are also being evaluated (see Chapter 1). These include clinical trials of zidovudine, HIV immune globulin, and vaccine in pregnant women as well as evaluation of different obstetric practices. Health care providers and public health professionals face considerable challenges in the coming decade to care for families affected by HIV disease and prevent future cases from occurring.

References

Allen, M., Weisman, C., Weedon, J. & Krasinski, K. (1993). Antepartum and intrapartum factors in perinatal HIV transmission [abstract PO-CO2–2594]. Berlin: IXth International AIDS Conference.

Ades, A. E., Davison C. F., Holland F. J., et al. (1993). Vertically transmitted HIV infection in the British Isles. British Medical Journal, 306, 1296–9.

American Academy of Pediatrics (1991). Committee on Child Abuse and Neglect. Guidelines for the evaluation of sexual abuse of children. Pediatrics, 87, 254–60.

American Public Health Association, American Academy of Pediatrics (1992). Caring for our children–national health and safety performance standards: guidelines for out-of-home child care programs. Washington, D.C: American Public Health Association, 24–8.

Auger, I., Thomas, P., de Grutola, V., et al. (1988). Incubation periods for pediatric AIDS patients. Nature, 336, 575–7.

Blanche, S., Rouzioux, C., Moscato, M.L., et al. (1989). A prospective study of infants born to women seropositive for HIV type 1. New England Journal of Medicine, 320, 1643–8.

Blanche, S., Tardieu, M., Duliege, A.-M., et al. (1990). Longitudinal study of 94 symptomatic infants with perinatally acquired human immunodeficiency virus infection. American Journal of Diseases of Children, 144, 1210–15.

Bryson, Y. J., Luzuriaga, K., Sullivan, J. L. & Wara, D. W. (1992). Proposed definitions for in utero versus intrapartum transmission of HIV-1. New England Journal of Medicine, 327, 1246–7.

Bryson, Y., Dillon, M., Garratty, E., et al. (1993). The role timing of HIV maternal-fetal transmission (in utero vs. intrapartum) and HIV phenotype on onset of symptoms in vertically infected infants (abstract WS-C10-2). Berlin: IXth International AIDS Conference.

Buehler, J. W., Berkelman, R. L. & Stehr-Green, J. K. (1992). The completeness of AIDS surveillance. Journal of Acquired Immunodeficiency Syndromes, 5, 257–64.

Caldwell, M. B., Fleming, P. L. & Oxtoby, M. J. (1992a). Estimated number of AIDS orphans in the United States (letter). Pediatrics, 90, 482.

Caldwell, M. B., Mascola, L., Smith, W., et al. (1992b). Biologic, foster, and adoptive parents: Care givers of children exposed perinatally to human immunodeficiency virus in the United States. Pediatrics, 90, 603–7.

Caldwell, B., Mascola, L., Lyon, L., et al. (1992c). Increasing PCP prophylaxis antiretroviral use and CD4 monitoring in HIV-infected children (abstract 907). Anaheim, CA: 32nd Interscience Conference on Antimicrobial Agents and Chemotherapy.

Castro, K. G., Lifson, A. R., White, C. R., et al. (1988). Investigations of AIDS patients with no previously identified risk factors. Journal of the American Medical Association, 259, 1338–42.

Centers for Disease Control (1982). Unexplained immunodeficiency and opportunistic infections in infants: New York, New Jersey, California. Morbidity and Mortality Weekly Report, 31, 665–7.

Centers for Disease Control (1985a). Education and foster care of children infected with human T-lymphotrophic virus type III/ lymphadenopathy-associated virus. Morbidity and Mortality Weekly Report, 34, 517–21.

Centers for Disease Control (1985b). Recommendations for assisting in the prevention of perinatal transmission of human T-lymphocyte type III lymphadenopathy-associated virus and acquired immunodeficiency syndrome. *Morbidity and Mortality Weekly Report*, **34**, 721–32.

Centers for Disease Control (1986). Apparent transmission of human T-lymphotropic virus type III/lymphadenopathy-associated virus from a child to a mother providing health care. *Morbidity and Mortality Weekly Report*, **35**, 76–9.

Centers for Disease Control (1987*a*). Classification system for human immunodeficiency virus (HIV) infection in children under 13 year of age. *Morbidity and Mortality Weekly Report*, **36**, 225–230, 235–6.

Centers for Disease Control (1987*b*). Revision of the CDC surveillance case definition for acquired immunodeficiency syndrome. *Morbidity and Mortality Weekly Report*, **36** (Suppl 1), 1S–15S.

Centers for Disease Control (1987*c*). Recommendations for prevention of HIV transmission in health-care settings. *Morbidity and Mortality Weekly Report*, **36** (Suppl 2S), 1–18S.

Centers for Disease Control (1988). Update: universal precautions for prevention of transmission of HIV, hepatitis B virus, and other bloodborne pathogens in health-care settings. *Morbidity and Mortality Weekly Report*, **37**, 377–82, 387–8.

Centers for Disease Control (1991). Guidelines for prophylaxis against *Pneumocystis carinii* pneumonia for children infected with human immunodeficiency virus. *Morbidity and Mortality Weekly Report*, **40** (RR-2), 1–13.

Centers for Disease Control (1992*a*). HIV infection in two brothers receiving intravenous therapy for hemophilia. *Morbidity and Mortality Weekly Report*, **41**, 228–31.

Centers for Disease Control (1992*b*). Projections of the number of persons diagnosed with AIDS and the number of immunosuppressed HIV-infected persons: United States, 1992–94. *Morbidity and Mortality Weekly Report*, **41** (RR-18), 1–29.

Centers for Disease Control (1992*c*). 1993 Revised classification system for HIV infection and expanded surveillance case definition for AIDS among adolescents and adults. *Morbidity and Mortality Weekly Report*, **41** (RR-17), 1–19.

Centers for Disease Control (1992*d*). Public health uses of HIV-infection reports: South Carolina. 1986–91. *Morbidity and Mortality Weekly Report*, **41**, 245–9.

Centers for Disease Control (1993*a*). Update: acquired immunodeficiency syndrome: United States, 1992. *Morbidity and Mortality Weekly Report*, **42**, 547–551, 557.

Centers for Disease Control (1993*b*). HIV transmission between two adolescent brothers with hemophilia. *Morbidity and Mortality Weekly Report*, **42**, 948–51.

Centers for Disease Control (1993*c*). Recommendations on prophylaxis and therapy for disseminated *Mycobacterium avium* complex for adults and adolescents infected with human immunodeficiency virus. *Morbidity and Mortality Weekly Report*, **42** (RR-9), 14–20.

Centers for Disease Control (1993*d*). 1993 Sexually transmitted diseases treatment guidelines. *Morbidity and Mortality Weekly Report*, **42**, 99–102.

Centers for Disease Control (1993*e*). Update: mortality attributable to HIV infection/AIDS among persons aged 25–44 years: United States, 1990 and 1991. *Morbidity and Mortality Weekly Report*, **42**, 481–86.

Centers for Disease Control (1993*f*). Update: barrier protection against HIV infection and other sexually transmitted diseases. *Morbidity and Mortality Weekly Report*, **42**, 589–91, 597.

Centers for Disease Control (1993g). National HIV serosurveillance summary, vol 3. Results through 1992. *Atlanta: U.S. Department of Health and Human Services, publication HIV/NCID/11–93/036.*

Centers for Disease Control (1994). Update: impact of the expanded AIDS surveillance case definition for adolescents and adults on case reporting: United States, 1993. *Morbidity and Mortality Weekly Report*, **43**, 160–1, 167–70.

Chu, S. Y., Buehler, J. W., Oxtoby, M. J. & Kilbourne, B. W. (1991). Impact of the human immunodeficiency virus epidemic on mortality in children, United States. *Pediatrics*, **87**, 806–10.

Commenges, D. Alioum, A., Lepage, P., *et al.* (1992). Estimating the incubation period of paediatric AIDS in Rwanda. *AIDS*, **6**, 1500–20.

Costagliola, D., Laporte, A., Chevret, S., *et al.* (1990.) Incubation time for AIDS among homosexual and pediatric cases (abstract Th.C.661). San Francisco: VIth International Conference on AIDS.

Conway, G. A., Epstein, M. R., Hayman, C. R., *et al.* (1992). Trends in HIV prevalence among disadvantaged youth. Survey results from a national job training program, 1988 through 1992. *Journal of the American Medical Association*, **269**, 2887–9.

Curran, J. W., Jaffe, H. W., Hardy, A. M., *et al.* (1988). Epidemiology of HIV infection and AIDS in the United States. *Science*, **239**, 610–16.

Dabis, F., Msellati, P., Dunn, D., *et al.* (1993). Estimating the rate of mother-to-child transmission of HIV. Report of a workshop on methodological issues Ghent (Belgium), 17–20 February 1992. *AIDS*, **7**, 1139–47.

Davis, S., Gwinn, M., Wasser, S., *et al.* (1993). *HIV prevalence among US childbearing women, 1989–92* (abstract 27). Washington, D. C.: First National Conference on Human Retroviruses and Related Infections.

Devash, Y., Calvelli, T. A., Wood, D. G., *et al.* (1990). Vertical transmission of human immunodeficiency virus is correlated with the absence of high-affinity/avidity maternal antibodies to the gp120 principal neutralizing domain. *Proceedings of the National Academy of Sciences, USA*, **87**, 3445–9.

Duliege, A.-M., Messiah, A., Blanche S., *et al.* (1992). Natural history of human immunodeficiency virus type 1 infection in children: prognostic value of laboratory test on the bimodal progression of the disease. *Pediatric Infectious Disease Journal*, **11**, 630–6.

Dunn, D. T., Newell, M. L., Ades, A. E. & Peckham, C. S. (1992). Risk of human immunodeficiency virus type 1 transmission through breastfeeding. *Lancet*, **340**, 585–7.

Ellerbrock, T. V., Bush, T. J., Chamberland, M. E. & Oxtoby, M. J. (1991) Epidemiology of women with AIDS in the United States, 1981 through 1990. *Journal of the American Medical Association*, **265**, 2971–5.

European Collaborative Study. (1992). Risk factors for mother-to child transmission of HIV-1. *Lancet*, **339**, 1007–12, 41.

Fitzgibbon, J. E., Gaur, S., Frenkel, L. D., *et al.* (1993). Transmission from one child to another of human immunodeficiency virus type 1 with a zidovidine-resistant mutation. *New England Journal of Medicine*, **329**, 1835–41.

Fleming, P. L. & Gwinn, M. (1994). Human immunodeficiency virus. In *From Data To Action: CDC's Public Health Surveillance for Women, Infants, and*

Children, ed. L. Wilcox & J. Marks. Public Health Service, US Dept of Health and Human Services (in press).

Fleming, P. L., Ward, J. W., Morgan, M. W., *et al.* (1993). Mandatory HIV reporting: characteristics of adults reported with HIV compared to AIDS in the United States (abstract WS-C17–2). Berlin: IX International Conference on AIDS.

Fricke, W., Augustyniak, L., Lawrence, D., *et al.* (1992). Human immunodeficiency virus infection due to clotting factor concentrates: results of the Seroconversion Surveillance Project. *Transfusion*, **32**, 707–9.

Friedland, G., Kahl, P., Saltzman, B., *et al.* (1990). Additional evidence for lack of transmission of HIV infection by close interpersonal (casual) contact. *AIDS*, **4**, 639–44.

Gabiano, C., Tovo, P. A., de Martino, M., *et al.* (1992). Mother-to-child transmission of human immunodeficiency virus type 1: risk of infection and correlates of transmission. *Pediatrics*, **90**, 369–74.

Gellert, G. A., Durfee, M. J. & Berkowitz, C. D. (1990). Developing guidelines for HIV antibody testing among victims of pediatric sexual abuse. *Child Abuse and Neglect*, **14**, 9–17.

Gellert, G. A., Durfee, M. J., Berkowitz, C. D., *et al.* (1993). Situational and sociodemographic characteristics of children infected with human immunodeficiency virus from pediatric sexual abuse. *Pediatrics*, **91**, 39–44.

Goedert, J. J., Mendez, H., Drummond, J. E., *et al.* (1989). Mother to infant transmission of human immunodeficiency virus type 1: Association with prematurity or low anti-gp120. *Lancet* **334**, 1351–4.

Goedert, J. J., Duliege, A. M., Amos, C. I., *et al.* (1991). High risk of HIV-1 infection for first born twins. *Lancet*, **338**, 1471–5.

Goedert, J. J., Amos, C. I., Willoughby, A., *et al.* (1993). Reduced risk of HIV-1 infection with cesarean delivery in singletons and first-born twins (abstract PO-C16–2986). Berlin: IXth International Conference on AIDS.

Grint, P. & McEvoy, M. (1985). Two associated cases of the acquired immune deficiency syndrome (AIDS). *Communicable Disease Report* **42**, 4.

Gutman, L. T., St Claire, K. K., Weedy, C., *et al.* (1991). Human immunodeficiency virus transmission by child sexual abuse. *American Journal of Diseases in Children*, **145**, 137–41.

Gwinn, M., Pappaionaou, M., George, J. R., *et al.* (1991). Prevalence of HIV infection in childbearing women in the United States: surveillance using newborn blood samples. *Journal of the American Medical Association*, **265**, 1704–8.

Halsey, N. A., Boulos, R., Holt, E., *et al.* (1990). Transmission of HIV-1 infections from mothers to infants in Haiti. Impact on childhood mortality and malnutrition. *Journal of the American Medical Association*, **264**, 2088–92.

Hammett, T. A., Bush, T. J., Ciesielski, C. A. (1993). *Pediatric AIDS cases reported with no identified risk* (session 1023). San Francisco: 121st meeting of the American Public Health Association.

Hira, S. K., Kamanga, J., Bhat, G. J., *et al.* (1989). Perinatal transmission of HIV-1 in Zambia. *British Medical Journal*, **299**, 1250–2.

Hoff, R., Beradi, V. P., Weiblen, B. J., *et al.* (1988). Seroprevalence of human immunodeficiency virus among childbearing women. *New England Journal of Medicine*, **318**, 525–30.

Horsburgh, C. R., Caldwell, M. B. & Simonds, R. J. (1993). Epidemiology of disseminated nontuberculous mycobacterial disease in children with acquired immunodeficiency syndrome. *Pediatric Infectious Disease Journal*, **12**, 219–22.

Hsu, H. Moye, J., Kunches, L., *et al.* (1992). Perinatally acquired human immunodeficiency virus infection: extent of clinical recognition in a population-based cohort. *Pediatric Infectious Disease Journal*, **11**, 941–5.

Hutto, C., Parks, W. P., Lai, S., *et al.* (1991). A hospital-based prospective study of perinatal infection with human immunodeficiency virus type 1. *Journal of Pediatrics*, **118**, 347–53.

Italian Multicentre Study (1988). Epidemiology, clinical features, and prognostic factors of paediatric HIV infection. *Lancet*, **ii**, 1043–6.

Jones, D. S., Byers, R. H., Bush, T. J., *et al.* (1992*a*). Epidemiology of transfusion-associated acquired immunodeficiency syndrome in children in the United States, 1981–89. *Pediatrics*, **89**, 123–127.

Jones, D. S., Malecki, J. M., Bigler, W. J., *et al.* (1992*b*). Pediatric tuberculosis and HIV infection in Palm Beach County, Florida. *American Journal of Diseases of Children*, **146**, 1166–70.

Karon, J. M., Buehler, J. W., Byers, R. H., *et al.* (1992). Projections of the numbers of persons diagnosed with AIDS and of immunosuppressed HIV-infected persons, United States, 1992–94; statistical methods and parameter estimates. Washington, D. C.: U.S. Department of Health and Human Services, publication HIV/NCID/10–92/028.

Koenig, R. E., Gautier, T. & Levy, J. A. (1986). Unusual intrafamilial transmission of human immune deficiency virus. *Lancet*, **ii**, 627.

Krugman, R. D. (1986). Recognition of sexual abuse in children. *Pediatric Review*, **8**, 25–30.

Lawrence, D. N., Jason, J. M., Bouhasin, J. D., *et al.* (1985). HTLV-III/LAV antibody status of spouses and household contacts assisting in home infusion of hemophilia patients. *Blood*, **66**, 703–705.

Lepage, P., van de Perre, P., Msellati, P., *et al.* (1993). Mother-to-child transmission of human immunodeficiency virus type 1 (HIV-1) and its determinants: a cohort study in Kigali, Rwanda. *American Journal of Epidemiology*, **137**, 589–99.

Lifson, A. R., Rogers, M. F., White, C., *et al.* (1987). Unrecognized modes of transmission of HIV: acquired immunodeficiency syndrome in children reported without risk factors. *Pediatric Infectious Disease Journal*, **6**, 292–3.

Lindgren, S., Anzen, B., Bohlin, A. B. & Lidman, K. (1991). HIV and child-bearing: clinical outcome and aspects of mother-to-infant transmission. *AIDS*, **5**, 1111–16.

Lyon, L., Obiri, G., Thomas, P., *et al.* (1993). An evaluation of the pediatric AIDS case definition (abstract PO-C01-2575). Berlin IXth International Conference on AIDS.

Matheson, P. B., Weedon, J., Cappelli, M., *et al.* (1993). Comparative methods of estimating mother-to-child HIV-1 transmission rate (MTCTR) (abstract PO-C16-2984). Berlin IXth International AIDS Conference.

Mayers, M. M., Davenny, K., Schoenbaum, E. E., *et al.* (1991). A prospective study of infants of human immunodeficiency virus seropositive and seronegative women with a history of intravenous drug use or of intravenous drug-using sex partners, in the Bronx, New York City. *Pediatrics*, **88**, 1248–56.

McDougal, J. S., Martin, L. S., Cort, S. P., *et al.* (1985). Thermal inactivation of the AIDS virus, HTLV-III/lymphadenopathy-associated virus, with special reference to antihemophilic factor. *Journal of Clinical Investigations*, **76**, 875–7.

Michaels, D. & Levine, C. (1992). Estimates of the number of motherless youth orphaned by AIDS in the United States. *Journal of the American Medical Association*, **268**, 3456–61.

Mofenson, L. M., Wright, P. F. & Fast, P. E. (1992). Summary of the working group on perinatal intervention. *AIDS Research and Human Retroviruses*, **8**, 1435–8.

Nair, P., Alger, L., Hines, S., *et al.* (1993). Maternal and neonatal characteristics associated with HIV infection in infants of seropositive women. *Journal of Acquired Immune Deficiency Syndromes*, **6**, 298–302.

National Center for Health Statistics. (1993). Advance report of final mortality statistics, 1991. *Monthly vital statistics report*, vol. 42, no. 2, (Suppl). Hyattsville, Maryland: Public Health Service.

Nicholas, S. W. & Abrams, E. J. (1992). The 'silent' legacy of AIDS. Children who survive their parents and siblings. *Journal of the American Medical Association*, **268**, 3478–9.

Novick, L. F., Glebatis, D. M., Stricof, R. L., *et al.* (1991). Newborn seroprevalence study: methods and results. *American Journal of Public Health*, **81** (Suppl), 15–21.

Pappaioanou, M., George, J. R., Hannon, W. H., *et al.* (1990a). HIV seroprevalence surveys of childbearing women: objectives, methods, and uses of the data. *Public Health Report*, **105**, 147–52.

Pappaioanou, M., Dondero, T. J., Petersen, L. R., *et al.* (1990b). The family of HIV seroprevalence surveys: objectives, methods, and uses of sentinel surveillance for HIV in the United States. *Public Health Report*, **105**, 113–19.

Parekh, B. S., Shaffer, N., Pau, C.-P., *et al.* (1991). Lack of correlation between maternal antibodies to V3 loop peptides of gp120 and perinatal HIV-1 transmission. *AIDS*, **5**, 1179–84.

Perinatal AIDS Collaborative Transmission Studies Group. (1992). Lack of increased risk of HIV perinatal transmission to subsequent siblings born to an HIV-infected mother (abstract WeC 1057). Amsterdam: VIII International AIDS Conference.

Petersen, L. R., Simonds, R. J. & Koistinen, J. (1993). HIV transmission through blood, tissues, and organs. *AIDS*, **7** (Suppl 1):S99–S107.

Pitt, J., Goldfarb, J., Schluchter, M., *et al.* (1993a) Transmission rate determinations are subject to differing definitions and therefore different rates. (abstract 662). Washington, D. C.: First National Conference on Human Retroviruses and Related Infections.

Pitt, J., Landay, A., McIntosh, K., *et al.* (1993b) Maternal CD4% and viral culture positivity interact to influence the risk of maternal-fetal HIV transmission (abstract 671). Washington D. C.: First National Conference on Human Retroviruses and Related Infections.

Pizzo, P. A. & Butler, K. M. (1991). In the vertical transmission of HIV, timing may be everything. *New England Journal of Medicine*, **325**, 652–3.

Report of a consensus workshop (1992). Maternal factors involved in mother-to-child transmission of HIV-1, Siena, Italy, 17–18 January 1992. *Journal of Acquired Immune Deficiency Syndromes*, **5**, 1019–29.

Rogers, M. F., White, C. R., Sanders, R., *et al.* (1990). Lack of transmission of human immunodeficiency virus from infected children to their household contacts. *Pediatrics*, **85**, 210–14.

Rolfs, R. T. & Nakashima, A. K. (1990). Epidemiology of primary and secondary syphilis in the United States, 1981–89. *Journal of the American Medical Association*, **264**, 1432–7.

Rosenblum, L., Buehler, J. W., Morgan, M. W., *et al.* (1992). The completeness of AIDS case reporting, 1988: A multisite collaborative project. *American Journal of Public Health,* **82,** 1495–9.

Rossi, P., Moschese, V., Broliden, P., *et al.* (1989). Presence of maternal antibodies to human immunodeficiency virus envelope glycoprotein gp120 epitopes correlates with the uninfected status of children born to seropositive mothers. *Proceedings of the National Academy of Sciences, USA,* **86,** 8055–58.

Rutstein, R. M., Cobb, P., McGowna, K. L., *et al.* (1993). *Mycobacterium avium* intracellular complex infection in HIV-infected children. *AIDS,* **7,** 507–12.

Ryder, R. W., Nsa, W., Hassig, S. E., *et al.* (1989). Perinatal transmission of the human immunodeficiency virus type 1 to infants of seropositive women in Zaire. *New England Journal of Medicine,* **320,** 1637–42.

Selik, R. M., Chu, S. Y., & Buehler, J. W. (1993*a*). HIV infection as leading cause of death among young adults in US cities and states. *Journal of the American Medical Association,* **269,** 2991–4.

Selik, R. M., Ward, J. W., & Buehler, J. W. (1993*b*). Trends in transfusion-associated AIDS in the U.S., 1982–91. *Transfusion,* **33,** 890–3.

Simonds, R. J. & Chanock, S. (1993). Medical issues related to caring for HIV-infected children in and out of the home. *Pediatric Infectious Disease Journal,* **12,** 845–52.

Simonds, R. J. & Rogers, M. F. (1993). HIV prevention: bringing the message home. *New England Journal of Medicine,* **329,** 1883–4.

Simonds, R. J., Holmberg, S. D., Hurwitz, R. L., *et al.* (1992). Transmission of human immunodeficiency virus type 1 from a seronegative organ and tissue donor. *New England Journal of Medicine,* **326,** 726–32.

Simonds, R. J., Oxtoby, M. J., Caldwell, M. B., *et al.* (1993). *Pneumocystis carinii* pneumonia among US children with perinatally acquired HIV infection. *Journal of the American Medical Association,* **270,** 470–3.

St Louis, M. E., Kamenga, M., Brown, C., *et al.* (1993). Risk for perinatal HIV-1 transmission according to maternal immunologic, virologic, and placental factors. *Journal of the American Medical Association,* **269,** 2853–9.

Sweeney, P. A., Onorato, I. M., Allen, D. M., *et al.* (1992). Sentinel surveillance of human immunodeficiency virus infection in women seeking reproductive health services in the United States, 1988–89. *Obstetrics and Gynecology,* **79,** 503–10.

Thomas, P., Weedon, J. & the New York City Perinatal HIV Transmission Collaborative Study group (1992). *Maternal predictors of perinatal HIV transmission* (abstract WeC 1059). Amsterdam: VIII International AIDS Conference.

Thomas, P. A., Weisfuse, I. B., Greenberg, A. E., *et al.* (1993). Trends in the first ten years of AIDS in New York City. *American Journal of Epidemiology,* **137,** 121–33.

Tibaldi, C., Tovo, P. A., Ziarati, N., *et al.* (1993). Asymptomatic women at high risk of vertical HIV-1 transmission to their fetuses. *British Journal of Obstetrics and Gynaecology,* **100,** 334–337.

Tovo, P. A. (1993). Caesarean section and perinatal HIV transmission: what next? *Lancet,* **342,** 630.

Tovo, P. A., de Martino, M., Gabiano, C., *et al.* (1992). Prognostic factors and survival in children with perinatal HIV-1 infection: *Lancet,* **339,** 1249–53.

US Department of Defense (1993). Prevalence of HIV-1 antibody in civilian applicants for military service. October 1985–December 1992. Selected tables prepared by the Division of HIV/AIDS, Centers for Disease Control and Prevention, Atlanta, GA.

Villari, P., Spino, C., Chalmers, T. C., *et al.* (1993). Cesarean section to reduce perinatal transmission of human immunodeficiency virus. *Online Journal of Current Clinical Trials*, July 8, 1993 (Doc. no. 74).

Wahn, V., Kramer, H. H., Voit, T., *et al.* (1986). Horizontal transmission of HIV infection between two siblings. *Lancet*, **ii**, 694.

Wasser, S. C., Gwinn, M. & Fleming, P. (1993*a*). Urban-nonurban distribution of HIV infection in childbearing women in the United States. *Journal of Acquired Immune Deficiency Syndromes*, **6**, 1035–1042.

Wasser, S., Gwinn, M., Rogers, M., *et al.* (1993*b*). Prevalence-based strategies for perinatal HIV screening in the United States (abstract PO-C16–2987). Berlin: IXth International Conference on AIDS.

William-Herman, D., Wara, D. Levy, J., *et al.* (1993). Risk factors for perinatal HIV-I transmission (abstract PO-B05–1064). Berlin: IXth International AIDS Conference.

Working Group on Antiretroviral Therapy, National Pediatric HIV Resource Center (1993). Antiretroviral therapy and medical management of the human immunodeficiency virus-infected child. *Pediatric Infectious Disease Journal*, **12**, 513–22.

Wortley, P., Diaz, T., Chu, S. (1993). Reasons for HIV testing among persons reported with AIDS. San Francisco: 121st American Public Health Association Meeting 1993, session 1132.

Addenda

The new classification for paediatric HIV infection, which is based on the infection status, clinical and immunological status, has now been published:

Centers for Disease Control (1994). 1994 revised classification system for human immunodeficiency virus infection in children less than 13 years of age. *Morbidity and Mortality Weekly Report*, **43**, RR-12: 1–10.

The paediatric AIDS definition remains unchanged for the time being, although laboratory evidence for HIV infection was updated. The definitions for HIV encephalopathy and wasting syndrome were revised to reflect advances in the understanding of their manifestations in children.

Given the results of the 076 zidovudine trial and the recommendations for the use of zidovudine (see Chapter 1), early identification of HIV-infected women will be critical.

Additional references:

Centers for Disease Control (1994). *HIV/AIDS Surveillance Report*, **6**, 1–27.

Hanson, I. C., Lindegren, M. L., Hammett, T. A., *et al.* (1994). Sexual transmission of HIV infection in children (≤13 years of age) reported with AIDS, USA (abstract PC0401). In: Xth International Conference on AIDS, Yokohama, Japan.

3

Classification of HIV infection and definition of AIDS

PIER-ANGELO TOVO

Introduction

The correct diagnosis and adequate treatment of any disease is based on a clear definition of diagnostic criteria, recognition of various clinical and laboratory features, and awareness of their prognostic significance. In this context, the puzzle of HIV infection in children has become clearer over time, though some pieces are still lacking. The diagnosis of paediatric AIDS, problematic in the early 1980s (Oleske *et al.*, 1983; Rubinstein *et al.*, 1983; Scott *et al.*, 1984), has been facilitated by the discovery of the virus and introduction of specific antibody tests. Meanwhile, the diverse manifestations of the disease have been recognised, and recently the impact on survival of some clinical signs and laboratory findings has been outlined. However, the early diagnosis of infection in infants born to sero-positive mothers is not yet a straightforward procedure, the predictive value of certain disorders remains doubtful, and the debate is still open as to the percentage or total number of CD4+ cells under which, depending on age, prognosis becomes poor. This makes the correct classification of HIV-infected children problematic, while increasing evidence highlights that some conditions listed in the AIDS definition are less indicative of full-blown disease than others excluded.

In 1987 the Centers for Disease Control and Prevention (CDC) in Atlanta, Georgia, first proposed a classification system for HIV infection in children under 13 years, including infants born to seropositive mothers (Centers for Disease Control, 1987*a*). This classification, though based on sparse data at that time, has been useful and widely employed, defining the diagnostic criteria for HIV infection in perinatally exposed children and associated clinical signs. In the same year, the CDC revised the case definition for paediatric AIDS (Centers for Disease Control, 1987*b*), which has been used world wide in surveillance systems implemented by most countries. With increasing knowledge, several problems and shortcomings have, however, emerged for

52

both the classification system and AIDS definition. The aim of this chapter is to highlight these limitations and to propose a simple disease staging of possible prognostic significance.

Current CDC classification system

Diagnosis of HIV infection

Perinatally HIV-infected children older than 15 months of age and those who acquired infection following administration of contaminated blood or blood products are easily diagnosed by common antibody tests (see Chapter 5).

Younger infants born to seropositive mothers are considered to be infected when: (1) HIV has been detected in blood or tissues, (2) immunological tests are abnormal, indicating both humoral and cellular immunodeficiency, and meet the clinical criteria listed under class P-2, or (3) they satisfy the case definition for paediatric AIDS.

Children under 15 months of age who were born to infected mothers and remain antibody-positive, but cannot be diagnosed as definitely infected, are classified in *class P-0*.

Clinical staging

Children fulfilling the definition of infection are classified in one of two mutually exclusive classes based on the presence or absence of clinical signs or symptoms.

Class P-1 includes asymptomatic children. According to their immune status, they are further subdivided as normal (A), abnormal (B) or indeterminate (C). It must be underlined that children who develop only one non-specific sign, listed in the P-2A subclass, are still categorised as P-1.

Class P-2 includes children who have developed HIV-associated signs or symptoms. They are further subclassified according to clinical manifestations (see Table 3.1), such as two or more non-specific findings (subclass A), progressive neurological disease (subclass B), lymphoid interstitial pneumonitis (subclass C), secondary infectious diseases (subclass D), cancers (subclass E), and other diseases possibly due to HIV infection (subclass F).

Secondary infectious diseases are subdivided in three categories: specific opportunistic infections (D-1), recurrent serious bacterial infections (D-2) and other infections (D-3); secondary cancers include those listed in the surveillance definition for AIDS (E-1), and those possibly associated with HIV infection (E-2).

Table 3.1. *Classification system for HIV infection in children under 13 years of age*

Class P-0. Indeterminate infection
Seropositive children <15 months born to infected mothers, but without definitive evidence of HIV infection

Class P-1. Asymptomatic infection

Subclass A.	No immune abnormalities
Subclass B.	One or more of the typical immune abnormalities: hyper-gammaglobulinaemia, CD4 lymphopenia, decreased CD4/CD8 ratio, absolute lymphopenia
Subclass C.	Immune function not tested

Class P-2. Symptomatic infection

Subclass A.	Non-specific findings (>2 for >2 months): fever, failure to thrive or weight loss (>10%), generalised lymphadenopathy, hepatomegaly, splenomegaly, parotitis, persistent or recurrent diarrhoea
Subclass B.	Progressive neurological disease: loss of developmental milestones or intellectual ability, impaired brain growth, or progressive symmetrical motor deficits
Subclass C.	Lymphoid interstitial pneumonitis
Subclass D.	Secondary infectious diseases
Category D-1.	Opportunistic infections listed in the CDC case definition for AIDS
Category D-2.	Recurrent, serious bacterial infections (2 or more in a 2 year period): sepsis, meningitis, pneumonia, abscess of an internal organ, bone or joint infections
Category D-3.	Other infectious diseases: persistent oral candidiasis (>2 months), recurrent herpes stomatitis (>2 episodes in 1 year), multidermatomal or disseminated herpes zoster
Subclass E.	Secondary cancers
Category E-1.	Cancers listed in the CDC case definition for AIDS
Category E-2.	Other malignancies possibly associated with HIV
Subclass F.	Other conditions possibly due to HIV infection: hepatitis, cardiopathy, nephropathy, haematological disorders, dermatological diseases

---

Centers for Disease Control (1987*a*).

Problems of the current classification system

Diagnostic criteria

The diagnosis of HIV infection in infants exposed to infected mothers in the perinatal period is mostly based on clinical findings and persistence of specific antibody beyond 18 months of age. The early identification of infection status through the appearance of clinical signs and typical immunological abnormalities has proved fairly sensitive. In fact, about half of infected infants have clinical manifestations within the first 6 months of life, and three-quarters by the age of 1 year (Scott *et al.*, 1989; Blanche *et al.*, 1990; European Collaborative Study, 1991; Tovo *et al.*, 1992). However, some seropositive children, initially classified as P-2A, seroreverted and symptoms resolved. Given the clinical and psychological impact of such a diagnosis, this reduced specificity can no longer be accepted.

The cut-off for passively acquired maternal antibodies has been set at 15 months. In contrast, it has been shown that these may persist, though in few cases, for up to 18 months (Mok *et al.*, 1987).

Clinical staging

A classification system must express the disease progression for distinct groups of children requiring the same monitoring and prophylactic or therapeutic intervention. The clinical categories must therefore be mutually exclusive and prognostic, whereas in the CDC classification system this occurs only between asymptomatic (P-1) and symptomatic (P-2) children. In addition, signs of different prognostic significance are grouped together in subclasses P-2A and P-2F. Thus, the system has little prognostic value and makes clinical follow-up difficult, with children falling into multiple subclasses.

Considerations for a new classification system

Diagnostic criteria

Given the aforementioned low specificity of minor clinical manifestations, only signs meeting the CDC case definition for AIDS can denote HIV infection in the absence of confirmatory laboratory assays.

Several tests for the early diagnosis of HIV infection in at-risk infants have become available, such as viral culture, polymerase chain reaction and p24 antigen assay, including serum acid pretreatment to dissociate immune complexes (Rogers *et al.*, 1989; Krivine *et al.*, 1990; Scarlatti *et al.*, 1991; Burgard *et al.*, 1992; Borkowsky *et al.*, 1992; Comau *et al.*, 1992; Palomba *et al.*, 1992, 1993; Miles *et al.*, 1993). Almost all children ultimately shown to be infected are identified through these assays by the age of 3–6 months (Consensus Workshop, 1992). Therefore, the diagnosis of HIV infection should rely much more on laboratory findings than on clinical signs or antibody kinetics. It must, however, be underlined that positive results in children who seroreverted have been observed with every assay (European Collaborative Study, 1992*a*; Borkowsky *et al.*, 1992;

Gabiano *et al.*, 1992; Miles *et al.*, 1993). A silent infection in perinatally exposed antibody-negative children cannot be ruled out. On the other hand, technical errors or contamination problems may have resulted in false positive results. Thus, two positive findings, obtained by different assays from the same sample or by the same assay in sequential samples, are necessary before giving a definitive diagnosis of HIV infection (Consensus Workshop, 1992).

In children older than 18 months, HIV-antibody tests repeatedly positive are sufficient to document their infection status.

Clinical staging

The predictive value of some clinical signs is well established. There is a general agreement that children who develop opportunistic infections or encephalopathy have shortened survival. In contrast, the influence on disease course of other manifestations, such as chronic sinusitis or cardiopathy, remains to be clarified. Hence, their place in a progressive classification is doubtful. Moreover, some clinical conditions, such as hepatitis, are characterised by chronic evolution, and may have a different predictive value as they progress. Consequently, the same disorder should be subclassified, depending on the degree of severity, but this would make the classification too complex.

The evolution of infection and frequency of single clinical patterns are expected to change as prophylactic measures and therapeutic interventions improve. The prognostic value of certain clinical signs may thus vary over time.

Information from the Italian Register on the prognostic value of single clinical patterns allows the identification of four progressive disease stages (Tovo *et al.*, 1992; Italian Register, 1994). This proposal is reported in Table 3.2.

A. Asymptomatic children

No study has clarified whether the course of HIV infection differs significantly between asymptomatic children and those with minor signs. It would seem reasonable to keep the former in a distinct category.

B. Mild clinical signs

Many investigators have highlighted the negative prognostic value of some HIV-related clinical manifestations. The only analysis addressing conditions associated with a better prognosis revealed that lymphadenopathy, hepatomegaly, splenomegaly, parotitis, skin diseases and recurrent upper

Table 3.2. *Clinical staging of HIV infection in children*

A.	No clinical manifestation
B.	Mild clinical signs
	Lymphadenopathy
	Hepatomegaly
	Splenomegaly
	Parotitis
	Dermatological diseases
	Recurrent upper respiratory tract infections, including otitis
C.	Intermediate conditions
	Lymphoid interstitial pneumonitis
	Growth failure
	Recurrent or persistent sinusitis
	Cardiopathy
	Nephropathy
	Hepatitis
	Haematological disorders, including thrombocytopenia, anaemia, neutropenia
D.	Severe clinical manifestations
	Opportunistic infections listed in the CDC case definition for paediatric AIDS[a]
	Recurrent, severe bacterial infections[a]
	Bronchiectasis
	Persistent oral candidiasis
	Recurrent herpes stomatitis
	Multidermatomal or disseminated herpes zoster
	Persistent or recurrent diarrhoea
	Fever of unknown origin
	Encephalopathy[a]
	Cancers[a]
	Wasting syndrome[a]

[a] See Table 3.3.

respiratory tract infections are the mildest disease patterns (Tovo *et al.*, 1992).

Generalised lymphadenopathy, hepatomegaly and splenomegaly are the most common HIV-associated signs, usually developing early in infancy, and thus represent the first clinical manifestations. The size significantly changes over time without a clear correlation with disease progression.

Parotitis is a less frequent condition, manifesting later on. Like lymphadenopathy, it seems to represent a positive response of the host against the virus, and is associated with a longer survival (Tovo *et al.*, 1992).

Several forms of *skin diseases* have been observed in HIV-infected children, though no specific picture has been described.

Recurrent upper respiratory tract infections are frequently found in HIV-infected as well as in non-infected children.

C. Intermediate disease forms

In contrast to other upper respiratory tract infections, *chronic or recurrent sinusitis* may be an indication of more severe immunosuppression predicting clinical deterioration. As sinusitis is also common in children without HIV infection, only chronic forms or a certain number of episodes (e.g. more than 3) can be negative prognostic markers.

Lymphoid interstitial pneumonitis (LIP) is a typical HIV-associated disease manifestation in perinatally infected children, characterised by diffuse interstitial and peribronchiolar infiltrates of lymphocytes and plasma cells (see Chapters 4 and 10). In the CDC classification, LIP is an AIDS-defining disease. However, children with LIP may have a well-preserved immune function, including higher CD4 cell counts and a longer survival, compared with those with other AIDS-defining conditions (Scott *et al.*, 1989; Thomas *et al.*, 1992; Tovo *et al.*, 1992, Turner *et al.*, 1993). Its evolution may be favourably influenced by antiretroviral and corticosteroid therapy.

Nephropathy and *cardiopathy* are HIV-related chronic conditions, the severity of which correlates with underlying disease progression. Retrospective reviews of children with these conditions would suggest an intermediate outcome (Connor *et al.*, 1988; Stewart *et al.*, 1988; Bharati *et al.*, 1989; Strauss *et al.*, 1989, Scott *et al.*, 1989; Glassock *et al.*, 1990). Current antiretroviral agents do not seem to influence the course of renal or cardiac disease.

Hepatitis caused by HIV varies greatly in severity in different patients or in the same patient over time (Duffy *et al.*, 1986; Kahn *et al.*, 1991; Persaud *et al.*, 1993). There is evidence that HIV can infect liver cells (Cao *et al.*, 1992). As a result, biochemical signs of hepatitis are found in most HIV-infected children. The increase in aminotransferase values appears very early, often before symptom onset, and tends to persist at variable levels (de Martino *et al.*, 1993). A fivefold increase in transferases has been found to be associated with a significantly shorter survival (Tovo *et al.*, 1992). Minor alterations in liver function may be included among intermediate disease forms.

Haematological disorders originate from bone marrow infection by either HIV or other agents, alterations in cytokine production or autoimmune phenomena (Donahue *et al.*, 1987; Stella *et al.*, 1987; McCance-Katz *et al.*, 1987; Van der Lelie *et al.*, 1987; Doweiko, 1993). Thrombocytopenia usually persists without severe bleeds, may resolve spontaneously or may require immunoglobulin or corticosteroid treatment (Rigaud *et al.*, 1992). It represents a form of intermediate disease, whereas marked anaemia (<8 g/dl) is associated with a poorer prognosis (Tovo *et al.*, 1992). Neutropenia is a rare disorder and data on affected patients are lacking. With these limitations it seems reasonable, for simplicity, to group together all haematological disorders in the intermediate category.

Apart from wasting syndrome, which represents the final outcome of HIV infection, *growth failure* is one of the most simple and sensitive predictors of clinical deterioration (Brettler *et al.*, 1990; Tovo *et al.*, 1992). The decrease in linear growth manifests earlier than weight loss, in contrast to that observed in psychosocial deprivation. Several mechanisms are likely to contribute to growth failure, such as inadequate nutrient intake, malabsorption due to HIV-induced enteropathy or secondary infections (Batman *et al.*, 1989; Ullrich *et al.*, 1989), increased resting energy expenditure (Grunfeld *et al.*, 1992) and hormonal alterations (Kaufman & Gomperts, 1989; Jospe & Powel, 1990; Laue *et al.*, 1990). Increase in appetite and recovery in body weight are among the earliest indications of response to antiretroviral treatment (see Chapter 10).

D. Severe disease patterns

With the exception of LIP, every condition listed in the CDC surveillance case definition for paediatric AIDS can be seen as an expression of profound immunodeficiency or severe viral damage resulting in serious morbidity and shortened survival (see Table 3.3).

Neurological disease is one of the most severe disorders directly induced by HIV (Belman *et al.*, 1988; Epstein *et al.*, 1988c; European Collaborative Study, 1990; Aylward *et al.*, 1992; Bale *et al.*, 1993). When it manifests in the first year of life it is often associated with opportunistic infections and wasting syndrome (see Chapter 4). It is a highly significant and independent negative marker for survival (Scott *et al.*, 1989; Krasinski *et al.*, 1989; Blanche *et al.*, 1990; Tovo *et al.*, 1992; Turner *et al.*, 1993).

There is general agreement that children developing *specific secondary infections*, in particular *Pneumocystis carinii pneumonia* (PCP), have the poorest prognosis (Rogers *et al.*, 1987; Bernstein *et al.*, 1989; Krasinski *et al.*, 1989; Scott *et al.*, 1989; Blanche *et al.*, 1990; Thomas *et al.*, 1992; Kline *et al.*, 1992; Tovo *et al.*, 1992; Turner *et al.*, 1993). PCP is the most frequent AIDS-specific opportunistic infection in both adults and children. In adults it is a reactivation and manifests in the final disease stages, when the CD4 cell number is markedly reduced (Phair *et al.*, 1990). In children it is a primary infection with its incidence highest in the first year of life, and may occur in infants whose CD4 cell count is not particularly decreased (Bernstein *et al.*, 1989; Leibovitz *et al.*, 1990; Connor *et al.*, 1991; Centers for Disease Control, 1991). Its incidence will presumably reduce with the early identification of infected infants and the prompt institution of specific prophylaxis.

Table 3.3. *Conditions listed in the CDC surveillance case definition for paediatric AIDS*

Opportunistic infections
Viral:
  Cytomegalovirus disease (other than liver, spleen, lymph nodes in a patient
    >1 month of age)
  Herpes simplex virus infection causing a mucocutaneous ulcer (>1 month
    duration) or bronchitis, pneumonitis or oesophagitis (for any duration in a
    patient >1 month of age)
  Progressive multifocal leucoencephalopathy
Bacterial:
  Mycobacterium tuberculosis, extrapulmonary
  Mycobacterium avium complex or *M. kansasii* disease or any other acid-fast
    infection, disseminated (at a site other than or in addition to lungs, skin,
    or cervical or hilar lymph nodes)
Fungal:
  Candidiasis (of the oesophagus, trachea, bronchi or lungs)
  Coccidioidomycosis or histoplasmosis, disseminated (at a site other than or in
    addition to lungs or cervical or hilar lymph nodes)
  Cryptococcosis, extrapulmonary
Parasitic:
  Pneumocystis carinii pneumonia;
  Cryptosporidiosis or isosporiasis (with diarrhoea persisting >1 month)
  Toxoplasmosis of brain (in a patient >1 month of age)
  Multiple or recurrent bacterial infections (at least 2 within a 2 year period):
    septicaemia, pneumonia, meningitis, bone or joint infection, abscesses of
    an internal organ or body cavity (excluding otitis media or superficial skin
    or mucosal abscesses)
  HIV encephalopathy: loss of developmental milestones or intellectual ability,
    impaired brain growth, or progressive symmetrical motor deficits
  Lymphoid interstitial pneumonitis
  Wasting syndrome due to HIV

Cancers
Kaposi's sarcoma
Lymphoma of the brain (primary)
Other non-Hodgkin's lymphoma of B-cell or unknown phenotype (small
  non-cleaved lymphoma, either Burkitt or non-Burkitt type, or immunoblastic
  sarcoma)

Centers for Disease Control (1987*b*).

Recurrent, serious bacterial infections, particularly pneumonia, sepsis, and meningitis due to encapsulated microorganisms can be observed in HIV-infected children following humoral immunodeficiency and alterations of phagocytic cells (Bernstein *et al.*, 1985; Borkowsky *et al.*, 1987; Ellis *et al.*, 1988; Murphy *et al.*, 1988). Prophylactic interventions can reduce their frequency, as observed with intravenous immunoglobulin infusions in children with CD4 cell counts >200/mm^3 and with trimethoprim–sulfamethoxazole administered for PCP prophylaxis (National Institute of Child Health, 1991; Mofenson *et al.*, 1992). Despite antimicrobial treatments, lower respiratory tract infections sometimes give rise to *bronchiectasis*, which is a severe prognostic indicator.

In contrast to opportunistic and recurrent bacterial infections, *other secondary infections*, such as persistent oral candidiasis, recurrent herpes stomatitis and multidermatomal herpes zoster infection, are not listed among AIDS-defining conditions. This may suggest that they are expressions of a less compromised immune response, whereas their impact on survival is comparable to that of recurrent bacterial infections (Tovo *et al.*, 1992), demonstrating that they should be grouped among the severe disease forms.

HIV-induced *wasting syndrome* has been defined as profound weight loss (>10% of baseline body weight) together with either chronic diarrhoea or fever or weakness (lasting >30 days). It is worth noting that *persistent or recurrent diarrhoea* and *fever of unknown origin* are also listed in subclass P-2A, suggesting mild signs when seen in isolation, whereas they are significant and independent negative predictors of survival (Tovo *et al.*, 1992).

Cancers are linked to a poor prognosis (Kamani, *et al.*, 1988; Epstein *et al.*, 1988*b*; Montalvo *et al.*, 1990; Arico' *et al.*, 1991).

Immunological classification

Data from HIV-infected adults indicate that loss of CD4 cells can be used as a surrogate marker for advanced disease (Hanson *et al.*, 1993; Easterbrook, *et al.*, 1993). Therefore, the CD4 cell count and percentage have been included in the adult HIV classification system (Centers for Disease Control, 1993). A correlation between a decline in CD4 cells and the development of PCP, neurological disorders and, in general, with rapid disease progression in children has been recorded in several studies (Leibovitz *et al.*, 1990; de Martino *et al.*, 1991; Connor *et al.*, 1991; Kovacs *et al.*, 1991; Butler *et al.*, 1992). Nevertheless, the cut-off values for distinguishing different degrees of immunosuppression (normal, moderate, severe) are still under debate. Since the physiological decrease in CD4 lymphocytes is less marked in percentage terms than in absolute number, the former may provide more reliable reference values. Data must be adjusted for age, since CD4 lymphocytes decline progressively from infancy to adulthood (Denny *et al.*, 1992; Erkeller-Yursel *et al.*, 1992; McKinney & Wilfert, 1992; European Collaborative Study, 1992*b*).

An attempt to set age-adjusted CD4 categories, encompassing most HIV-infected children at-risk for developing PCP, has led to specific guidelines for PCP prophylaxis (Centers for Disease Control, 1991). Lower

Table 3.4 *Guideline values for CD4 T-lymphocyte categories*

	Age			
	<12 months	12–23 months	24 months– 6 years	>6 years
PCP prophylaxis[a]	<1500 (20%)	<750 (20%)	<500	<200
Antiretroviral treatment guidelines[b]	<1750 (30%)	<1000 (25%)	<750 (20%)	<500
CDC proposed categories[c]				
Moderate depletion	<1500 (<35%)	<750 (<30%)	<500[d] (<30%)	
Severe depletion	<750 (<20%)	<500 (<20%)	<200[d] (<20%)	

[a] Centers for Disease Control (1991).
[b] National Pediatric HIV Resource Center, September 1992 Workshop (USA).
[c] Caldwell *et al.* (1993), M.F. Rogers (personal communication).
[d] Including children >6 years.

threshold values have been chosen in the proposed guidelines for antiretroviral therapy (see Table 3.4), based on the consideration that treatment should start before reaching levels of immunosuppression associated with increased risk of opportunistic infections. Still different CD4 categories have emerged from data collected by the CDC for the continuing revision of the current classification system (Caldwell *et al.*, 1993).

Values indicative of profound immunodeficiency do not seem, however, to correlate with the course of infection in older children. Results from the Italian Register for HIV infection in children highlight that the annual rate of CD4 cell loss is lower in children surviving beyond 5 years of age than in those dying before, but the proportion of children with CD4 cell counts $<200/mm^3$ rises progressively with age in long-term survivors (Italian Register, 1994). At 8 years of age, 40% of infected children have a CD4 cell count $<200/mm^3$. The rate of loss of CD4 cells early in life rather than static values later seems more predictive of outcome. Therefore, the use of an immunological classification of HIV-infected children based on the CD4 cell count or percentage is warranted, but further information is needed to set definite threshold values reflecting the degree of immunosuppression at different ages.

Other potential markers of disease progression

Other markers of disease activity have been proposed, such as β_2-microglobulin and neopterin levels (Chan *et al.*, 1990; Ellaurie & Rubinstein, 1990; Ellaurie, *et al.*, 1992, Siller *et al.*, 1993), serum tumour necrosis factor alpha and interleukin 1-beta concentrations (Arditi *et al.*, 1991), antibodies mediating cellular cytotoxicity and neutralisation (Ljunggren *et al.*, 1990), and helper T cell responses (Roilides *et al.*, 1991; Clerici *et al.*, 1992). Their use has, however, been limited and none has proved highly specific or with reliable threshold values for distinguishing different stages of disease.

Quantification of virus burden would be useful to predict the evolution of infection. Although HIV replication is initially greater in lymphoid tissues (Pantaleo *et al.*, 1993), in practice only peripheral blood samples can be used to obtain prognostic information. Several methods are available to measure levels of serum and plasma viraemia or to quantitate cell-associated virus DNA or RNA. Among these, p24 antigenaemia is at present the only marker that could be used for a classification system. Its prognostic significance, however, remains questionable (Epstein *et al.*, 1988a; Borkowsky *et al.*, 1989; Ellaurie & Rubinstein, 1991; Butler *et al.*, 1992; Bollinger *et al.*, 1992; Tudor-Williams *et al.*, 1992).

Variations of virulence among different HIV strains might precede attrition of the immune system and ultimately clinical deterioration. Assessment of virus characteristics, such as replicative capacities (rapid/high versus slow/low), cellular tropism (lymphocytic versus monocytic) and drug resistance, will presumably offer useful and early indications for disease progression. On the other hand, the evaluation of these parameters requires adequate laboratory facilities, is time consuming and costly. It is therefore unsuitable for routine purposes.

Case definition for paediatric AIDS

The CDC case definition for paediatric AIDS (see Table 3.3) has been adopted for epidemiological purposes. Since this definition includes severe disease, AIDS has been taken to be synonymous with full-blown disease. In many studies it has been used as a starting point for survival estimates or, conversely, an endpoint to assess the efficacy of therapeutic interventions. Application of the definition in children differs from that in adults because it includes multiple or recurrent severe bacterial infections and lymphoid interstitial pneumonitis. As previously mentioned, the latter does not represent a severe disabling condition and is associated with a better prognosis than other signs which are not included. If AIDS is to represent end-stage disease, its definition should be integrated with the classification system and mirror its most severe manifestations, both clinical and immunological. Apart from doubts regarding some markers of full-blown disease, a crucial point to be taken into account is that a

Table 3.5. *World Health Organization case definitions for paediatric AIDS*

Definition (1986)
Major signs
   Weight loss or failure to thrive
   Chronic diarrhoea (>1 month)
   Prolonged fever (>1 month)
Minor signs
   Generalised lymphadenopathy
   Oropharyngeal candidiasis
   Repeated common infections
   Persistent cough
   Generalised dermatitis
   Confirmed maternal HIV infection

Modified definition (1989)
Major signs
   Weight loss or failure to thrive
   Chronic diarrhoea (>1 month)
   Prolonged fever (>1 month)
   Severe or repeated pneumonia
Minor signs
   Generalised lymphadenopathy
   Oropharyngeal candidiasis
   Repeated common infections
   Generalised pruritic dermatitis
   Confirmed maternal HIV infection

With both definitions, paediatric AIDS is suspected in a child presenting with at least two major signs and two minor signs in the absence of known causes of immunosuppression.

modified AIDS definition would result in a reduced possibility of comparing future data with historical data. This discrepancy between clinical and epidemiological needs should lead to a clear distinction between the classification system and case definition for paediatric AIDS. While clinicians seek a comprehensive clinical staging, epidemiologists will wish to preserve the ability to estimate the prevalence of cases in individual countries over time.

Another definition for paediatric AIDS is also in use, with a subsequent revision (WHO, 1986, 1989). This is targeted at developing countries, has low specificity and is not widely used. In this case, the aim of surveillance, independent from clinical staging, is evident (see Table 3.5).

Conclusion

The prognostic value of most HIV-associated clinical manifestations in infancy and childhood has been clearly demonstrated. This facilitates the revision of the current classification system for HIV infection in children for clinical purposes. Doubts remain regarding an immunological classification that can predict the velocity of disease progression. Threshold values of CD4 cells to define the degree of immunosuppression at different ages have been proposed. Their accuracy seems, however, greater in younger than in older children. Other prognostic markers have been identified, but their application in a classification system is premature.

Prophylactic measures may reduce the frequency of opportunistic infections, but it remains questionable whether children susceptible to these infections will present a different clinical evolution. Antiretroviral therapy is expected to reduce the loss of CD4 cells, to modify the frequency and time of appearance of clinical manifestations, and to prolong survival in HIV-infected children (see Chapters 12 and 13).

It is clear that the CDC AIDS-defining conditions do not reflect the final disease stage completely. This does not imply that the definition must be changed, bearing in mind that it should be used for epidemiological, not clinical purposes.

References

Aylward, E. H., Butz, A. M., Hutton, N., Joyner, M. L. & Vogelhut, J. W. (1992). Cognitive and motor development in infants at-risk for human immunodeficiency virus. *American Journal of Diseases of Children*, **146**, 218–22.

Arditi, M., Kabat. W. & Yogev, R. (1991). Serum tumor necrosis factor alpha, interleukin 1-beta, p24 antigen concentrations and CD4+ cells at various stages of human immunodeficiency virus 1 infection in children. *Pediatric Infectious Disease Journal*, **10**, 450–5.

Arico', M., Caselli, D., D'Argenio, P., *et al.* (1991). Malignancies in children with human immunodeficiency virus type 1 infection. *Cancer*, **68**, 2473–7.

Bale, J. F., Contant, C. F., Garg, B., Tilton, A., Kaufman, D. M. & Wasiewski, W. (1993). Neurologic history and examination results and their relationship to human immunodeficiency virus type 1 serostatus in hemophilic subjects: Results from the hemophilia growth and development study. *Pediatrics*, **91**, 736–41.

Batman, P. A., Miller, A. R., Forster, S. M., Harris, J. R., Pinching, A. J. & Griffen, G. E. (1989). Jejunal enteropathy associated with human immunodeficiency virus infection: a quantitative histology. *Journal of Clinical Pathology*, **42**, 275–81.

Belman, A., Diamond, G., Dickson, D., *et al.* (1988). Pediatric acquired immunodeficiency syndrome: neurologic syndromes. *American Journal of Diseases of Children*, **142**, 29–35.

Bernstein, L., Bye, M. R. & Rubinstein, A. (1989). Prognostic factors and life expectancy in children with acquired immunodeficiency syndrome and *Pneumocystis carinii* pneumonia. *American Journal of Diseases of Children*, **143**, 775–8.

Bernstein, L. J., Ochs, H. D., Wedgwood, R. J., *et al.* (1985). Defective humoral immunity in pediatric acquired immunodeficiency syndrome. *Journal of Pediatrics*, **107**, 352–7.

Bharati, S., Joshi, V. V., Connor, E. M., Oleske J. M. & Lev, M. (1989). Conduction system in children with acquired immunodeficiency syndrome. *Chest*, **96**, 406–13.

Blanche, S., Tardieu, M., Duliege, A-M., *et al.* (1990). Longitudinal study of 94 symptomatic infants with perinatally acquired human immunodeficiency virus infection. *American Journal of Diseases of Children*, **144**, 1210–5.

Bollinger, R. C., Kline, R. L., Francis, H. L., Moss, M. W., Bartlett, J. G. & Quin, T. C. (1992). Acid dissociation increases the sensitivity of p24 antigen detection for the evalutation of antiviral therapy and disease progression in asymptomatic human immunodeficiency virus-infected persons. *Journal of Infectious Diseases*, **165**, 913–16.

Borkowsky, W., Krasinski, K., Paul, D., *et al.* (1989). Human immunodeficiency virus type 1 antigenemia in children. *Journal of Pediatrics*, **114**, 940–5.

Borkowsky, W., Krasinski, K., Pollack, H., Hoover, W., Kaul, A. & Ilmet-Moore, T. (1992). Early diagnosis of human immunodeficiency virus infection in children <6 months of age: comparison of polymerase chain reaction, culture, and plasma antigen capture techniques. *Journal of Infectious Diseases*, **166**, 616–19.

Borkowsky, W., Steele, C. J., Grubman, S., Moore, T., La Russa, P. & Krasinski, K. (1987). Antibody responses to bacterial toxoid in children infected with human immunodeficiency virus. *Journal of Pediatrics*, **110**, 563–6.

Brettler, D. B., Forsberg, A., Bolivar, E., Brewster, F. & Sullivan, J. (1990). Growth failure as a prognostic indicator for progression to acquired immunodeficiency syndrome in children with hemophilia. *Journal of Pediatrics*, **117**, 584–88.

Burgard, M., Mayaux, M. J., Blanche, S., *et al.* (1992). The use of viral culture and p24 antigen testing to diagnose human immunodeficiency virus infection in neonates. *New England Journal of Medicine*, **327**, 1192–7.

Butler, K. M., Husson, R. N., Lewis, L. L., Mueller, B. U., Venzon, D. & Pizzo, P. A. (1992). CD4 satus and p24 antigenemia. Are they useful predictors of survival in HIV-infected children receiving antiretroviral therapy? *American Journal of Diseases in Children*, **146**, 932–6.

Caldwell, B., Oxtoby, M. & Rogers, M. (1993). Proposed CDC pediatric classification system: Evaluation in an active surveillance system (abstract WS-Co1-2P-41). Berlin: IXth International Conference on AIDS.

Cao, Y., Dieterich, D., Thomas, P. A., Huang, Y., Mirabile, M. & Ho, D. D. (1992). Identification and quantification of HIV in the liver of patients with AIDS. *AIDS*, **6**, 65–70.

Centers for Disease Control (1987*a*). Classification system for human immunodeficiency virus (HIV) infection in children under 13 years of age. *Morbidity and Mortality Weekly Report*, **36**, 225–35.

Centers for Disease Control (1987*b*). Revision of the CDC surveillance case definition for acquired immunodeficiency syndrome. *Morbidity and Mortality Weekly Report*, **36**, 1S–13S.

Centers for Disease Control (1991). Guidelines for prophylaxis against *Pneumocystis carinii* pneumonia for children infected with human immunodeficiency virus. *Morbidity and Mortality Weekly Report*, **40**, 1–13.

Centers for Disease Control (1993). 1993 revised classification system for HIV infection and expanded surveillance case definition for AIDS among adolescents and adults. *Morbidity and Mortality Weekly Report*, **41**, 1–17.

Chan, M. M., Campos, J. M., Josephs, S. & Rifai, N. (1990). β₂-microglobulin and neopterin: Predictive markers for human immunodeficiency virus type 1 infection in children? *Journal of Clinical Microbiology*, **28**, 2215–19.

Clerici, M., Roilides, E., Butler, K. M., DePalma, L., Shearer, G. M. & Pizzo, P. A. (1992). Changes in T-helper cell function in human immunodeficiency virus-infected children during didanosine therapy as a measure of antiretroviral activity. *Blood*, **80**, 2196–202.

Comau, A. M., Harris, J., McIntosh, K., Weiblen, B. J., Hoff, R. & Grady, G. F. (1992). Polymerase chain reaction in detecting HIV infection among seropositive infants: relation to clinical status and age and to results of other assays. *Journal of Acquired Immunodeficiency Syndromes*, **5**, 271–8.

Connor, E., Bagarazzi, M., McSherry, G., *et al.* (1991). Clinical and laboratory correlates of *Pneumocystis carinii* pneumonia in children infected with HIV. *Journal of the American Medical Association*, **265**, 1693–7.

Connor, E., Gupta, S., Joshi, V., *et al.* (1988). Acquired immunodeficiency syndrome-associated renal disease in children. *Journal of Pediatrics*, **113**, 39–44.

Consensus Workshop, Siena, Italy (1992). Early diagnosis of HIV infection in infants. *Journal of Acquired Immunodeficiency Syndromes*, **5**, 1169–78.

Denny, T., Yogev, R., Gelman, R., *et al.* (1992). Lymphocyte subsets in healthy children during the first 5 years of life. *Journal of the American Medical Association*, **267**, 1484–8.

de Martino, M., Tovo, P. A., Galli, L., *et al.* (1991). Prognostic significance of immunologic changes in 675 infants perinatally exposed to human immunodeficiency virus. *Journal of Pediatrics*, **119**, 702–9.

de Martino, M., Tovo, P. A., Zuccotti, G. V., *et al.* (1993). Transaminase values in infants at-risk from human immunodeficiency virus type 1 perinatal infection. *Pediatric Infectious Disease Journal*, **12**, 248–50.

Donahue, R. E., Johnson, M. M. & Zon, L. I. (1987). Suppression of *in vitro* hematopoiesis following human immunodeficiency virus infection. *Nature*, **326**, 200–3.

Doweiko, J. P. (1993). Hematologic aspect of HIV infection. *AIDS*, **7**, 753–7.

Duffy, L. F., Daum, F., Kahn, E., *et al.* (1986). Hepatitis in children with acquired immune deficiency syndrome. *Gastroenterology*, **90**, 173–81.

Easterbrook, P. J., Emami, J. & Gazzard, B. (1993). Rate of CD4 cell decline and prediction of survival in zidovudine-treated patients. *AIDS*, **7**, 959–67.

Ellaurie, M., Calvelli, T. & Rubinstein, A. (1992). Neopterin concentrations in pediatric human immunodeficiency virus infection as predictor of disease activity. *Pediatric Infectious Disease Journal*, **11**, 286–9.

Ellaurie, M. & Rubinstein, A. (1990). Beta-2-microglobulin concentrations in pediatric human immunodeficiency virus infection. *Pediatric Infectious Disease Journal*, **9**, 807–9.

Ellaurie, M. & Rubinstein, A. (1991) Correlation of serum antigen and antibody concentration with clinical features in HIV infection. *Archives of Disease in Childhood*, **66**, 200–3.

Ellis, M., Gupta, S., Galant, S., *et al.* (1988). Impaired neutrophil function in patients with AIDS or AIDS related complex: a comprehensive evaluation. *Journal of Infectious Diseases*, **158**, 1268–75.

Epstein, L. G., Boucher, C. A., Morrison, S. H., *et al.* (1988a). Persistent human immunodeficiency virus type 1 antigenemia in children correlates with disease progression. *Pediatrics*, **82**, 919–24.

Epstein, L. G., DiCarlo, F. J., Joshi, V. V., *et al.* (1988*b*). Primary lymphoma of the central nervous system in children with acquired immunodeficiency syndrome. *Pediatrics*, **82**, 255–62.

Epstein, L. G., Sharer, L. R. & Goudsmit, J. (1988*c*). Neurological and neuropathological features of human immunodeficiency virus infection in children. *Annals of Neurology*, **23**(Suppl), S19–23.

Erkeller-Yursel, F. M., Deneys, V., Yursel, B. *et al.* (1992). Age-related changes in human blood lymphocyte sub-populations. *Journal of Pediatrics*, **120**, 216–22.

European Collaborative Study (1990). Neurologic signs in young children with human immunodeficiency virus infection, *Pediatric Infectious Disease Journal*, **9**, 402–6.

European Collaborative Study (1991). Children born to women with HIV-1 infection: natural history and risk of transmission. *Lancet*, **337**, 253–60.

European Collaborative Study (1992*a*). Risk factors for mother-to-child transmission of HIV-1. *Lancet*, **339**, 1007–12.

European Collaborative Study (1992*b*). Age-related standards for T lymphocyte subsets based on uninfected children born to human immunodeficiency virus 1-infected mothers. *Pediatric Infectious Disease Journal*, **11**, 1018–26.

Gabiano, C., Tovo, P. A., de Martino, M., *et al.* (1992). Mother-to-child HIV transmission: risk of infection and correlates of transmission. *Pediatrics*, **90**, 369–74.

Glassock, R. J., Cohen, A. H., Danovitch, G. & Parsa, K. P. (1990). Human immunodeficiency virus (HIV) infection and the kidney. *Annals of Internal Medicine*, **112**, 35–49.

Grunfeld, C., Pang, M., Shimitzu, L., Shigenaga, J. K., Jensen, P. & Feingold, K. R. (1992). Resting energy expendidure, caloric intake, and short-term weight change in human immunodeficiency virus infection and acquired immunodeficiency syndrome. *American Journal of Clinical Nutrition*, **55**, 455–60.

Hanson, D. L., Horsburgh, C. R., Fann, S. A., Halvik, J. A. & Thomson, S. E. (1993). Survival prognosis of HIV-infected patients. *Journal of Acquired Immune Deficiency Syndromes*, **6**, 624–9.

Italian Register for HIV Infection in Children (1994). Features of children perinatally infected with HIV-1 surviving longer than 5 years. *Lancet*, **343**, 191–5.

Jospe, N. & Powel, K. R. (1990). Growth hormone deficiency in an 8-year-old girl with human immunodeficiency virus infection. *Pediatrics*, **86**, 309–12.

Kahn, E., Greco, A. M., Daum, F., *et al.* (1991). Hepatic pathology in pediatric acquired immunodeficiency syndrome. *Human Pathology*, **22**, 1111–19.

Kamani, N., Kennedy, J. & Brandsma, J. (1988). Burkitt lymphoma in a child with human immunodeficiency virus infection. *Journal of Pediatrics*, **112**, 241–4.

Kaufman, F. R. & Gomperts, E. D. (1989). Growth failure in boys with hemophilia and HIV infection. *American Journal of Pediatric Hematology/Oncology*, **11**, 292–4.

Kline, M. W., Bohannon, B., Kozinetz, C. A., Rosenblatt, H. M. & Shearer, W. T. (1992). Characteristics of human immunodeficiency virus-associated mortality in pediatric patients with vertically transmitted infection. *Pediatric Infectious Disease Journal*, **11**, 676–7.

Kovacs, A., Frederick, T., Church, J., Eller, A., Oxtoby, M. & Mascola, L. (1991). CD4 T-lymphocyte counts and Pneumocystis carinii pneumonia in pediatric HIV infection. *Journal of the American Medical Association*, **265**, 1698–703.

Krasinski, K., Borkowsky, W. & Holzman, R. S. (1989). Prognosis of human immunodeficiency virus infection in children and adolescents. *Pediatric Infectious Disease Journal*, **8**, 216–20.

Krivine, A., Yakudima, A., Le May, M., Pena-Cruz, V., Huang, A. S. & McIntosh, K. (1990). A comparative study of virus isolation, polymerase chain reaction, and antigen detection in children of mothers infected with human immunodeficiency virus. *Journal of Pediatrics*, **116**, 372–6.

Laue, L., Pizzo, P. A., Butler, K. & Cutler, G. B. (1990). Growth and neuroendocrine dysfunction in children with acquired immunodeficiency syndrome. *Journal of Pediatrics*, **117**, 541–5.

Leibovitz, E., Rigaud, M., Pollack, H., et al. (1990) *Pneumocystis carinii* pneumonia in infants infected with the human immunodeficiency virus with more than 450 CD4 T lymphocytes per cubic millimeter. *New England Journal of Medicine*, **323**, 531–3.

Ljunggren, K., Moschese, V., Broliden P.-A., et al. (1990). Antibodies mediating cellular cytoxicity and neutralization correlate with a better clinical stage in children born to human immunodeficiency virus-infected mothers. *Journal of Infectious Diseases*, **161**, 198–202.

McCance-Katz, E. F., Hoecker, J. L., & Vitale N. B. (1987). Severe neutropenia associated with anti-neutrophil antibody in a patient with the acquired imunodeficiency syndrome-related complex. *Pediatric Infectious Disease Journal*, **4**, 417–8.

McKinney, R. E. & Wilfert, C. M. (1992) Lymphocyte subsets in children younger than 2 years old: normal values in a population at-risk for human immunodeficiency virus infection and diagnostic and prognostic application to infected children. *Pediatric Infectious Disease Journal*, **11**, 639–44.

Miles, S. A., Balden, E., Magpantay, L., et al. (1993). Rapid serologic testing with immune-complexed-dissociated HIV p24 antigen for early detection of infection in neonates. *New England Journal of Medicine*, **328**, 297–302.

Mofenson, L. M., Moye, J.Jr., Bethel, J., et al. (1992). Prophylactic intravenous immunoglobulin in HIV-infected children with CD4-counts of 0.02×10^9/L or more. Effect on viral, opportunistic, and bacterial infections. *Journal of the American Medical Association*, **268**, 483–8.

Mok, J. Q., Giaquinto, C., De Rossi, A., Gross-Worner, I., Ades, A. E. & Peckham, C. S. (1987) Infants born to HIV-positive mothers. Preliminary findings from a multicentre European study. *Lancet*, **i**, 1164–8.

Montalvo, F., Casanova, R., Clavell, L., et al. (1990). Treatment outcome in children with malignancies associated with human immunodeficiency virus infection. *Journal of Pediatrics*, **116**, 735–8.

Murphy, P. M., Lane, C., Fauci, A. & Gallin J. I. (1988). Impairment of neutrophil bactericidal capacity in patients with AIDS. *Journal of Infectious Diseases*, **158**, 627–30.

National Institute of Child Health and Human Development Intravenous Immunoglobulin Study Group (1991). Intravenous immune globulin for the prevention of bacterial infections in children with symptomatic human immunodeficiency virus infection. *New England Journal of Medicine*, **325**, 73–80.

Oleske, J., Minnefor, A., Cooper, R., et al. (1983). Immune deficiency in children. *Journal of the American Medical Association*, **249**, 2345–9.

Palomba, E., Gay, V., de Martino, M., Fundaro', C., Perugini, L. & Tovo, P. A. (1992). Early diagnosis of human immunodeficiency virus infection in infants by detection of free and complexed p24 antigen. *Journal of Infectious Diseases*, **165**, 394–5.

Palomba, E., Gay, V., Galli, L., de Martino, M., Perugini, L. Tovo, P. A. (1993). Sensitivity and specificity of complexed p24 antigen assay for early diagnosis of perinatal HIV-1 infection. AIDS, 7, 1391–3.

Pantaleo, G., Graziosi, C. & Fauci, A. S. (1993). The immunopathogenesis of human immunodeficiency virus infection. New England Journal of Medicine, 328, 327–35.

Persaud, D., Bangaru, B., Greco, A., et al. (1993). Cholestatic hepatitis in children infected with the human immunodeficiency virus. Pediatric Infectious Disease Journal, 12, 492–8.

Phair, J., Munoz, A., Detels, R., et al. (1990) The risk of Pneumocystis carinii pneumonia among men infected with human immunodeficiency virus type 1. New England Journal of Medicine, 322, 161–5.

Rigaud, M., Leibovitz, E., Quee, C. S., et al., (1992). Thrombocytopenia in children infected with human immunodeficiency virus: long-term follow-up and therapeutic considerations. Journal of Acquired Immune Deficiency Syndromes, 5, 450–5.

Rogers, M. F., Ou, C. Y., Rayfield, M. et al. (1989). Use of the polymerase chain reaction for early detection of the proviral sequences of human immunodeficiency virus in infants born to seropositive mothers. New England Journal of Medicine, 320, 1649–54.

Rogers, M. F., Thomas, P. A., Starcher, E. T., et al. (1987). Acquired immunodeficiency syndrome in children: report of the Centers for Disease Control national surveillance, 1982–85. Pediatrics, 79, 1008–14.

Roilides, E., Clerici, M., De Palma, L., Rubin, M., Pizzo, P. A. & Shearer, G. M. (1991). Helper T-cell responses in children infected with human immunodeficiency virus type 1. Journal of Pediatrics, 118, 724–30.

Rubinstein, A., Sicklick, M., Gupta, A., et al. (1983) Acquired immunodeficicincy with reversed T4/T8 ratios in infants born to promiscuous and drug-addicted mothers. Journal of the American Medical Association, 249, 2350–6.

Scarlatti, G., Lombardi, V., Plebani, A., et al. (1991). Polymerase chain reaction, virus isolation and antigen assay in HIV-antiboby-positive mothers and their children. AIDS, 5, 1173–8.

Scott, G. B., Buck, B. E., Leterman, J. G., Bloom, F. L. & Parcks, W. P. (1984) Acquired immunodeficiency syndrome in infants. New England Journal of Medicine, 310, 76–81.

Scott, G. B., Hutto, C., Makuck, R. W., et al. (1989). Survival in children with perinatally acquired human immunodeficiency virus type 1 infection. New England Journal of Medicine, 321, 1791–6.

Siller, L., Martin, N. L., Kostuchenko, P., Beckett, L., Rautonen, J., Cheng, S. C. & Wara, D. W. (1993). Serum levels of soluble CD8, neopterin, β-2 microglobulin and p24 antigen as indicators of disease progression in children with AIDS on zidovudine treatment. AIDS, 7, 369–74.

Stella, C. C., Ganser, A., & Hoelzer, D. (1987). Defective in vitro growth of the hematopoietic progenitor cells in the acquired immunodeficiency syndrome. Journal of Clinical Investigation, 80, 286–93.

Stewart, J. M., Kaul, A., Gromish, D. S., Reyes, E., Woolf, P. K. & Gowitz, M. H. (1988). Symptomatic cardiac dysfunction in children with human immunodeficiency syndrome. American Heart Journal, 117, 140–4.

Strauss, J., Abitbol, C., Zilleruelo G., et al. (1989). Renal disease in children with the acquired immunodificiency syndrome. New England Journal of Medicine, 321, 625–30.

Thomas, P., Singh, T., Williams, R. & Blum, S. (1992). Trends in survival for children reported with maternally transmitted acquired immunodeficiency syndrome in New York City, 1982 to 1989. *Pediatric Infectious Disease Journal*, **11**, 34–9.

Tovo, P. A., de Martino, M., Gabiano, C., *et al.* (1992). Prognostic factors and survival in children with perinatal HIV-1 infection. *Lancet*, **339**, 1249–53.

Tudor-Williams, G., StClair, M., McKinney, R. E., *et al.* (1992). HIV-1 sensitivity to zidovudine and clinical outcome in children. *Lancet*, **339**, 15–9.

Turner, B. J., Dennison, M., Eppes, S. C., Houchens, R., Fanning, T. & Markson, L. E. (1993). Survival experience of 789 children with the acquired immunodeficiency syndrome. *Pediatric Infectious Disease Journal*, **12**, 310–20.

Ullrich, R., Zeitz, M., Heise, W., L'age, M., Hoffken, G. & Rieken, O. (1989). Small intestinal structure and function in patients infected with human immunodeficiency virus (HIV): evidence for HIV-induced enteropathy. *Annals of Internal Medicine*, **111**, 15–21.

Van der Lelie, J., Lange, J. M., Vos, J. J., *et al.* (1987). Autoimmunity against blood cells in human immunodeficiency-virus (HIV) infection. *British Journal of Haematology*, **67**, 109–14.

World Health Organization (1986). Acquired immunodeficiency syndrome (AIDS): WHO/CDC case definition for AIDS. *Weekly Epidemiological Record*, **61**, 69–73.

World Health Organization Global Program on AIDS (1989). Report of the Meeting of the Technical Working Group on HIV/AIDS in Childhood. Geneva: WHO (WHO/GPA/SFI/89.2AF).

Addenda

In late 1994 the CDC published a new classification system for paediatric HIV infection. Infected children are grouped into one of 12 classes based on clinical (N, A, B, C) and immunological (1, 2, 3) findings. Class N includes asymptomatic children; class A mildly symptomatic, with two or more non-specific findings; class B moderately symptomatic, including children with LIP; and class C denotes severely symptomatic children (AIDS defining). Each clinical class can be divided into three immunological groupings. The absolute cut-off points, based on CD4 count or percentage, vary with age (see Table 3.4: CDC proposed categories).

Centers for Disease Control (1994). 1994 revised classification system for human immunodeficiency virus infection in children less than 13 years of age. *Morbidity and Mortality Weekly Report*, **43**, RR-12: 1–10.

4

Natural history of HIV infection in children

STÉPHANE BLANCHE

Introduction

Information on the natural history of vertically acquired HIV infection is becoming available from the various prospective cohorts of infants born to HIV-seropositive women that have been set up worldwide (Boylan & Stein, 1991; Dabis *et al.*, 1993). The main advantage of prospective studies is that infected children are monitored from birth, enabling identification of prognostic factors. The drawback of these studies is their logistics: as the mother-to-child transmission rate is about 20% and a definitive serological diagnosis cannot be made before 18 months, a large number of infants has to be included to obtain a sufficient number of infected cases. In addition, the first prospective cohorts began in 1985–6, which means that the oldest children are now only 7 or 8 years old, and their long-term prognosis thus remains to be established. National AIDS registries (Auger *et al.*, 1988; Tovo *et al.*, 1992) and series of symptomatic children in large centres (Scott *et al.*, 1989; Blanche *et al.*, 1990) also provide useful data, particularly on older children, but carry a major risk of bias.

Industrialised countries

Global analyses of the frequency of the various manifestations are of little value, as HIV infection is a progressive disease, the course of which can vary widely from one child to the next. Furthermore, some signs and symptoms can resolve: for example, 90% of infected children develop lymphadenopathy and/or hepatosplenomegaly before the age of 18 months, yet 30% of children are without clinical signs at the age of 3–4 years (Blanche *et al.*, unpublished data; European Collaborative Study 1994).

The age distribution of the two most severe manifestations of HIV disease in children, i.e. opportunistic infections and specific encephalopathy, shows two distinct phases (Fig. 4.1). The risk of developing either or both manifestations increases rapidly to between 15% and

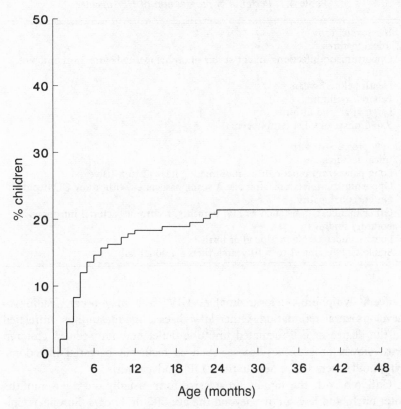

Fig. 4.1. Cumulative curve (Kaplan–Meier) of opportunistic infection and/or specific encephalopathy in 196 infected children. French prospective study, August 1993.

20% in the first 12 months of life, and far more slowly thereafter, by about 3–4% per year. As HIV encephalopathy is a non-infectious condition and biological parameters are also affected, these two phases are not due simply to changes in susceptibility to infections with age or to environmental conditions, but rather to two distinct modes of disease progression (Table 4.1). It is estimated that between 15% and 20% of infants develop an early and severe immune deficiency associated with opportunistic infections and, in most cases, encephalopathy. In contrast, HIV disease progresses less rapidly in the remaining infants who, following generalised lymphadenopathy in the first few months of life, remain without clinical manifestations for long periods. The immune deficiency develops gradually, over 2–10 years or more. These children have no signs of encephalopathy, although neurological manifestations related to opportunistic agents such as cytomegalovirus or toxoplasma,

Table 4.1. *Patterns of progression of HIV disease*

Early, severe form
Clinical features
Opportunistic infections and/or severe encephalopathy before 18 months of life
Death before 5 years
Laboratory findings
Large viral load at birth
Rapid onset of CD4 lymphopenia
Slowly progressive form
Clinical features
Long paucisymptomatic or asymptomatic phase (2 to >10 years)
Opportunistic infections after age 2 years, associated with a low CD4 count
No encephalopathy
Other manifestations such as LIP, parotitis, recurrent bacterial infections
Laboratory findings
Low or undetectable viral load at birth
Stable CD4 count (2 to >10 years), then a gradual fall

cancers (lymphoma, leiosarcoma) or HIV itself may occur, leading to developmental retardation. Other HIV disease manifestations, unrelated to the degree of cell-mediated immune deficiency, are seen in children with slowly progressive disease, such as recurrent bacterial infections, lymphoid interstitial pneumonitis (LIP) and parotitis.

Children with the rapidly progressive form usually die a few months after birth, and few survive beyond the age of 3 or 4 years (European Collaborative Study, 1994). In contrast, the long-term prognosis for children with slowly progressive disease remains to be established. Thus, in Fig. 4.2, the majority of the deaths in the first few years of life are in children with rapidly progressive disease. In the French prospective cohort, as in other prospective studies, the cumulative mortality rate at 18 months is about 10%; it then increases by 3% or 4% per year. At the age of 6 years about 70% of children are still alive. This implies that some children will live to reach adulthood.

The pattern of rapid progression is typical for vertically infected children, whereas a significant risk of opportunistic infections and/or death only appears in adults at least a year after infection (Lui *et al.*, 1988). However, the slowly progressive form in children resembles the course of the disease in adults.

This bimodal age distribution is also consistent with the information from AIDS registries. It is estimated that 20% of children in the New York register are diagnosed with AIDS before the age of 1 year and that the yearly risk thereafter is about 8% (Auger *et al.*, 1988). However, a large

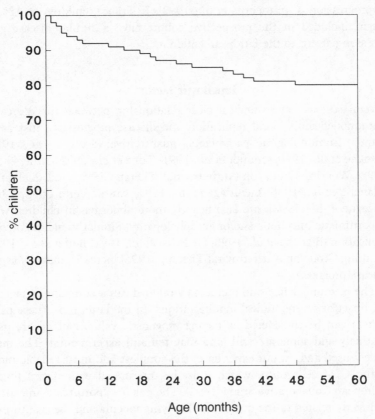

Fig. 4.2. Survival curve (Kaplan–Meier) in 196 infected children. French prospective study, August 1993.

proportion of AIDS cases notified after the age of 3–4 years had LIP, which although an AIDS-defining disease in the Centers for Disease Control and Prevention (CDC) classification, is not associated with an increased risk of death (Blanche *et al.*, 1990) (see Chapter 3). Data based on such AIDS registers therefore almost certainly overestimate the risk of AIDS in older children.

Developing countries

Data from developing countries are difficult to interpret because of diagnostic and therapeutic problems with both HIV infection itself and its infectious complications. Also, different definitions of AIDS are in use, and excess mortality may be due to causes other than AIDS. An analysis of data from an AIDS register in Rwanda also showed a bimodal pattern of progression (Commenges *et al.*, 1992). In France, children of African origin included in the prospective cohort have a similar disease progression pattern to the European children.

Prognostic factors

Several studies have shown a clear relationship between the degree of immunodeficiency, viral replication and disease progression, just as in adults. Immunological parameters, quantitative (Scott *et al.*, 1989; Blanche *et al.*, 1990; Connor *et al.*, 1991; Tovo *et al.*, 1992; Butler *et al.*, 1992; Working Group on Antiretroviral Therapy 1993) and qualitative (Blanche *et al.*, 1986; Luzuriaga *et al.*, 1991; van de Perre *et al.*, 1992; Buzeyne *et al.*, 1993), are significantly more abnormal in children with opportunistic infections and/or encephalopathy. Similarly, indices of viral replication (Blanche *et al.*, 1990; De Rossi *et al.*, 1991; Butler *et al.*, 1992; Working Group on Antiretroviral Therapy, 1993) increase gradually as the disease progresses.

The immune deficit and increased viral load can accompany or precede the onset of severe clinical manifestations. In the latter case, these parameters can be considered as having prognostic value. Not all are used routinely and some are still (and may remain) experimental. The most widely used and, in our experience, the simplest and most reliable index is the CD4 cell count, which must be interpreted with regard to age (European Collaborative Study, 1992). The risk of opportunistic infections is directly related to the degree of CD4 lymphopenia and the risk thresholds established by the CDC (1991), although not fully specific, can be useful for the day-to-day follow-up and therapeutic management of these children (see Chapters 3 and 10). It is important to note, however, that some children (especially after the age of 5–6 years) can survive for several years with very low CD4 cell counts (Butler *et al.*, 1992).

p24 antigenaemia is also widely used, but its predictive value is less reliable at the individual level than that of the CD4 cell count (Blanche *et al.*, 1990). Finally, other indirect prognostic markers such as serum β_2-microglobulin and neopterin levels, have been evaluated. Although they may have some predictive value, this is more limited than the CD4 cell count and of no practical use.

In addition to these laboratory indicators of progression, it is useful to identify as early as possible those children who will have rapidly progressive disease. Contrary to what is observed later, positive virological tests at birth have high prognostic value although limited diagnostic sensitivity (Consensus Workshop, 1992). Based on small numbers, it has been suggested that the risk of the early, severe form of HIV disease is twice as high when culture (or polymerase chain reaction) is positive at birth (Rogers *et al.*, 1989; Burgard *et al.*, 1992), and 3–4 times higher if p24 antigen is detected at birth (Burgard *et al.*, 1992; Blanche *et al.*, 1994), compared with infants in whom positive results are obtained only after a few weeks or months of life. This is generally taken to represent early intrauterine infection, and could reflects intense viral replication that started *in utero*. The CD4 cell count is also lower than normal in these infants, although the wide variation of CD4 values at birth makes analysis of each case difficult. By repeating the test a few weeks after birth and then every 2 or 3 months for the first year of life, it is possible to detect a sharp drop in the CD4 cell count which is associated with the early, severe form.

More recently, it has been possible to establish a correlation between maternal immunological and virological parameters at delivery and the pattern of HIV disease progression in the infant (Blanche *et al.*, 1994; Tovo *et al.*, 1994). The risk of the early, severe form was higher if the mother has AIDS at the time of delivery, and there was a strong correlation between immunological and virological parameters (p24 antigen and the CD4 cell count) in the mother and infant.

Hypothesis

The reason for this bimodal disease pattern in children remains to be determined. The most common hypothesis involves the timing of transmission from the mother to the fetus (or newborn). Early transmission, *in utero*, would be associated with rapid disease progression due to an interaction of the virus with the developing immune system and/or central nervous system, while in the case of later (perinatal) transmission, the neonate's cellular and humoral immune response is closer to that of the adult. This view is supported by the fact that most children who develop the early, severe form have a large viral load and relative CD4 lymphopenia at birth. However, other factors are no doubt involved, because children infected perinatally by blood transfusion can also develop early opportunistic infections with encephalopathy (Jones *et al.*, 1992). In addition, in a recent study of length of time for the production of infant specific anti-HIV antibodies (Rouzioux *et al.*, 1993), the early, severe form was not restricted to those children supposed to be infected *in utero*, although the risk of early progression was greater. Finally, some infants develop the rapidly progressive form despite a normal CD4 count and undetectable virus at birth. Factors such as the viral inoculum and the HIV phenotype may also play a role. The recently identified association between the mother's disease status at the time of delivery and the disease course in the infant does not provide the answer. Indeed, a mother at an advanced stage of the disease and with a large cellular and plasma viral load could transmit a larger inoculum, or transmit the virus earlier in gestation, and/or transmit a highly virulent strain.

Conclusion

Although HIV disease is generally considered more severe in children than in adults, most children in fact show the adult pattern of disease progression. With regard to the minority of infants who develop the early, severe form of HIV disease, optimal management requires diagnosis at birth and identification of the causes of this disease pattern typical of vertically infected children.

References

Auger, I., Thomas, P., De Gruttola, V., *et al.* (1988). Incubation periods for paediatric AIDS patients. *Nature*, **336**, 575–7.

Blanche, S., Le Deist, F., Fischer, A., *et al.* (1986). Longitudinal study of 18 children with perinatal LAV-HTL VIII infection. *Journal of Pediatrics*, **109**, 965–70.

Blanche, S., Mayaux, M. J., Rouzioux, C., *et al.* (1994). Relationship between maternal status at delivery and disease progression in vertically HIV-1 infected children. *New England Journal of Medicine*, **330**, 308–12.

Blanche, S., Tardieu, M., Duliege, A. M., *et al.* (1990). Longitudinal study of 94 symptomatic infants with perinatal acquired HIV infection. *American Journal of Diseases of Children*, **144**, 1210–5.

Boylan, L., Stein, Z. A. (1991) The epidemiology of HIV infection in children and their mothers. *Epidemiological Review*, **13**, 143–77.

Burgard, M., Mayaux, M. J., Blanche, S., *et al.* (1992). The use of viral culture and p24 antigen testing to diagnose HIV infection in neonates. *New England Journal of Medicine*, **327**, 1192–7.

Butler, K. M., Husson, R. N., Lewis, L. L., *et al.* (1992). CD4 status and p24 antigenemia. Are they useful predictors of survival in HIV-infected children receiving antiretroviral therapy. *American Journal of Diseases of Children*, **146**, 932–6.

Buzeyne, F., Blanche, S., Schmitt, D., Griscelli, C., Riviere, Y. (1993). Detection of HIV specific cell-mediated cytotoxicity in the peripheral blood from infected children. *Journal of Immunology*, **150**, 3569–74.

Centers for Disease Control (1991). Guidelines for prophylaxis against *Pneumocystis Carinii* pneumonia for children infected with HIV. *Mortality and Morbidity Weekly Report*, **40**, RR-2.

Commenges, D., Alioum, A., Lepage, P., *et al.* (1992). Estimating the incubation period of paediatric AIDS in Rwanda. *AIDS*, **6**, 1515–20.

Connor, E., Bagarazzi, M., McSherry, G., *et al.* (1991). Clinical and laboratory correlates of *Pneumocystis carinii* in children infected with HIV. *Journal of the American Medical Association*, **265**, 1693–7.

Consensus Workshop (1992). Early diagnosis of HIV infection in infants. Siena, Italy, 17–18 January. *AIDS*, **5**, 1169–78.

Dabis, F., Msellati, P., Dunn, D., *et al.* (1993). Estimating the rate of mother-to-child transmission of HIV. Report of a workshop on methodological issues. Ghent (Belgium) 17–20 Feb 1992. *AIDS*, 7, 1139–48.

De Rossi, A., Plasti, M., Mammano, F., *et al.* (1991). Perinatal infection by HIV-1: Relationship between proviral copy, number in vivo, viral properties in vitro and clinical outcome. *Journal of Medical Virology*, 35, 283–89.

European Collaborative Study (1992). Age related standards for T lymphocyte subsets based on uninfected children born to HIV-1 infected mothers. *Pediatric Infectious Disease Journal*, 11, 1018–26.

European Collaborative Study (1994). Natural history of vertically acquired HIV infection. *Pediatrics* (in press).

Jones, D. S., Byers, R. H., Bush, T. J., *et al.* (1992). Epidemiology of transfusion acquired immunodeficiency syndrome in children in the United States 1981 through 1989. *Pediatrics*, 89, 123–7.

Lui, K., Darrow W. W., Rutherford, G. W. (1988). A model-based estimate of the mean incubation period for AIDS in homosexual men. *Science*, 240, 1333–5.

Luzuriaga, K. R. A., Koup, C. A., Pikora, D. B., *et al.* (1991). Deficient HIV-1 specific cytotoxic T cell responses in vertically infected children. *Journal of Pediatrics*, 119, 230–4.

Rogers, M. F., Ou C. Y., Rayfield, M., *et al.* (1989). Use of the polymerase chain reaction for early detection of the proviral sequences of HIV in infants born to seropositive mothers. *New England Journal of Medicine*, 320, 1649–54.

Rouzioux, C., Costagliola, D., Burgard, M., *et al.* (1993). Timing of mother-to-child HIV-1 transmission depends on maternal status. *AIDS*, 7 (Suppl. 2), 549–52.

Scott, G. B., Hutto, C., Makuch, R. W., *et al.* (1989). Survival in children with perinatally acquired HIV-1 infection. *New England Journal of Medicine*, 321, 1791–6.

Tovo, P., De Martino, M., Gabiano, C., *et al.* (1992). Prognostic factors and survival in children with perinatal HIV-1 infection. *Lancet*, 339, 1249–53.

Tovo, P., De Martino, M., Gabiano, C., *et al.* (1994). AIDS appearance in children is associated with the velocity of disease progression in their mothers. *Journal of Infectious Diseases*, 170, 1000–2.

Van de Perre, P., Lepage, P., Simonon, A., *et al.* (1992). Biological markers associated with prolonged survival in African children maternally infected by the HIV-1. *AIDS Research and Human Retroviruses*, 8, 435–41.

Working Group on Antiretroviral Therapy: National Pediatric HIV Resource Center (1993). Antiretroviral therapy and medical management of the HIV-infected child. *Pediatric Infectious Disease Journal*, 12, 513–22.

5

Diagnosis of HIV infection

ANITA DE ROSSI

Introduction

An early diagnosis of HIV infection in infants is crucial for parental aware-ness, medical intervention and social care; moreover, highly sensitive tests to detect the infection as early as possible may be useful for understanding the timing of transmission and the natural history of vertical infection. This information is mandatory for the development of strategies aimed at preventing mother-to-child HIV transmission, and for designing anti-retroviral drug and/or vaccine trials in infected children. The diagnosis of HIV infection in infants born to seropositive mothers has been problem-atic, because all newborns are seropositive at birth due to the presence of maternal immunoglobulin G (IgG) antibodies which cross the placenta. The persistence of these maternal antibodies in infants, often up to 18 months of age (European Collaborative Study, 1988; Rogers *et al.*, 1991), means that an early identification of infected children cannot be achieved by the conventional IgG antibody assays that have been successfully applied to the diagnosis of HIV in adults.

In the last few years, alternative antibody assays that allow the child's autochthonous antibodies to be detected have been developed and evalu-ated in terms of their application to the diagnosis of HIV infection in infants. Since IgA and IgM do not cross the placenta, their detection could be used as a marker of infection; however, reliable tests for HIV-specific IgM have not yet been developed, and the HIV-specific IgA approach, although much more promising, has a low sensitivity in young infants (Weiblen *et al.*, 1990a; Landesman *et al.*, 1991). The *in vitro* antibody production (IVAP) assay, which is based on evidence that B lymphocytes of HIV-infected subjects spontaneously secrete HIV-specific antibodies *in vitro* (Amadori *et al.*, 1988), also permits the identification of infected children according to the capacity of their B cells to produce antibodies *in vitro*; however, this procedure is also not reliable in very young infants (Amadori *et al.*, 1990).

Because none of the alternative HIV-antibody assays guarantees high specificity and sensitivity in infants under 3–6 months of age, early diagnosis should be based on direct identification of the virus or its components, such as antigens or nucleic acid. In this setting, modifications in the virus culture technique have led to increased sensitivity in detecting the virus from cells and plasma of infected children (Burgard *et al.*, 1992). However, this assay remains expensive and time-consuming. The technique of treating plasma to dissociate antigen–antibody immunocomplexes that are present in most infants in the first few months of life because of maternal antibodies in circulation, has improved the diagnostic value of serum antigen detection (Miles *et al.*, 1993). Moreover, the introduction of the polymerase chain reaction (PCR) technique to amplify specific nucleic acid sequences (Erlich *et al.*, 1991) has greatly contributed to the identification of viral sequences in patient samples.

This chapter reviews the advantages and drawbacks of these assays in diagnosing paediatric HIV infection, and focuses on recent findings that are shedding light on the pathogenesis of vertically acquired HIV infection.

HIV life cycle

Efforts to understand the biology and molecular biology of HIV have led to remarkable advances in diagnostic assays, and in the critical evaluation of tests results.

HIV, a lentivirus, belongs to the family of retroviruses (Wong-Staal & Gallo, 1985), so called because of their ability to retrotranscribe their RNA genome into viral DNA (Warmus, 1988). The genetic organisation of HIV is shown schematically in Fig. 5.1. The characteristic retroviral genes *gag*, *pol* and *env* encode for the nucleocapsid proteins, the reverse transcriptase, protease and integrase enzymes, and the envelope proteins, respectively. HIV also contains a number of accessory genes delegated to the control of viral replication, virion maturation and morphogenesis (Cullen, 1991). After virus entry into human cells (a process that involves several steps after the binding of gp120 envelope viral protein to its specific cellular CD4 receptor) single-stranded genomic RNA is retrotranscribed into double-stranded viral DNA by the RNA/DNA-dependent DNA polymerase and ribonuclease H activities of the reverse transcriptase enzyme. Viral DNA (provirus) then migrates to the nucleus and is integrated randomly into host DNA by the endonuclease activity of viral integrase. In addition to the crucial activities of the viral enzymes, both reverse transcription and provirus integration processes involve several cellular factors, and occur mainly in activated cells (Zach *et al.*, 1990).

The HIV genome in its proviral form is flanked by characteristic long

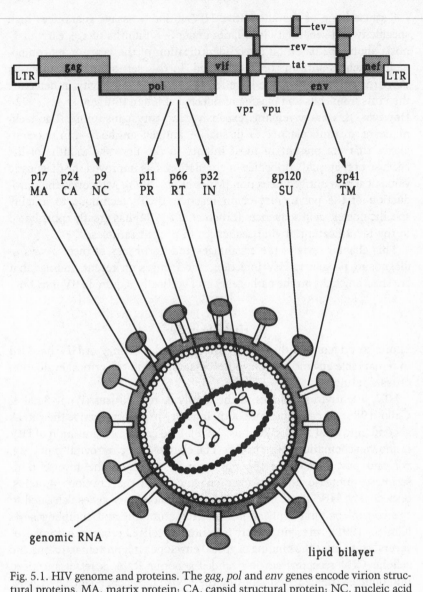

Fig. 5.1. HIV genome and proteins. The *gag*, *pol* and *env* genes encode virion structural proteins. MA, matrix protein; CA, capsid structural protein; NC, nucleic acid
associated protein; PR, protease; RT, reverse transcriptase; IN, integrase; SU,
envelope surface protein; TM, envelope transmembrane protein. *vif, tev, rev, tat* and
nef encode for the corresponding regulatory proteins. LTR, long terminal repeat.

terminal repeats (LTRs) generated during the reverse transcription that contain control elements which direct and regulate viral expression. HIV gene expression is controlled by cellular and viral *trans*-regulatory proteins acting on *cis*-regulatory elements located in the viral LTR (Felber & Pavlakis, 1993), and proceeds via synthesis of viral transcripts using host cell RNA polymerase II. Full-length mRNA transcripts encode for *gag*, *gag–pol* precursor, and genomic RNA found in the virion; singly-spliced transcripts encode for the envelope components, and multiple-spliced transcripts generate the viral regulatory proteins, which are usually detectable in infected cells but not in the mature virion. Retroviral assembly involves the formation of an RNA dimer complexed with *gag* and *gag–pol* polyprotein precursors. This core structure buds from the cellular membrane, acquiring a coat of virus envelope glycoprotein and cellular lipid bilayer components. During this process, the viral-coded protease cleaves the core precursors to generate mature core proteins, thus completing the morphological maturation of virions prior to the next cycle of infection (Vaishnav & Wong-Staal, 1991).

It was recognised that primary HIV infection in adults is associated with high levels of plasma viraemia (Tindall & Cooper, 1991), and dissemination of the virus to lymphoid organs (Pantaleo *et al.*, 1993). Within 1–3 months the emergence of cellular and humoral immune responses to HIV contribute to curtailing viral replication, and a variable period of clinical latency is established. A true viral latency phase, however, does not seem to occur in HIV-infected individuals, since viral RNA can be found in the plasma of patients at all stages of infection, including the asymptomatic phase, albeit at different levels (Piatak *et al.*, 1993).

The HIV assays described below allow the detection of virus in one or more steps of the HIV life cycle (Fig. 5.2); a combination of the diagnostic results might help in characterising the phase of infection.

HIV detection assays

Polymerase chain reaction

The PCR technique was developed to provide highly efficient amplification of target DNA sequences (Saiki *et al.*, 1988). It consists of repeated three-step cycles of: (1) DNA template denaturation at high temperature; (2) annealing of two oligonucleotide primers to complementary sequences on each DNA strand template, and (3) extension of the annealed primers on the DNA template driven by a thermostable DNA polymerase in the presence of the four deoxyribonucleotide triphosphates (dNTP). These three-step cycles are carried out in an automated thermal cycler that ensures

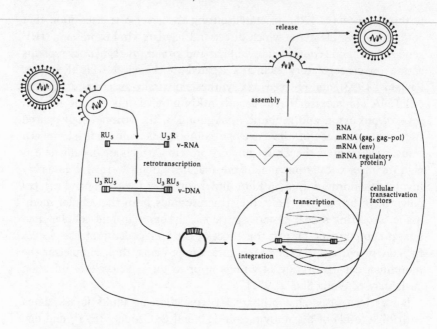

HIV cycle step

Methods of detection

retrotranscription
integration

virus culture
DNA-PCR
(cells)

transcription
replication

virus culture
RNA-PCR
(cells)

extracellular virus/
release of viral
components

virus culture
RNA-PCR
p24 antigen
(biological fluids)

Fig. 5.2. HIV biological cycle and methods of HIV detection.

the temperature and the timing of each step, and after 20 cycles, which take place in 1–3 hours, DNA target molecules are virtually amplified 1 million times. The amplified products can be visualised on agarose or acrylamide gel using a simple staining procedure, or can be detected with radiolabelled probes by the southern blot or liquid hybridisation procedure. The recent introduction of immunoenzymatic systems for PCR product analysis using non-isotopic labelled probes and/or primers will, it is hoped, provide an additional advantage in terms of feasibility and assay cost (Ou, *et al.*, 1990; Whetsell *et al.*, 1992).

Due to its amplification property, PCR currently constitutes the most sensitive method for detecting specific nucleic acid sequences, even if they are present in a low number of copies and in a small number of cells. Since provirus originated by reverse transcription of viral RNA into DNA is a fundamental step in the HIV life cycle, DNA-PCR should in theory permit the identification of all infections. PCR assay does not require a highly purified starting DNA as template; thus it can be directly performed on freshly isolated cells, on dried cell pellets stored at −80 °C or cryopreserved in liquid nitrogen, and on DNA recovered from blood spots dried on filter paper (Cassol *et al.*, 1992).

Amplification can also be carried out with RNA as the initial template (RT-PCR). Prior to amplification, the RNA is converted *in vitro* to DNA (cDNA) using the reverse transcriptase enzyme. RT-PCR can be performed starting from cells, plasma, or other body fluids.

The specificity of the PCR reaction is dictated by the primers which usually anneal the sequences flanking the region to be amplified; thus, the selection of the primers and the template to employ in the reaction (cellular DNA or RNA, extracellular RNA) determines what is actually amplified. The use of specifically designed primers allows determination of the extent of the reverse transcription process as well as the integrated and unintegrated forms of viral DNA (Zach *et al.*, 1990) – aspects which are relevant to the understanding of the molecular mechanisms that underlie infection in target cells. Moreover RNA-PCR provides information regarding viral activation replication, and offers an effective tool for investigating the state of viral infection in patients.

To diagnose HIV infection, DNA-PCR is routinely performed in 10^5 lysed peripheral blood mononuclear cells (PBMC) previously separated from blood by Ficoll gradient centrifugation, or using directly lysed PBMC starting from 0.5 ml of blood (Table 5.1). Primer pairs selected from the constant regions of the viral genes are used to avoid the possibility of false negative results due to HIV variability (Krivine *et al.*, 1990; De Rossi *et al.*, 1991*a*; Scarlatti *et al.*, 1991; Comeau *et al.*, 1992). Primers SK 29/30 (spanning LTR sequences), SK 38/39 and 101/145 (spanning *gag* sequences) and SK 68/69 (spanning *env* sequences) (Ou *et al.*, 1988) consistently amplify specific sequences of viral strains from American and European patients, but their efficiency is lower in cases from African countries (Candotti *et al.*, 1991).

The sensitivity of PCR allows the detection of as few as 1–5 copies of HIV present in the specimen to be amplified; in a few cases, a very low

Table 5.1. *Laboratory assays for HIV-1 detection*

Tests	Specimens (amount)	Target	Time to results	Standardisation	Advantages	Disadvantages
DNA-PCR	PBMC ($1-10 \times 10^5$ PBMC) Blood (500 µl)	Proviral DNA	1–2 days	++	Small sample required; rapid	Requires different working area to process preamplified and postamplified samples; expensive
RNA-PCR	PBMC ($1-10 \times 10^5$ PBMC) Plasma/serum (100–500 µl)	Viral RNA; viral mRNA Viral RNA	1–2 days 1–2 days	In progress In progress		
Virus culture	PBMC ($2-5 \times 10^6$ PBMC) Blood (500 µl) Plasma/serum (1000 µl)	Whole virus	15–30 days	++	Provides virus isolation; allows biological studies of HIV isolates	Time-consuming; expensive; laborious; requires biosafety laboratory
p24 antigen	Plasma/serum (<500 µl)	Free p24 viral antigen	1 day	+++	Simple; rapid; low cost	Lower sensitivity than PCR and virus culture
p24 IC antigen	Plasma/serum (<500 µl)	Immunocomplexed p24 viral antigen	1 day	+++		
IgG (ELISA, WB)	Plasma/serum	HIV-specific antibodies	2 hours–1 day	+++	Simple; rapid; low cost	Not suitable in infants <18 months of age
IgA	Plasma/serum	HIV-specific IgA antibodies	1–2 days	++	Simple; rapid; low cost	Low sensitivity in infants <6 months of age
IVAP	PBMC (2×10^6)	HIV-specific IgG antibodies	7–8 days	++	Simple; moderate cost	Low specificity in infants <3 months of age; requires biosafety laboratory
ELISPOT	PBMC (<1×10^6)	Cells producing HIV antibodies	1–3 days	–	Simple; moderate cost	Specificity not well known; requires biosafety precautions

viral burden (less than 1 copy per 10^5–10^6 cells) may lead to a false negative result (Table 5.2). In addition, although high-quality DNA is not required for amplification, some inhibitors, such as haemoglobin, may reduce the thermostable DNA polymerase activity. The quality of the DNA to be amplified can be controlled by using primers specific for a cellular gene, such as β-globin. The high levels of amplification, however, constitute the major drawback to the PCR technique, as contaminant DNA sequences that are not detectable with other procedures may be amplified and produce false positive results (Kwok & Higuchi, 1989). The amplified products of a previously amplified sample constitute the most important source of exogenous DNA contamination (DNA carry-over), but recent improvements in PCR methodology have helped to minimise false positive results thus obtained. One method uses dUTP instead of dTTP in the PCR reaction mixture, so the amplified product will contain uracil instead of thymidine. By treating the sample with uracil-*N*-glycosylase enzyme prior to amplification, any DNA product with the uracil substitution will be degraded, while the template DNA will remain unaffected (Lango, Beringer & Hartley, 1990).

Since the HIV genome shares a partial homology with human endogenous retroviral-like sequences (Horwitz, Boyce-Jacino & Faras, 1992), the possibility exists that some primers will amplify HIV-related genomic sequences. The use of a specific HIV probe to identify the amplified product of the expected size will increase the specificity of the results.

A recent technique combines PCR methodology with *in situ* hybridisation (Patterson *et al.*, 1993). This approach allows a single-copy proviral DNA or low levels of viral mRNA to be identified directly in cells that preserve their morphology. It appears to be an extremely interesting and useful procedure for directly investigating the *in vivo* distribution of the virus in the target cells, although at present it is suitable only for research purposes.

Virus culture

Virus culture is generally performed by culturing a patient's cells, usually PBMC, with an equal number of PBMC from healthy donors that have been pre-stimulated for 48 hours with phytohaemagglutinin. The co-cultures are incubated for at least 15 days, more often 30 days, in the presence of T-cell growth factor (interleukin-2). Culture supernatants are collected twice weekly and assayed for p24 antigen or reverse transcriptase activity. For diagnostic purposes, 2–5 × 10^6 cells are usually co-cultured with indicator cells; microculture can be performed in 12- or 24-well microtitre plates, but sensitivity might be lower depending on the number

Table 5.2. *Sensitivity and specificity of diagnostic assays*

Tests	Sensitivity of the assay	Factors affecting sensitivity	Factors affecting specificity
DNA-PCR	1–10 DNA target molecule per 10^6 cells	DNA not suitable for amplification; HIV variability; extremely low viral burden in patient PBMC	Contamination by exogenous DNA; primer hybridisation with genomic retrovirus-like sequences
RNA-PCR	1–10 cDNA target molecule per 10^6 cells	Extremely low rate of viral replication	
Virus culture	1–10 cDNA target molecule/ml 1–100 virus particles per 1×10^6 cells	Susceptibility of indicator cells to HIV infection; low viral burden in patient PBMC; sample storage conditions	
p24 antigen	10 pg/ml	Low/absent rate of HIV replication in patient; high level of anti-p24 antibodies	Carry-over of maternal p24 antigen (newborn); non-specific binding of plasma factors to p24 antibody-coated well
p24 IC antigen	10 pg/ml	Low/absent rate of HIV replication in patient	
IgG	>95% in adults and children >18 months of age	Advanced impairment of the immune system	Presence of maternal antibodies (infants <18 months); partial cross-reactivity against cellular antigens
IgA	10–90% (age and disease status dependent)	High level of IgG; low affinity	
IVAP	Age dependent	Low number of HIV antibody committed B cells; hypogammaglobulinaemia	Carry-over of maternal cytophilic IgG (newborn)
ELISPOT	Age dependent	Low number of HIV antibody committed B cells; hypogammaglobulinaemia	

of infected cells present in the initial inoculum. HIV culture can be also performed starting from plasma, again using PBMC from healthy donors as target cells (Table 5.1).

Virus culture is the most specific assay for detecting HIV, and the only one which provides isolation of whole virus. The isolation of naturally occurring infecting strains allows investigation of their biological features, i.e. tropism, replication rate and cytopathic activity, which have been reported to play a role in disease outcome (Cheng-Mayer *et al.*, 1988; Fenyo *et al.*, 1988; Tersmette *et al.*, 1989; Schuitemaker *et al.*, 1992), and therefore may also help in formulating the prognosis.

However, the use of virus culture as a diagnostic test has several restrictions. Cultures must be performed in laboratories with special biosafety precautions to prevent exposure of laboratory personnel. The culture technique is expensive, laborious, time-consuming and requires from 15 to 30 days for results. The sensitivity of this assay is lower than that of the PCR assay (Table 5.2). Several factors may influence its sensitivity; these include the initial viral burden in the patient, the sample storage conditions, the target cells used in the culture and the biological properties of the virus being cultured. Recent improvements in methodology, such as the addition of polybrene and anti-alpha-interferon to the culture medium, and ultracentrifugation to concentrate viral particles in the culture supernatants, increase its sensitivity – which may reach 100% when fresh patient PBMC are employed (Burgard *et al.*, 1992; De Rossi *et al.*, 1992). Cryopreservation of the PBMC prior to culture seems to reduce the sensitivity of the virus assay (personal observations). The sensitivity of HIV detection in plasma is greatly influenced by the rate of HIV replication in the patient. The use of plasma instead of cells may be particularly helpful for monitoring antiretroviral therapy, but it is less sensitive for diagnostic purposes (Coombs *et al.*, 1989; Escaich *et al.*, 1991). The indicator cells used may also affect assay sensitivity. Although PBMC from healthy donors are the best indicator cells, these may differ from one donor to another in their susceptibility to HIV infection, thereby affecting the virus yield in culture (Williams & Cloyd, 1991). Although this aspect does not seem to impair the diagnostic result, it may assume importance when quantitative examination of sequential samples is required, for example to monitor the course of infection and/or therapy; in this case pooled cells from multiple donors may be useful.

p24 antigen

p24 antigen assay is a simple, rapid and quantitative immunoenzymatic procedure for detecting free p24, the major structural core protein of HIV.

Several commercially available kits employ high-affinity monoclonal antibodies bound to microtitre plastic wells to capture the p24 antigen. In addition to monitoring HIV in culture, this assay detects free p24 in plasma or serum (Table 5.1). Therefore, it may be useful for diagnosis of HIV infection, but its sensitivity is lower than that of virus culture or PCR, since it detects only virions released from infected cells (De Rossi et al., 1991a; Burgard et al., 1992; Borkowsky et al., 1992).

The major drawback of the p24 antigen assay is its inability to detect p24 immunocomplexed (p24IC) with anti-p24 antibodies – a common finding in young infants due to the presence of maternal antibodies (Table 5.2). Acid hydrolysis pretreatment of plasma/serum dissociates these immunocomplexes (Nishanian et al., 1990) and greatly increases the diagnostic value of the assay (Miles et al., 1993; Palomba et al., 1993; Schupbach et al., 1994). Nevertheless, reactivity above the cut-off value may be due to non-specific binding of plasma components to the antibody-coated plastic wells, especially if the plasma was subjected to acid hydrolysis. Therefore, reactive samples should be confirmed by a neutralisation test with specific anti-24 antibodies, particularly when p24 antigen is the only evidence of HIV infection.

Moreover, in a few cases, positive results in the p24 assay in newborns were not correlated with a true HIV infection (De Rossi et al., 1991a; Simon et al., 1993). Transplacental passage of some viral proteins without an ensuing viral infection could possibly explain these findings, which demand caution and a highly critical interpretation of test results obtained in the first days after birth.

Quantitation of HIV infection

All of the assays employed to identify HIV have also been set up to quantify HIV: virus culture and DNA-PCR can be employed to evaluate the cell viral burden, while p24 antigen assay, RT-PCR and virus culture from plasma quantitate HIV release into blood. Quantitative virus culture discloses the number of infectious viral particles, while all the other assays detect specific viral components. Due to their different sensitivities, quantitative values obtained by different assays in the same sample may vary, while maintaining similar trends during the course of infection.

p24 antigen assay is the simplest, although the least sensitive, method for quantitating both free and (after acid hydrolysis) immunocomplex-associated p24 antigen in blood. Studies to optimise quantitative DNA-PCR to evaluate the number of proviral copies in cells, and RT-PCR to estimate the viral copies in blood, are in progress (Michael et al., 1992; Piatak et al., 1993). It was estimated that the virus number per 10^6 PBMC varied from 1 to 10 000 as evaluated by virus culture (Ho *et al.*, 1989; Connor *et al.*, 1993) and from 1 to 100 000 by DNA-PCR (Simmonds *et al.*, 1990; De Rossi *et al.*, 1991b; Jurrians *et al.*, 1992; Michael *et al.*, 1992), according to the status of infection, and was at least 10- to 100-fold lower in asymptomatic subjects.

During primary HIV infection in adults, the p24 antigen level in the blood rises to more than 1 ng/ml plasma and up to 20×10^6 HIV copies per millilitre of plasma can be detected by RT-PCR (Piatak *et al.*, 1993). Circulating virus decreases after the onset of an adequate immune response and during the clinically latent phase. During this period, viral nucleic acid in the plasma can be detected by RNA-PCR, but p24 antigen assay and plasma virus culture usually give negative results. Deterioration of the immune system and onset of symptoms are usually accompanied by an increase in the number of infected cells and circulating virus. During the symptomatic phase, HIV levels are comparable to or higher than those recorded during the primary acute infection (Ho *et al.*, 1989; Connor *et al.*, 1993).

HIV antibody detection

The most common antibody tests are the enzyme-linked immunosorbent assay (ELISA) and Western blot (WB) assays (Table 5.1). In ELISA microtitre wells are coated with viral antigen (whole virus and/or recombinant viral proteins), while in Western blot assay the viral proteins are separated by electrophoresis and transferred to a filter paper strip. The wells or strips are incubated with patient plasma/serum and the resulting antigen–antibody complexes evidenced by adding enzyme-linked anti-human antibodies followed by the appropriate substrate. Both assays are simple, commercially available and well standardised. Moreover, the criteria for interpreting results have been established by the Centers for Disease Control and Association of State and Public Health Laboratory Directors (Centers for Disease Control, 1989) and WHO (World Health Organization, 1990, 1992). Their sensitivity and specificity reach 99%; both require only small amounts of plasma/serum (5–20 μl), and both have been adapted to test saliva and urine specimens from infected patients (Connell *et al.*, 1990; Croft *et al.*, 1991; Frerichs *et al.*, 1992). However, these assays detect HIV-specific IgG antibodies, and therefore cannot usefully be employed for diagnosis in infants up to 18 months of age born to seropositive mothers (Table 5.2).

Alternative serological assays

Since IgA and IgM do not usually cross the placenta, their detection in infants could be used as a marker of infection. HIV-specific IgM antibody detection is difficult, and lacks sensitivity and specificity. In addition to technical difficulties, its poor diagnostic value arises from the fact that IgM antibodies are produced transiently and at varying periods following infection (Schupbach *et al.*, 1989; Weiblen *et al.*, 1990*b*).

In contrast, HIV-specific IgA detection is much more specific and sensitive as a diagnostic assay (Weiblen *et al.*, 1990*a*; Martin *et al.*, 1991; Quinn *et al.*, 1991) (Table 5.1). As IgG may compete with IgA for binding sites to viral antigens, its removal from serum by absorption with protein G-coated beads increases the sensitivity and specificity of the assay (Weiblen *et al.*, 1990*b*). However, some positive IgA results obtained in newborns were not correlated with a true HIV infection (Connell *et al.*, 1992), and sensitivity of this assay is still highly variable, depending on the infant's age at testing and disease status. Indeed, assay sensitivity is very low in newborns, though it reaches 90% in children over 6 months of age (Table 5.2). Given its low cost and feasibility, this assay may be appropriate for large-scale screening of infant populations, particularly when other more sophisticated technologies, such as PCR and virus culture, are not available.

New and simpler tools for early serological diagnosis are emerging from studies concerning the immune response to specific epitopes of HIV, and the HIV-specific IgG subclass. By means of an immunoenzymatic assay using peptides designed from the V3 region of gp120 viral protein as antigen, it was demonstrated that maternal IgG antibodies to the V3 domain were lost soon after birth, within the first 2–4 months of life (Jansson *et al.*, 1992; De Rossi *et al.*, 1993*c*). This finding implies that their detection in children over 4 months of age might be highly predictive of infection. Moreover, it was also reported that the clearance of IgG3 HIV-specific antibodies occurred earlier than that of IgG1 (14 weeks versus 7–18 months) (Arico' *et al.*, 1991). Therefore, the search for IgG3 HIV-specific antibodies in infants over 4 months of age may be useful to discrimimate between infected and uninfected infants. However, further studies are needed to define the specificity and sensitivity of these serological approaches.

In vitro HIV-specific antibody production/secretion

The rationale of this assay is based on the fact that B cells from infected individuals produce HIV-specific antibodies spontaneously *in vitro*. This antibody production is modified by exposure of the B cells to some mitogens *in vitro*, and is dependent on interleukin-6 (IL-6) but not IL-1 and IL-2, thus indicating the presence of terminally committed differentiated HIV-specific B cells.

In the IVAP assay, 2×10^6 unstimulated PBMC are cultured for 7 days *in vitro*, and culture supernatants analysed for the presence of HIV-antibody by Western blot or ELISA (Amadori *et al.*, 1988; Pahwa *et al.*, 1989) (Table 5.1). In the ELISPOT (enzyme-linked immunospot) procedure, PBMC are not cultured but placed directly on viral antigen-coated nitrocellulose filters. The addition of anti-human immunoglobulin enables the visualization of HIV-antibody-secreting cells (Lee *et al.*, 1989) (Table 5.1). While the sensitivity of ELISPOT is largely influenced by the antigen used to coat the nitrocellulose filters, and ranges from 60% to 80%, the sensitivity of the IVAP assay ranges from 90% to 95% when performed in children over 3 months of age (Amadori *et al.*, 1990). However, the assay is not reliable in infants under this age since its specificity is low due to the carry-over of maternal cytophilic antibodies that bind to Fc receptor-bearing cells (Indraccolo *et al.*, 1993) (Table 5.2).

Pattern of HIV infection in the newborn and sensitivity of diagnostic assays

The sensitivity of the diagnostic assays varies significantly according to the age at testing (Fig. 5.3). At birth, even the most sensitive assays, such as virus culture and DNA-PCR, will identify only 10–50% of infected children (Borkowsky *et al.*, 1992; Burgard *et al.*, 1992; De Rossi *et al.*, 1992; Krivine *et al.*, 1992); their sensitivity increases with increasing age of the child, and reaches more than 95% in infants older than than 2 months (Burgard *et al.*, 1992; De Rossi *et al.*, 1992; Krivine *et al.*, 1992; Kline *et al.*, 1994). On the whole, p24IC antigen detection assay is more sensitive than p24 antigen assay; its sensitivity increases in the first 2 months of life, as observed with the PCR and virus culture procedures, but remains consistently lower, depending on the phase and rate of active HIV replication. After 3 months of age, several assays allow detection of the child's autochthonous antibodies, and after 6 months of age both IVAP and ELISPOT have more than 90% sensitivity.

These findings may be relevant to diagnostic strategies aimed at identifying vertical infection as early as possible. Since screening at birth identifies only a proportion of the infected children, the cost–benefit ratio of newborn screening programmes should be analysed. On the other hand, positive and negative findings at birth might reflect different times and/or modes of mother-to-child HIV transmission, and could possibly have some prognostic value. Indeed, the poor sensitivity of both PCR and virus culture procedures at birth clearly demonstrates that most infected children have very low HIV levels or no HIV in their peripheral blood cells at this time.

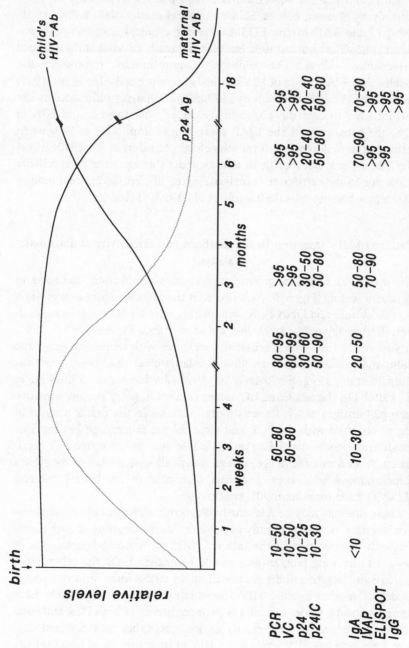

Fig. 5.3. Sensitivity of the HIV-1 tests according to age. VC, virus culture.

Several hypotheses had been advanced to explain this finding: (1) positive and negative detection of HIV at birth might correspond to HIV transmission *in utero* and during the intrapartum period, respectively; (2) HIV transmission *in utero* may occur in organs other than the peripheral blood compartment, such as thymus, spleen and lymph nodes; (3) HIV infection may remain latent before birth due to the lack of antigenic stimuli and/ or the presence of maternal factors which contribute to restricting viral expression. Reports concerning the presence of HIV in fetal tissue are inconclusive; some investigators detected proviral DNA in a high percentage of cases (Courgnaud *et al.*, 1991; Mano & Chermann, 1991), while others have obtained completely negative results (Ehrnst *et al.*, 1991). Recent evidence that caesarean delivery might reduce the risk of transmission suggests that transmission is likely to take place during delivery (European Collaborative Study, 1994; Gabiano *et al.*, 1992), but these data have not been conclusively confirmed. It is also likely that the time and mode of HIV transmission may largely depend on the mother's virological, immunological and clinical status (see Chapter 1).

However, regardless of the reason for the lack of HIV in PBMC at birth in a large proportion of infected children, it is clear that HIV spreads to the PBMC during the first weeks of life, and after 2 months of age virtually all infected infants can be identified by PCR and virus culture performed on PBMC. Concomitantly, the p24IC assay allows an increase in blood p24 antigen levels to be detected, and most infants who are p24-negative at birth will show high blood levels of p24 at 1–2 months of age (De Rossi *et al.*, 1993*b*; Miles *et al.*, 1993). In most cases antigenaemia will successively decline markedly or disappear. Moreover, sequential studies in infants who were antibody-negative at birth to several HIV epitopes disclosed that seroconversion occurs from 4 to 10 weeks after birth (De Rossi *et al.*, 1993*b,c*), thus supporting the concept of transmission during the intrapartum period in a large percentage of cases. This time course of antigenaemia and seroconversion appears to be superimposable on that observed during acute infection in adults (Horsburgh *et al.*, 1989; Tindall & Cooper, 1991). Therefore, it is likely that the pattern observed in neonates reflects the earliest phase of the primary infection.

Prognostic value of virological parameters

Different patterns of clinical outcome have been discerned among infected children: some develop AIDS within their first months of life, in others disease progresses more slowly, and some remain clinically asymptomatic for several years (Scott *et al.*, 1989; Blanche *et al.*, 1989; European Collaborative Study, 1991; Tovo *et al.*, 1992; Turner *et al.*, 1993). The timing of HIV transmission, the child's immunocompetent status, the primary cell/organ target of infection, as well as the viral burden and phenotype, are all factors which probably play a role in disease outcome (De Rossi et al., 1994; Verhofstede et al., 1994). Transmission of HIV during gestation may cause a more extensive infection due to the fetus's inability to mount an adequate cellular and humoral immune response to curtail viral replication. It has been suggested that detection of virus within the first 48 hours after birth might reflect intrauterine HIV transmission (Bryson et al., 1992). In a recent study of 74 mother-infant pairs, it appeared that early positive PCR findings correlated with early onset of AIDS (Bryson et al., 1993), while other data obtained in 181 mother-infant pairs did not reveal this relationship (Burgard et al., 1992). It is also possible that viral detection at birth might be due, at least in some cases, to the transmission of a high number of HIV particles during the intrapartum period.

Whatever the time of transmission, the infection of immune progenitor cells, such as thymic cells (De Rossi et al., 1990; Schnittman et al., 1990), may contribute to the depletion of immunocompetent cells, and compromise the infant's immune response, thus contributing to the rapidity of disease progression. Peripheral blood measurements may not accurately reflect the total-body burden of HIV infection, since lymphoid organs may constitute the major virus reservoir and sites of viral replication (Pantaleo et al., 1993). However, a body of evidence indicates that an increase in the viral burden in blood mirrors the disease onset and outcome. In adults, primary infection is associated with high levels of viraemia, followed by the cellular and immune responses which restrict viral replication, and a period of clinical latency can then be established. Anecdotal reports of some adult cases suggest that high levels of circulating virus during the primary infection and failure of the immune system to control virus replication after the initial infection may be associated with a negative prognosis (Salk et al., 1993). Preliminary data on infants also suggest that a high viral burden at 1–2 months of age is associated with persistently high plasma p24 antigen levels and early onset of AIDS (De Rossi et al., 1993a). Confirmation of this observation in a larger study would imply that early paediatric AIDS is an acute manifestation of the primary HIV infection.

In addition to the initial viral burden and immune factors, the intrinsic genetic and biological characteristics of the infecting strain are likely to contribute to the rate of viral replication and disease progression, as documented in adults (Cheng-Meyer et al., 1988; Fenyo et al., 1988; Tersmette et al., 1989; Fiore et al., 1990; Schuitemaker et al., 1992). Preliminary findings suggest that infection with a syncytium-inducing virus does not appear to be more strongly associated with a negative prognosis than infection with a non-syncytium-inducing virus (Bryson et al., 1993), but further studies are needed to investigate the relationship between viral phenotype and the course of infection.

Conclusions and perspectives

The development of new molecular techniques and the acquisition of further knowledge about HIV in the last few years has had a great impact on the field of paediatric AIDS diagnosis. Several assays guarantee more than 99% specificity, with sensitivity strictly dependent on the infant's age. Only a percentage of infected children can be identified at birth, but virtually all can be diagnosed within the first 3 months of life by the virus culture and DNA-PCR procedures. After this time, alternative HIV-antibody assays also provide high specificity, although they are less sensitive than PCR and virus culture techniques. However, it is important to stress that although early diagnosis of infection will be more available in developed countries, it remains problematic in developing nations, where the spread of paediatric AIDS is striking. Here the costs of molecular biology and viral culture techniques, and the lack of necessary equipment and trained laboratory personnel, place these assays out of reach. Every effort should be made to simplify the available tests and/or to set up alternative less expensive and more feasible diagnostic methods.

Moreover, further studies are needed to clarify the meaning of positive and negative HIV detection at birth; whether or not these findings depend on HIV transmission during the intrauterine or intrapartum periods is relevant to the development of strategies aimed at preventing mother-to-child transmission, as well as to the design of chemo- or immunoprophylactic protocols (see Chapter 1). Studies of HIV expression in cells and blood, as well as analysis of the child's autochthonous cellular and humoral immune response, are needed for better understanding of the course of infection in newborns. It is hoped that these investigations may help to elucidate the timing of HIV transmission and the relevance of the early phase of primary infection to the subsequent disease outcome. Several sensitive assays, such as DNA-PCR and RNA-PCR, are being standardised; the quantitative assessment of viral burden *in vivo*, besides providing insight into the mechanisms of HIV infection, may have important implications for the prognosis of HIV-infected infants.

References

Amadori, A., De Rossi, A., Chieco-Bianchi, L., Giaquinto, C., De Maria, A. & Ades, A. E. (1990). Diagnosis of HIV-1 infection in infants: *in vitro* production of virus specific antibody in lymphocytes. *Pediatric Infectious Diseases Journal*, **9**, 26–30.

Amadori, A., De Rossi, A., Giaquinto, C., Faulkner-Valle, G., Zacchello, F. & Chieco-Bianchi, L. (1988). In vitro production of HIV specific antibody in children at-risk of AIDS. *Lancet*, **i**, 852–4.

Arico', M., Caselli, D., Marconi, M., *et al.* (1991). Immunoglobulin G3-specific antibodies as a marker for early diagnosis of HIV infection in children. *AIDS*, **5**, 1315–18.

Blanche, S., Rouzioux, C., Guihard-Moscato, M. L., *et al.* (1989). A prospective study of infants born to women seropositive for human immunodeficiency virus type 1. *The New England Journal of Medicine*, **320**, 1643–1648.

Borkowsky, W., Krasinski, K., Pollack, H., Hoover, W., Kaul, A. & Ilmet-Moore, T. (1992). Early diagnosis of human immmunodeficiency virus infection in children 6 months of age: comparison of polymerase chain reaction, culture, and plasma antigen capture techniques. *Journal of Infectious Diseases*, **166**, 616–19.

Bryson, Y. I., Luzuriaga, K., Sullivan, J. L. & Wara, D. W. (1992). Proposed definition for *in utero* versus intrapartum transmission of HIV-1. *New England Journal of Medicine*, **337**, 1246–1247.

Bryson, Y., Dillon, M., Garratty, E., Dickover, R., Keller, M. & Deveikis, A. (1993). The role of timing of HIV maternal-fetal transmission (in utero vs intrapartum) and HIV phenotype on onset of symptoms in vertically infected infants. (abstract, vol. I, WS-C10–2, 91) Berlin: IXth International Conference on AIDS.

Burgard, M., Mayaux, M. J., Blanche, S., *et al.* (1992). The use of virus culture and p24 antigen testing to diagnose human immunodeficiency virus infection in neonates. *New England Journal of Medicine*, **327**, 1192–97.

Candotti, D., Jung, M., Kerouedan, D., *et al.* (1991). Genetic variability affects the detection of HIV by polymerase chain reaction. *AIDS*, **5**, 1003–7.

Cassol, S. A., Lapointe, N., Salas, T., *et al.* (1992). Diagnosis of vertical HIV-1 transmission using the polymerase chain reaction and dried blood spot specimens. *Journal of Acquired Immune Deficiency Syndromes*, **5**, 113–19.

Centers for Disease Control (1989). Interpretation and use of the Western blot assay for serodiagnosis of human immunodeficiency virus type 1 infections. *Morbidity and Mortality Weekly Report*, **38**, S1–S7.

Cheng-Meyer, C., Seto, D., Tateno, M. & Levy, J. A. (1988). Biological features of HIV-1 that correlate with virulence in the host. *Science*, **240**, 80–82.

Comeau, A. M., Harris, J.-A., McIntosh, K., Weiblen, B. J., Hoff, R. & Grady, G. F. (1992). Polymerase chain reaction in detecting HIV infection among seropositive infants: relation to clinical status and age and to results of other assays. *Journal of Acquired Immunodeficiency Syndromes*, **5**, 271–8.

Connell, J. A., Parry, J. V., Mortimer, P. P. *et al.* (1990). Preliminary report of accurate assays for anti-HIV in urine. *Lancet*, **335**, 1366–9.

Connell, J. A., Parry, J. V., Mortimer, P. P., *et al.* (1992). HIV antibodies in babies. *British Medical Journal*, **305**, 367.

Connor, R. I., Mohri, H., Cao, Y. & Ho, D. D. (1993). Increased viral burden and cytopathicity correlate temporally with CD4+ T-lymphocyte decline and clinical progression in human immunodeficiency virus type 1-infected individuals. *Journal of Virology*, **67**, 1772–7.

Coombs, R. W., Collier, A. C., Allain, J. P., *et al.* (1989). Plasma viremia in human immunodeficiency virus infection. *New England Journal of Medicine*, **321**, 1626–31.

Courgnaud, V., Laure', F., Brossard, A. *et al.* (1991). Frequent and early *in utero* HIV-1 infection. *AIDS Research and Human Retroviruses*, **7**, 337–341.

Croft, N., Nicholson, S., Coghlan, P. & Gust, I. D. (1991). Testing for antibodies to HIV-1. *AIDS*, **5**, 561–3.

Cullen, B. R. (1991). Human immunodeficiency virus as a prototypic complex retrovirus. *Journal of Virology*, **65**, 1053–6.

De Rossi, A., Calabro', M. L., Panozzo, M., *et al.* (1990). In vitro studies of HIV-1 infection in thymic lymphocytes: a putative thymus role in AIDS pathogenesis. *AIDS Research and Human Retroviruses*, **3**, 287–98.

De Rossi, A., Ades, A. E., Mammano, F., *et al.* (1991a). Antigen detection, virus culture, polymerase chain reaction, and in vitro antibody production in the diagnosis of vertically transmitted HIV-1 infection. *AIDS*, **5**, 15–20.

De Rossi, A., Pasti, M., Mammano, F., Ometto, L., Giaquinto, C. & Chieco-Bianchi, L. (1991b). Perinatal infection by human immunodeficiency virus type 1 (HIV-1): Relationship between proviral copy number in vivo, viral properties *in vitro*, and clinical outcome. *Journal of Medical Virology*, **35**, 283–9.

De Rossi, A., Ometto, L., Mammano, F., Zanotto, C., Giaquinto, C. & Chieco-Bianchi, L. (1992). Vertical transmission of HIV-1: lack of detectable virus in peripheral blood cells of infected children at birth. *AIDS*, **6**, 1117–20.

De Rossi, A., Giaquinto, C., Ometto, L., *et al.* (1993a). Replication and tropism of human immunodeficiency virus type-1 as predictors of disease outcome in infants with vertically acquired infection. *Journal of Pediatrics*, **123**, 930–6.

De Rossi, A., Ometto, L., Mammano, F., *et al.* (1993b). Time course of antigenaemia and seroconversion in infants with vertically acquired HIV-1 infection. AIDS, **7**, 1528–9.

De Rossi, A., Zanotto, C., Mammano, F., Ometto, L., Del Mistro, A. & Chieco-Bianchi, L. (1993c). Pattern of antibody response against the V3 loop in children with vertically acquired immunodeficiency virus type 1 (HIV-1) infection. *AIDS Research and Human Retroviruses*, **9**, 221–8.

Ehrnst, A., Lindgren, S., Dictor, M. *et al.* (1991). HIV in pregnant women and their offsprings: evidence for late transmission. *Lancet*, **338**, 203–7.

Erlich, H. E., Gelfand, D. & Sninsky, J. J. (1991). Recent advances in the polymerase chain reaction. *Science*, **252**, 1643–56.

Escaich, S., Ritter, J., Rougier, P., *et al.* (1991). Plasma viraemia as a marker of viral replication in HIV-infected individuals. *AIDS*, **5**, 1189–94.

European Collaborative Study (1988). Mother-to-child transmission of HIV infection. *Lancet*, **332**, 1039–42.

European Collaborative Study (1991). Children born to women with HIV-1 infection: natural history and risk of transmission. *Lancet*, **337**, 253–260.

European Collaborative Study (1992) Risk factors for mother-to-child transmission of HIV. *Lancet*, **339**, 1007–12.

Felber, B. K. & Pavlakis, G. N. (1993). Molecular biology of HIV-1: positive and negative regulatory elements important for virus expression. *AIDS*, **7**, S51–S62.

Fenyo, E. M., Morfeldt-Manson, L., Chiodi, F. *et al.* (1988). Distinct replicative and cytopathic characteristics of human immunodeficiency virus isolates. *Journal of Virology*, **62**, 4414–19.

Fiore, J. R., Calabro', M. L., Angarano, G., *et al.* (1990). HIV-1 variability and progression to AIDS: a longitudinal study. *Journal of Medical Virology*, **32**, 252–6.

Frerichs, R. R., Htoon, M. T., Eskes, N. & Lwin, S. (1992). Comparison of saliva and serum for HIV surveillance in developing countries. *Lancet*, **340**, 1496–9.

Gabiano, C., Tovo, P. A., De Martino, M. *et al.* (1992). Mother-to-child transmission of HIV: risk of infection and correlates of transmission. *Pediatrics*, **90**, 362–74.

Ho, D. H., Moudgil, T. & Alam, M. (1989). Quantitation of Human immunodeficiency virus type 1 in the blood of infected persons. *New England Journal of Medicine*, **321**, 1621–5.

Horsburgh, C. R., Jason, J., Longini, I. M., *et al.* (1989). Duration of human immunodeficiency virus infection before detection of antibody. **ii**, 637–40.

Horwitz, M. S., Boyce-Jacino, M. T. & Faras, A. J. (1992). Novel human endogenous sequences related to human immunodeficiency virus type 1. *Journal of Virology*, **66**, 2170–9.

Indraccolo, S., Zamarchi, R., Veronese, M. L., *et al.* (1993). Standardization of in vitro synthesis and detection of HIV-1-specific antibodies. *Journal of Immunological Methods*, **157**, 105–15.

Jansson, M., Wahren, B., Scarlatti, G., *et al.* (1992). Patterns of immunoglobulin G subclass reactivity to HIV-1 envelope peptides in children born to HIV-1-infected mothers. *AIDS*, **6**, 365–371.

Jurrians, S., Dekker, J. T. & de Ronde, A. (1992). HIV-1 viral DNA load in peripheral blood mononuclear cells from seroconverters and long-term infected individuals. *AIDS*, **6**, 635–41.

Krivine, A., Yakudima, A., LeMay, M., Pena Cruz, V., Huang, A. S. & McIntosh, K. (1990). A comparative study of virus isolation, polymerase chain reaction, and antigen detection in children of mothers infected with human immunodeficiency virus. *Journal of Pediatrics*, **116**, 372–6.

Krivine, A., Firtion, G., Cao, L., Francoual, C., Henrion, R., & Lebon, P. (1992). HIV replication during the first weeks of life. *Lancet*, **339**, 1187–9.

Kwok, S. & Higuchi, R. (1989). Avoiding false positive with PCR. *Nature*, **339**, 237–8.

Landesman, S. H., Weiblen, B. J., Mendez H. *et al.* (1991). Clinical utility of HIV-IgA immunoblot assay in the early diagnosis of perinatal HIV infection. *Journal of the American Medical Association*, **266**, 3443–6.

Lango, M. C., Beringer, M. S. & Hartley, J. L. (1990). Use of uracil DNA glycosylase to control carry-over contamination in polymerase chain reaction. *Gene*, **93**, 125–8.

Lee, F. K., Nahmias, A. J., Lowery, S., *et al.* (1989). Elispot: a new approach to studying the dynamics of virus immune system interaction for diagnosis and monitoring of HIV infection. *AIDS Research and Human Retroviruses*, **5**, 517–23.

Mano, H. & Chermann, J. C. (1991). Fetal human immunodeficiency virus type 1 infection of different organs in the second trimester. *AIDS Research and Human Retroviruses*, **7**, 83–8.

Martin, N. L., Levy, J. A., Legg, H., Weintrub, P. S., Cowan, M. J. & Wara, D. W. (1991). Detection of infection with human immunodeficiency virus (HIV) type 1 in infants by an anti-HIV immunoglobulin A assay using recombinant proteins. *Journal of Pediatrics*, **118**, 354–8.

Michael, N. L., Vahey, M., Burke, D. S. & Redfield, R. R. (1992). Viral DNA and mRNA expression correlate with the stage of human immunodeficiency virus (HIV) type 1 infection in humans: evidence for viral replication in all stages of HIV disease. *Journal of Virology*, **66**, 310–16.

Miles, S. A., Balden, E., Magpantay, L., *et al.* (1993). Rapid serologic testing with immune-complex-dissociated HIV p24 antigen for early detection of HIV infection in neonates. *New England Journal of Medicine*, **328**, 297–302.

Nishanian, P., Huskin, K. R., Stehn, S., Detels, R., & Fahey, J. L. (1990). A simple method for improved assay demonstrates that HIV p24 antigen is present as immune complexes in most sera from HIV-infected individuals. *Journal of Infectious Diseases*, **162**, 21–8.

Ou, C. Y., Kwok, S., Mitchell, S. W., *et al.* (1988). DNA amplification for direct detection of HIV-1 in DNA of peripheral blood mononuclear cells. *Science*, **239**, 295–7.

Ou, C. Y., McDonough, S. H. & Cabanas, D. (1990). Rapid and quantitative detection of enzymatically amplified HIV-1 DNA using chemiluminescent oligonucleotide probes. *AIDS Research and Human Retroviruses*, **6**, 1323–1329.

Pahwa, S., Chimurle, N., Leombruno, C., *et al.* (1989). *In vitro* synthesis of human immunodeficiency virus-specific antibodies in peripheral blood lymphocytes of infants. *Proceedings of the National Academy of Science, USA*, **86**, 7532–6.

Palomba, E., Gay, V., Galli, L., De Martino, M., Perugini, L. & Tovo, P. A. (1993). Sensitivity and specificity of complexed p24 antigen assay for early diagnosis of perinatal HIV-1 infection. *AIDS*, **7**, 1391–2.

Pantaleo, G., Graziosi, C. & Fauci, A. S. (1993). The immunopathogenesis of human immunodeficiency virus infection. *New England Journal of Medicine*, **328**, 327–335.

Patterson, B. K., Till, M., Otto, P., *et al.* (1993). Detection of HIV-1 DNA and messenger RNA in individual cells by PCR-driven *in situ* hybridization and flow cytometry. *Science*, **260**, 976–9.

Piatak, M., Saag, M. S., Yang, L. C., *et al.* (1993). High levels of HIV-1 in plasma during all stages of infection determined by competitive PCR. *Science*, **259**, 1749–54.

Quinn, T. C., Kline, R. L., Halsey, N., *et al.* (1991). Early diagnosis of perinatal HIV infection by detection of viral-specific IgA antibodies. *Journal of the American Medical Association*, **266**, 3439–42.

Rogers, M. F., Ou C-Y., Kilbourne, B. & Schochetman, G. (1991). Advances and problems in the diagnosis of human immunodeficiency virus infection in infants. *Pediatric Infectious Disease Journal*, **10**, 523–31.

Saiki, R. H., Gelfand, D. H., Stoffel, S., *et al.*, (1988). Primer-directed enzymatic amplification of DNA with a thermostable DNA polymerase. *Science*, **239**, 487–91.

Salk, J., Bretscher, P. A., Salk, P. L., Clerici, M. & Shearer, G. M. (1993). A strategy for prophylactic vaccination against HIV. *Science*, **260**, 1270–2.

Scarlatti, G., Lombardi, V., Plebani, A., *et al.*, (1991). Polymerase chain reaction, virus isolation, and antigen assay in HIV-1 antibody positive mothers and their children. *AIDS*, **5**, 1173–8.

Schnittman, S. M., Denning, S. M., Greenhouse, J. J., *et al.* (1990). Evidence for susceptibility of intrathymic T-cell precursors and their progeny carrying T-cell antigen receptor phenotypes TCR+ and TCR+ to human immunodeficiency virus infection: a mechanism for CD4+ (T4) lymphocyte depletion. *Proceedings of the National Academy of Science, USA*, **87**, 7727–31.

Schuitemaker, H., Koot, M., Koostra, N. A., *et al.* (1992). Biological phenotype of human immunodeficiency virus type 1 clones at different stages of infection: progression of disease is associated with a shift from monocytotropic to T-cell-tropic virus populations. *Journal of Virology*, **66**, 1354–60.

Schupbach, J., Wunderli W., Kind, C, Kernen, R., Baumgartner, A. & Tomasik, Z. (1989). Frequent detection of HIV positive and IgG-specific IgM and IgA antibodies in HIV-positive cord-blood sera: fine analysis by Western blot. *AIDS*, **3**, 583–9.

Scott, G. B., Hutto, C., Makuch, R. W., *et al.* (1989). Survival in children with perinatally acquired human immunodeficiency virus type 1 infection. *New England Journal of Medicine*, **321**, 1791–6.

Simmonds, P., Balfe, P., Peutherer, J. F., Ludlam, C. A., Bishop, J. O. & Leigh Brown, A. J. (1990). Human imunodeficiency virus-infected individuals contain provirus in small numbers of peripheral mononuclear cells and at low copy numbers. *Journal of Virology*, **64**, 864–72.

Simon, F., Rahimy, C., Krivine, A., *et al.* (1993). Antibody avidity measurement and immune complex dissociation for serological diagnosis of vertically acquired HIV-1 infection. *Journal of Acquired Immune Deficiency Syndromes*, **6**, 201–7.

Tersmette, M., Gruters, R. A., de Wolf, F. *et al.* (1989). Evidence for a role of virulent human immunodeficiency virus (HIV) variants in the pathogenesis of acquired immunodeficiency syndrome: studies on sequential HIV isolates. *Journal of Virology*, **63**, 2118–25.

Tindall, B. & Cooper, D. A. (1991). Primary HIV-infection: host responses and intervention strategies. *AIDS*, **5**, 1–14.

Tovo, P. A., De Martino, M., Gabiano, C., *et al.* (1992). Prognostic factors and survival in children with perinatal HIV-1 infection. *Lancet*, **339**, 1249–53.

Turner, B. J., Eppes, S. C., Houchens, R., Fanning, T. & Markson, L. E. (1993). Survival experience of 789 children with the acquired immunodeficiency syndrome. *Pediatric Infectious Disease Journal*, **12**, 310–320.

Vaishnav, Y. N. & Wong-Staal, F. (1991). The biochemistry of AIDS. *Annual Review of Biochemistry*, **60**, 577–630.

Warmus, H. (1988). Retroviruses. *Science*, **240**, 1427–35.

Weiblen, B. J., Lee, F. K., Cooper, E. R., *et al.* (1990*a*). Early diagnosis of HIV infection in infants by detection of IgA antibodies. *Lancet*, **335**, 988–990.

Weiblen, B. J., Schumacher, R.I & Hoff, R. (1990*b*). Detection of IgM and IgA HIV antibodies after removal of IgG with recombinant protein G. *Journal of Immunological Methods*, **126**, 199–204.

Whetsell, A. J., Drew, J. B., Milman, G., *et al.* (1992). Comparison of three non-radioisotopic polymerase chain reaction-based methods for detection of human immunodeficiency virus type 1. *Journal of Clinical Microbiology*, **30**, 845–853.

Williams, L. M. & Cloyd, M. W. (1991). Polymorphic human gene(s) determines differential susceptibility of CD4 lympohocytes to infection by certain HIV-1 isolates. *Virology*, **184**, 723–8.

Wong-Staal, F. & Gallo, R. C. (1985). Human T-lymphotropic retroviruses. *Nature*, **317**, 395–403.

World Health Organization (1990). Proposed WHO criteria for interpreting results from Western blot assays for HIV-1, HIV-2, and HTLV-I/HTLV-II. *Weekly Epidemiological Records*, **37**, 281–3.

World Health Organizacion Global Programme on AIDS (1992). Recommendations for the selection and use of HIV-antibody tests. *Weekly Epidemiological Records*, **67**, 145–9.

Zach, J. A., Arrigo, S. J., Weitsman, S. R., Go, S. A., Haislip, A., & Chen, I. S. Y. (1990). HIV-1 entry into quiescent primary lymphocytes: molecular analysis reveals a labile, latent viral structure. *Cell*, **61**, 213–2.

Addenda

Additional references which are relevant to the discussion of the early diagnosis of HIV infection in children born to HIV-infected women include:

De Rossi, A., Ometto, L., Zanotto, C., Salvatori, F., *et al.* (1994). Mother-to-child HIV transmission: quantitative assessment of viral burden as a diagnostic tool and prognostic parameter in HIV-1 infected children. *Acta Paediatrica*, **400**, s25–8.

European Collaborative Study (1994). Caesarean section and risk of vertical transmission of HIV-1 infection. *Lancet*, **343**, 1464–7.

Kline, M. W., Lewis, D. E., Hollinger, F. B., *et al.* (1994). A comparative study of human immunodeficiency virus culture, polymerase chain reaction and anti-human immunodeficiency virus immunoglobulin A antibody detection in the diagnosis during early infancy of vertically acquired human immunodeficiency virus infection. *Pediatric Infectious Disease Journal*, **13**, 90–4.

Schupbach, J., Boni, J., Tomasik, Z., Jendis, J., Seger, R. & Kind, C. (1994). Sensitive detection and early prognostic significance of p24 antigen in heat-denatured plasma of human immunodeficiency virus type 1 infected infants. *Journal of Infectious Diseases*, **170**, 318–24.

Verhofstede, C., Reniers, S., Van Wanzeele, F. & Plum, J. (1994). Evaluation of proviral copy number and plasma RNA levels as early indicators of progression in HIV-1 infection: correlation with virological and immunological markers of disease. *AIDS*, **8**, 1421–7.

6

Immunology of paediatric HIV Infection

A. GRAHAM BIRD

Introduction

With the progressive increase in the prevalence of adult HIV infection in the world population, the impact of this new cause of immunodeficiency in children is being increasingly recognised. Although many of the principles of the immunology of HIV infection are shared between adults and children with the disease, the effects of HIV on the developing immune system of the newborn provide additional challenges. In addition, HIV can cause diagnostic confusion in children with suspected primary immunodeficiency disease, particularly in the rare instance in which infected children fail to make specific HIV antibodies, a situation not encountered in adults.

Severe impairment of host defences in children can result from either early HIV infection or primary immunodeficiency disorders, and careful clinical and laboratory evaluation is required to establish the diagnosis, monitor progress and avoid some of the early and predictable complications of the developing immunodeficiency. Improvements in management will be critically reliant on an understanding both of the normal development of host immune responses in children and of the mechanisms by which HIV produces immune damage and the host immune responses that can slow the progress of virally induced damage.

This chapter begins by summarising aspects of relevant knowledge before examining in detail the effects of HIV on the neonatal immune system and some of the clinical implications of the damage which results.

Ontogeny of the human immune system and implications for HIV infection in neonates

The immune system of the human fetus develops early and by full-term birth is almost fully functionally mature. However, both B and T cell repertoires are virgin, being comprised of unprimed cells that have not yet undergone antigen-induced clonal expansion or maturation. Bone-marrow-derived lymphocyte stem cells colonise the thymus and fetal liver and in these primary lymphoid organs T and B lymphocyte repertoire generation commences. Later in fetal life, B cell development moves to the bone marrow. In the primary lymphoid organs, germ line DNA rearrangement and splicing result in the generation of random specificity repertoires and, during cell maturation, contact with antigen (usually auto-antigen) results in tolerance induction. Appropriately rearranged T and B lymphocytes leave the primary lymphoid organs to recirculate continuously through the secondary lymph nodes and spleen via blood and thoracic duct (lymph nodes) until activated by specific antigen.

At birth, repertoire generation of both B and T cells is complete and secondary lymphoid organs are populated with cells that are functional. Whilst the B cell repertoire is fully functional at day 1, the T cell repertoire is still somewhat functionally immature, particularly with regard to cytokine (especially gamma interferon) production (Wagasugi & Virelizier, 1985), but this reaches full maturity soon after delivery. Although B cells are mature and functional, their ability to make some specialised antibodies, especially immunoglobulins A and G2 (IgA and IgG2), matures late and the ability to produce satisfactory titres of polysaccharide antibodies protective against some encapsulated bacterial infections is only complete by 18 months of age in many normal infants (Leinonen *et al.*, 1986).

Whilst maturation progresses, placental transfer of maternal IgG during the last trimester provides the neonate with some protection for the first 6 months of life. Low titres of specific maternally derived antibody can occasionally be detected up to 18 months after delivery and this can cause difficulties in the early diagnosis of vertically acquired HIV infection.

The timing of HIV infection is critical in predicting likely consequences of infection. Early transmission (12–24 weeks) could result in rapidly progressive HIV infection resulting from a combination of immature specific immune responses and longer exposure to virus. In addition, very early infection could induce HIV tolerance with complete failure of immune recognition. Since many researchers believe that immune activation is required for HIV replication, very early infection could result in low levels of replication and lack of specific antiviral immune responses.

Despite the obvious importance of these considerations, studies to identify evidence of early vertical infection have been few. Epidemiological evidence suggests that a substantial proportion of infection occurs during parturition, but other clinical studies do suggest evidence of early infection in a number of cases (see Chapters 1, 4 and 5). A recent study of thymus glands from 37 mid-trimester abortuses from HIV-infected mothers did show evidence of lymphoid depletion and epithelial abnormalities in three cases, consistent with early HIV infection (Papiernik *et al.*, 1992). The oldest affected fetus had the most extensive lesions, suggesting progressive disease. Thus a subgroup of neonates (8%) could have acquired infection early in gestation and some of these may present with the rapid development of immunodeficiency seen in a proportion of vertically acquired cases. In contrast, perinatal infection against the background of a relatively mature immune system would be expected to result in a disease natural history closer to that seen in adults, perhaps accounting for the bimodal incubation distribution of disease (Auger *et al.*, 1988).

Since HIV infection induces not only T cell immunodeficiency but also B cell dysregulation and impaired specific antibody production, particularly to polysaccharides, it is important to appreciate that the neonate born to an HIV-infected mother does not receive maternal passive immunoglobulin of the same quality as that of the normal infant. Moreover, maternal hyperimmunoglobulinaemia will result in hypercatabolism of all IgG in the HIV-exposed neonate, resulting in the more rapid disappearance of any specific protective antibody than would be expected in infants born to non-infected mothers. Finally, although the neonate's immune system is mature at birth it is unprimed, in contrast to that of the older infant or adult who subsequently acquires HIV infection. Consequently, the primary immune response against any new pathogen, as well as to re-infection with the same pathogen, will be less effective compared with that of a recall memory response anticipated in an older child or adult. This differential sensitivity to new pathogens due to the compromise HIV imposes on initial clonal expansion explains the preferential vulnerability of the neonate to primary viral infections (such as measles). It may also contribute to the apparent lack of correlation of CD4 count with vulnerability to new opportunistic pathogens such as *Pneumocystis carinii*, since these infections represent primary exposures in immunologically naive subjects without prior expanded memory populations.

Overview of the pathogenesis of HIV infection

Knowledge of the means by which HIV infection results in immunodeficiency and disease is as essential as the fine structural and regulatory details of the virus itself. Whereas knowledge of the latter is extensive and represents a remarkable testimony of the power of molecular technology, understanding of the former lags far behind. Without firmer details about the precise way in which HIV interacts with key elements of the immune system, to induce both pathology and partial but temporary down-regulation of viral replication, the strategies for control of viral replication and protective immunisation will remain speculative.

Further understanding is particularly important for the implications of HIV infection in children, since the impact of the viral infection is different on the developing rather than the developed immune system of adults, and the prospect of intervention to prevent infection presents a more immediate challenge for the HIV-infected pregnant mother.

The following is a brief résumé of current knowledge about the natural history and immunopathology of HIV infection that will allow interpretation of many of the clinical observations described later.

Primary HIV infection

The first encounter with HIV infection resembles that of many human or animal infections. Initial viral infection is probably established mainly via the primary tropic receptor CD4 itself, but other routes into CD4 lymphocytes and macrophages are also possible.

Infection in adults results in viraemia, detectable by viral isolation or polymerase chain reaction (PCR), and this probably results in widespread systemic dissemination of virus to further macrophages and CD4 lymphocytes. However, in most individuals observed during early infection, significant depletion of blood CD4 lymphocytes is not a feature, probably because of the relatively short duration of this phase, the ability of the thymus to replace lost lymphocytes and, perhaps, the initiation of infection by viral strains that are less cytopathic to CD4 T lymphocytes at this stage (Groenink *et al.*, 1993).

In adults, this phase of uncontrolled viral replication and viraemia may be associated with symptoms of primary infection which include a febrile illness, sore throat, lymphadenopathy, transient erythematous skin rash and occasionally mild encephalitis, resembling that of many other primary virus illnesses. The primary infection is terminated by the appearance of specific host immune responses and detection of specific antibody which allows reliable routine diagnosis of viral exposure. As with most other viral infections, initial control of HIV replication and viraemia is due to the destruction of viral replication sites by class I MHC restricted CD8 cytotoxic cells specific for peptides derived from viral structural and regulatory proteins. Antibody appears a little later and, whilst probably exerting little impact on viral replication, is of critical importance in the rapid clearance of viral particles from the blood by the formation of viral immune complexes with antibody.

The importance of this event has been re-emphasised by recent studies which have shown that, after clearance of blood viraemia, HIV can be found in significant concentrations in the reticulo-endothelial system as sequestered immune complexes, particularly in the germinal centres of lymph nodes (Panteleo *et al.*, 1993; Embretson *et al.*, 1993).

In most cases this phase of primary infection is short-lived, self-terminating and usually asymptomatic.

Asymptomatic HIV replication

HIV infection does not establish true latency as defined by down-regulation of viral gene replication within cells following a host immune response. Instead, viral replication continues, in some cells at least, throughout the duration of disease (see Chapter 5). This ability of HIV to continue to replicate in the face of an immune response that in other viral infections would result in either elimination or latency is probably the key to its destructive capacity. The slow continuous replication of the virus in lymph nodes, combined with its apparently infinite capacity to mutate viral sequences, allows the virus progressively to escape from selective pressures exerted upon it by immune responses or administered antiviral drugs (Philips *et al.*, 1991).

Throughout the asymptomatic stage in both HIV-infected children and adults studied, specific cytotoxic T cells capable of killing HIV-infected cells and antibody capable of neutralising at least some of the divergent viral isolates persist at high levels but fail to silence viral replication (Nixon & McMichael, 1991; Cheynier *et al.*, 1992). Moreover, during this phase of infection, slow destruction of the specific T cell immune system is accelerating as a consequence of the selective tropism of HIV for CD4 cytokine-secreting T cells. CD4 T cells are essential for the co-ordination of new and memory-specific immune responses to a range of intracellular viral, bacterial, fungal and parasitic infections. The cytokines released (principally interferon gamma, interleukins 2, 4, 5 and 10, and tumour necrosis factor beta) activate macrophages and natural killer cells, thereby permitting the more effective phagocytosis and killing of such organisms. Interleukin 2 (IL2) is also essential for the proliferation of CD8 viral cyto-toxic cells vital for the control of primary viral infections and the containment of persistent or latent viral infections such as the herpes species and HIV itself.

During this silent phase of HIV infection, qualitative and then quantitative T cell defects are observed. The first clinical evidence of immuno-deficiency may precede an overt reduction in blood CD4 populations since functional immunodeficiency can be detected by laboratory investigations early in the second stage of HIV infection (Meynard *et al.*, 1993). Primary immune responses are more vulnerable to deficiency of CD4-driven cytokine release. IL2 in particular is critical for early T and B lymphocyte clonal expansion and maturation following first exposure to infection. Thus extreme susceptibility to first exposure to a pathogen can be seen even in early infection, whereas immunological memory and pre-existing antibody can protect against re-infection or reactivation for a much longer duration in the natural history of HIV disease. This consideration is particularly relevant in children since HIV infection will often predate all initial immune experience and clonal expansion of specific memory cells. This may explain why *Pneumocystis carinii* infection can present with devastating illness even in young HIV-infected children with normal CD4 cell counts for age, since it represents a primary infection in many infants, in contrast to the reactivation in late stage disease in adults.

It is probable that the early functional T cell immunodeficiency is not explicable purely on the basis of CD4 depletion by HIV since the CD4 cells that remain are unresponsive even to non-specific stimuli in early infection. It is likely that inadequacy of antigen presentation, perhaps because such cells are HIV infected, combined with suboptimal availability of essential cytokines, contributes to this early immunodeficiency.

In addition to subclinical or early clinical immunodeficiency, this mid-stage of HIV infection is also paradoxically associated with a high level of immune activation. A number of different parameters are involved in this heightened activation including increased expression of lymphocyte activation markers, hyperimmunoglobulinaemia and an increase in serum markers including neopterin and β_2-microglobulin. Neopterin is the product of activated macrophages whereas β_2-microglobulin is released from activated and dividing lymphocytes. The cause of this hyperactivation is still uncertain. A part at least is explained by the very high levels of specific HIV immunity seen in this stage of the disease but, since such elevated levels may persist into the later stages of disease, other explanations must also be involved.

The hypergammaglobulinaemia, also a consistent feature of mid-stage disease and a particular feature of HIV infection in children, remains similarly unexplained. Levels rise too early in the disease to be the consequence of secondary infection and are unlikely to be the result of HIV infection alone. A derangement in normal immunoregulation appears more likely, particularly since the elevated levels are deficient in specific antibodies and fail to reflect current antigenic exposure or challenge (Bernstein *et al.*, 1985*b*).

Clinical immunodeficiency

The prolonged subclinical disease is abruptly terminated by the appearance of opportunistic infections which, in their increasing range and

Table 6.1. *Postulated mechanisms involved in CD4 T cell depletion in HIV infection*

	Infected CD4 T cells	Bystander CD4 killing
HIV cytopathic effect	Yes	No
Syncytia formation	Yes	Yes
Antibody-dependent cellular cytotoxicity	Yes	Yes
CD4 HIV-specific cytotoxicity	Yes	Possibly
CD8 HIV-specific cytotoxicity	Yes	No
Inappropriate CD4 signalling and apoptosis	Yes	Yes
Superantigen action of HIV	Yes	Yes

severity, reflect the underlying increased pace of progressive cellular immunodeficiency. Controversy exists over whether the change from sub-clinical to clinical disease reflects a smooth progressive transition or an abrupt change in disease tempo. In most individuals, levels of plasma virus rise and CD4 cells fall, reflecting a return to earlier blood viraemia now accompanied by overt laboratory and clinical evidence of T helper cell destruction.

Increasing evidence suggests that this change is reflected in many cases by a trend towards the isolation of higher levels of more cytopathic HIV strains which are also more tropic to CD4 cells rather than macrophages (Groenink *et al.*, 1993). Coincident with this finding is the uniform obser-vation of the disappearance of previously high levels of specific anti-HIV CD8 cytotoxicity, partially explaining the acceleration of virus replication (Nixon & McMichael, 1991). Whether the apparent change in virus behaviour is the result of a dynamic change in virus selection, resulting in increased immunological destruction, or whether it is the direct result of immunological exhaustion, is a matter for debate. Similar controversy continues over the exact mechanism of CD4 cell destruction, fuelled in part by the realisation that only a small proportion of blood T cells are infected. This debate is less now that the scale of viral infection in lymph nodes is accepted, along with the acknowledged importance of macrophage infection in early disease. A number of pathogenic mechanisms, probably acting in concert, combine to cause the destruction of infected and prob-ably some uninfected CD4 lymphocytes (Table 6.1). A key determinant in entry into the final stages of disease is probably the failure of specific T cell control over HIV replication that characterises the mid-stage of dis-ease. It is reasonable to envisage how viral mutational escape results in progressive immunodeficiency and further loss of viral control, resulting in a rapid cycle of deterioration (Philips *et al.*, 1991).

Two key features emerge from studies of animal models of retroviral infection. In chimpanzees with HIV and African green monkeys with simian immunodeficiency virus (SIV), a combination of low levels of macrophage infection and high levels of specific CD8 antiviral cytotoxicity combine to keep virus replication low and immune responses normal, and appear to be associated with long-term survival.

In humans, factors associated with rapid deterioration include HLA haptotype (HLA A1, B8, DR3) and a severe acute seroconversion illness. The latter may denote a higher initial viral replicative load and the former less efficient T cell control. Factors determining long-term survival are less clear, but increasingly such individuals are being identified. From analogies with other infections, it is probable that certain HLA genotypes will also influence outcome favourably. It is likely that viral substrains may also determine outcome. A recently described cluster of infection associated with favourable outcome, linked with blood transfusion from a single infected donor, is a pointer to the importance of viral strain influences (Learmont *et al.*, 1992).

Immunological changes

Early cross-sectional studies suggested that HIV infection was associated with consistent and early evidence of a range of immunological abnormalities affecting virtually all aspects of immune phenotype and function. However, it is now clear that all these studies were subject to considerable ascertainment bias toward infants with symptomatic disease (Oleske *et al.*, 1983; Rubinstein *et al.*, 1983; Blanche *et al.*, 1986).

More recent studies involving complete prospective cohorts of infants born to HIV-infected mothers reveal a much more heterogeneous picture, with some infants showing little evidence of overt early immunological disturbance (Blanche *et al.*, 1989; de Martino *et al.*, 1991). The differences not only reflect different rates of disease progression in individual infants but also differences in incubation time (see Chapter 4).

Lymphocyte subpopulation markers

Studies agree that at birth CD4 lymphocyte distributions are marginally lower in children subsequently confirmed as infected than in uninfected children (Blanche *et al.*, 1989; de Martino *et al.*, 1991). Similarly, CD8 counts are slightly higher in the same studies. These findings provide evidence that the majority of vertically acquired HIV infection occurs either very late in pregnancy or around the time of delivery. If infection occurred *in utero*, CD8 counts in response to primary viral infection would be expected to be elevated in at least a proportion of cases. Risk factors responsible for maternal acquisition of HIV infection do not appear to be reflected in lymphocyte phenotype profiles of infected or non-infected infants at birth (Froebel et al., 1991).

Immunoglobulin levels are also broadly comparable between infected and uninfected infants at birth, although studies show a slight increase in IgM and IgA levels in those showing subsequent infection. Once again, this small overall rise is probably accounted for by a small group of infants experiencing early intrauterine infection (Blanche et al., 1989; de Martino et al., 1991). Sequential follow-up of infants in one study illustrates that a subgroup with low CD4 counts and high IgM levels at birth are all later found in the P-2 symptomatic group of patients, suggesting that this group includes some infants preferentially disadvantaged by early HIV infection prior to birth (Johnson et al., 1989).

Following birth, changes in routine immunological markers closely reflect the clinical evolution of HIV-associated immunodeficiency in cohorts of infected children. In the subgroup eventually developing symptomatic disease, CD4 counts fall progressively after birth so that by the age of 6 months the mean count for this population is approximately half that of age-matched control populations. The importance of adequate reference ranges from matched control populations cannot be overstated because of the physiological fall in both CD4 and CD8 absolute counts over the first year of life, which is the result of a falling absolute lymphocyte count (Niven et al., 1990; European Collaborative Study, 1992). These physiological changes, combined with the wide normal range and marked biological variation of individual lymphocyte counts, obscure an otherwise consistent trend towards falling CD4 cell counts and rising CD8 populations in individual children developing symptomatic disease. The determination of such trends in individual children requires the performance of repeated analyses taken in optimal conditions (same time of day, rapid laboratory analysis) and at times when infants are free of other intercurrent infections (Bird, 1992).

In children remaining asymptomatic, CD4 counts remain broadly comparable to those in age-matched control infants for the first 6 months of life and then fall slowly, but at a slower rate than that seen in the symptomatic infected group. The retained CD4 count, combined with a smaller rise in CD8 count in such infants, results in a CD4/CD8 ratio above 1.0 in most infants remaining well for the first year after birth (Johnson et al., 1989; European Collaborative Study, 1991).

However, in the assessment of individual children, overall lymphocyte subset levels are poorly discriminating in establishing either early infection or predisposition to clinical immunodeficiency – in marked distinction to the situation in adults with HIV infection. Indeed, in the European

Collaborative Study (1991), a low CD4/CD8 ratio was only apparent *after* a diagnosis of AIDS in 44% of infants. Clinical signs such as lymphadenopathy or splenomegaly or features of immunodeficiency such as candidiasis appear earlier than lymphocyte population changes. The greatest value of stable CD4 counts is probably in identifying the subgroup of infected children with apparently slowly progressive disease and favourable medium-term clinical outcome.

It is possible that the determination of selective subpopulations of T cells may prove of more prognostic value than total CD4 or CD8 numbers. For example, the early co-expression of CD8 and CD45RO, a marker of memory populations, reliably identifies the population of HIV-infected children, including those with normal CD4 cell counts (Froebel *et al.*, 1991).

Immunoglobulin levels

A similar divergence in immunoglobulin levels is seen between those infected infants developing symptomatic disease (P-2) and those who remain well (P-1). Total IgG, IgA and IgM levels rise progressively in virtually all infants developing symptomatic disease within the first 2 years of life, whereas such progressive rises are not so apparent in asymptomatic children (de Martino, 1991; Johnson *et al.* 1989). Once again interpretation of data is critically dependent on age-related reference ranges. Hypergammaglobulinaemia is apparent in about 50% of infected children at 4 months of age and in 75% or more by 9 months (Johnson *et al.*, 1989; European Collaborative Study, 1991) and is often an earlier and more reliable marker of infection than a reduction in CD4 cells (Falloon *et al.*, 1989) or clinical features (European Collaborative Study, 1991) in individual infants.

Age-related hypergammaglobulinaemia combined with low CD4 counts and a CD4/CD8 ratio below 1 in an infant aged less than 6 months born to an HIV-infected mother is diagnostic of infection and medium-term clinical progression likely at an age when serological or virological determination of HIV infection can still be problematical. However, these markers together have less sensitivity and identify infection in only 83% of infected infants at 6 months of age. Hyperimmunoglobulinaemia is a poor predictor of short-term progress to AIDS (European Collaborative Study, 1991) but may prove to be a more accurate marker of medium- to long-term progression, as it has done in adults.

A further complicating factor in the assessment of HIV infection in children is the rare but described variant of the disease in which infection is associated with the development of hypogammaglobulinaemia or hypergammaglobulinaemia with HIV-negative serology. This presentation was not a feature of any of the 64 infected children identified by the European Collaborative Study but has been described uncommonly by others (Maloney *et al.*, 1987; Pahwa *et al.*, 1987; Blanche *et al.*, 1989; Johnson *et al.*, 1989). Clearly other forms of primary or acquired immunodeficiency need to be excluded. Definitive attempts to isolate HIV or to detect the genome by molecular techniques including PCR are also required.

Two subgroups of disease expression following vertical HIV infection

Increasing evidence from cohort studies suggests a bimodal incubation period of disease in HIV infection (see Chapter 4). Whilst vertically acquired infection results in clinical or laboratory evidence of immunodeficiency in about 80–90% of infants by 1 year of age, in the remainder little evidence of further clinical or immunological deterioration is apparent over longer periods of up to 3 years or more. Moreover, even the symptomatic group is not homogeneous since a subgroup of children present with lymphocytic interstitial pneumonitis or bacterial pneumonia which are clinical features not associated with major laboratory evidence of immunodeficiency nor with further disease progression or early death over the medium term (Blanche *et al.*, 1990; European Collaborative Study, 1991). These clinical descriptions agree with incubation distribution statistical models which point to a second peak of AIDS cases at 6.1 years after birth (Auger *et al.*, 1988), corresponding more closely to the observed incubation distribution of adult cases. Whether this second delayed peak of incubation is the result of viral substrains, timing of infection or genetic population differences in host responses is not yet clear from available data.

Additional functional markers of specific immunodeficiency

By analogy with the classification and investigation of primary immunodeficiency in children, it is likely that evaluation of specific aspects of immunocompetence will be of more relevance in assessment. Better clues to progress will be provided by assessment of function rather than by the quantitation of total components of the cellular and humoral immune systems as exemplified by lymphocyte phenotype enumeration and measurement of immunoglobulin levels.

A large number of experimental studies have been performed assessing individual aspects of specific immune function but few have been added to prospective cohort studies; the specificity and sensitivity of these investigations are thus uncertain, as is their role in management. Properly evaluated, some of these markers may serve as important indicators of prognosis and as surrogate markers for trial outcome. More work in this area in children is urgently required.

Functional T cell evaluation

Increasing evidence suggests that adults with HIV infection can be further subdivided during the long asymptomatic phase of disease (Miedema *et al.* 1988; Clerici *et al.*, 1989). Assays examining specific T cell responses to non-specific activators, recall antigens or components of HIV itself have been extensively evaluated in adults but less so in children. However, the data available are encouraging. Blanche *et al.* (1990) showed that most HIV-infected infants with absent proliferative responses showed evidence of rapid disease progression, whereas the majority (28 of 33) who gave responses were associated with a slow rate of disease progression. A study of haemophiliac children infected post natally confirmed these findings and showed a correlation between impaired T lymphocyte function, assessed by tetanus toxoid proliferation, and clinical severity of disease (Petersen *et al.*, 1989, 1992). Borkowsky *et al.* (1992), who looked at proliferative responses to tetanus and diphtheria toxoids prospectively, showed that some infected children respond well initially following immunisation but lose responses in parallel with deteriorating clinical immunocompetence.

An extensive study of HIV-infected children aged between 17 months and 18 years (Roilides *et al.*, 1991) confirmed that a spectrum of functional deficiency exists similar to that seen in adults. A higher proportion of non-responsive children (79%) was found, probably reflecting the earlier and more severe progression associated with childhood disease. A history of opportunistic infections was seen almost exclusively in children with T cell dysfunction, suggesting that functional assays may be more sensitive than T cell phenotype changes in detecting significant immunodeficiency (Blanche *et al.*, 1990) (see Chapter 4). More minor but significant *in vitro* dysfunction was associated with increased susceptibility to bacterial rather than major opportunistic infections. Similar findings have been previously described by Krasinski and co-workers (1988).

These studies provide compelling evidence that wider introduction of such assays would be valuable in the staging and assessment of disease progression in HIV infection. Moreover, a preliminary report suggests that their use may give additional information to CD4 count changes in clinical trials of nucleoside analogues, where preferential improvement in these parameters was seen in children with early HIV disease (Clerici *et al.*, 1992).

Specific anti-HIV immunity

Probably the most important immune responses of all (in HIV infection) are directed against HIV itself. There is increasing evidence in adults that high levels of CD8 cytotoxic T lymphocyte (CTL) responses are associated with early and stable disease, whereas levels are lost in later progressive cases. However, little information is available in children, largely owing to the technical complexity and relatively large blood volume required. Preliminary evidence suggests that, as in adults, CD8 cytotoxic activity is reliably detected in children with vertically acquired HIV infection who survive for five years or longer, but is rarely seen in younger children with advanced disease (Luzuriaga & Sullivan, 1993). In limited studies, a strong CTL response correlated with a more favourable clinical course and in one study three children with documented CTL appeared to become HIV seronegative, although one child had symptoms consistent with HIV immunodeficiency at 5 months of age (Cheynier *et al.*, 1992). The intriguing possibility that high levels of CTL may occasionally result in complete suppression, or perhaps even elimination, of HIV received some support from a single very well documented case report of a child subsequently proven to be uninfected at 18 months of age (Rowland-Jones *et al*, 1993).

Defects in other effector cells

In addition to the previously described deficits in specific elements of immune recognition in children, HIV infection can also be responsible for a range of defects in non-specific effector mechanisms which could contribute to the severity of the observed immunodeficiency in children. Natural killer (NK) cells provide an early immune response which appears important in experimental systems in the early defence against viral infections and certain neoplastic disease, particularly in infections at the stage before appropriate specific responses can be mobilised. NK cell function is below the adult level at birth but rises rapidly to equal or exceed this level by 5 months of age. In HIV-infected adults a number of studies (Rook *et al.*, 1983; Lifson *et al.*, 1984; Bonavida, *et al.*, 1986) have demonstrated impairment of function which appears to result largely from the lack of cytokine production, especially IL2 and interferon gamma, usually produced by CD4 cells. Studies in children are few but a recent report suggests that deficiency of NK cell function is a generalised feature of paediatric HIV infection and occurs early and throughout the natural history in infants (Bonagura, *et al.*, 1992). Such deficiency is likely to be more clinically significant in HIV-infected children than in adults in view of the lack of development of the specific recognition memory compartment of the immune system at this age.

Defects in neutrophil chemotactic and bacteriocidal activity have also been identified in HIV-infected children (Roilides *et al.*, 1990, 1993), perhaps contributing to the increased susceptibility to bacterial infection seen in this population (Bernstein *et al.*, 1985a).

Use of CD4 counts to predict risk of Pneumocystis carinii pneumonia

Pneumocystis carinii is a major cause of morbidity and mortality in HIV-infected children. Effectiveness of prophylaxis has been accompanied by marked reductions in the frequency with which this opportunist pathogen causes clinical disease in adults. Since adults with CD4 counts below 200/mm^3 (0.2 × 10^9/l) have been shown in prospective trials to be at highest risk of this complication, prophylaxis is usually recommended once the CD4 count has fallen consistently below this level (Phair *et al.*, 1990). Higher normal reference ranges for CD4 cells in young children suggest that adult thresholds for CD4 would be inappropriate for children (European Collaborative Study, 1992). However, even adjusting for this, CD4 count thresholds are still unreliable predictors of susceptibility to *Pneumocystis*, especially in children below the age of 1 year (Leibovitz *et al.*, 1991; Rutstein, 1991; European Collaborative Study, 1992). Since it is these children who are at highest risk of fulminant *Pneumocystis* infection, often at an age when HIV status may still be unclear, a pragmatic approach would be to offer prophylaxis to all HIV-infected children below the age of 1 year and to children with CD4 counts below 0.3–0.4 × 10^9/l above the age of 1 year (see Chapters 9 and 10).

As indicated previously, the poor correlation between low absolute CD4 count and *Pneumocystis* infection in very young children may be because *Pneumocystis* represents primary infection where severe disease occurs earlier. Similar considerations will probably apply to the effective prophylaxis against other bacterial, fungal and protozoal infections in HIV-infected children.

Surrogate markers

The identification of surrogate markers to assess the response of HIV infection to therapy has been dictated by the prolonged natural history of the disease, necessitating large trials conducted over many years. Indeed the value of advanced disease as an end-point has been eroded with the success of clinical management, particularly with antimicrobial prophylaxis, which has advanced the AIDS diagnosis to a stage in the disease

Table 6.2. *Requirements for the ideal surrogate marker*

	Marker performance			
	CD4	β₂M	p24	Viral load
Natural history				
Progressive change with disease stage	✓	✗	✗	?
Biologically plausible	✓	✗	✓	✓
Not influenced significantly by other disease factors	✓	✗	✓	✓
Treatment response				
Rapid predictable change if short-term benefit	✓	✓	Occas.	?
Predicts drug failure	✓	?	✓	?
Reproducible with other drugs	?	?	?	?
Similar predictive power on or off therapy	✗	?	?	?
Technical factors				
Standardised methodology	✓	✓	✓	✗
Quality assurance	✓	✓	✓	✗
Inexpensive and easy to perform	✓	✓	✓	✗

Occas., occasional; ✓, valid; ✗, invalid; ?, uncertain; β₂M, β₂-microglobulin.

virtually coincident with death. Thus clinical advance has resulted in the phenomenon of 'vanishing', or at least retreating, clinical end-points initially employed for clinical trials.

Surrogate markers are biological indicators that should reflect the natural history of HIV disease and be prognostic of and reflect the improvement resulting from drug therapy. Such markers should be biologically plausible to the understanding of disease pathogenesis and should have been validated against clinical end-points, including death, in natural history studies. The key properties of an optimal surrogate marker are given in Table 6.2.

Some of the confusion and uncertainty surrounding the current critical reassessment of surrogate markers arises from a lack of confidence in current understanding of HIV pathogenesis and thus the parameters that reflect progressive disease. To date the CD4 lymphocyte count has been relied upon as the pioneer surrogate marker, principally because it remains a sensitive and accurate disease staging marker in adults, has biological plausibility and showed early promise in reflecting the clinical efficacy of nucleoside analogue antivirals in trials. Later it was used as a basis for the licensing approval of two agents: didanosine (ddI) and dideoxycytidine (ddC).

More recently it has become more apparent that the CD4 count is an incomplete marker and models suggest that it explains only part of the efficacy of nucleoside analogues (Lagakos & Hoth, 1992). Preliminary results of the randomised placebo-controlled Concorde trial suggest that CD4 improvements in response to nucleoside analogues may not be translated into long-term survival advantage (Aboulker & Swart, 1993). Other immunological markers of immune activation predict risk for clinical progression and appear to respond favourably to therapy, but their full value in predicting drug efficacy is unclear.

Quantification of viral load is attracting increasing attention as a direct reflection of antiviral activity. The viral subunit p24 is present too infrequently in the serum of asymptomatic individuals to prove a reliable marker, but assays of quantitative viraemia or molecular techniques such as PCR hold much promise. However, to date these markers have not been evaluated against clinical end-points. Moreover, a recent report suggesting that viral replicative activity or phenotype does not directly correlate with cytopathic potential for the CD4 population indicates that uncertainties over pathogenesis continue to complicate surrogate marker assessment of disease progression, and raises questions over the ability of molecular techniques to quantitate relevant viral burden (Mosier *et al.*, 1993).

Implications for trials in children

In trials of antiviral therapy in children, the role of surrogate markers is even more problematic. Since the CD4 count is a less certain predictive marker in paediatric disease and information about its behaviour in large clinical trials more difficult to define, its value as a single marker to assess drug efficacy is highly questionable. Quantitation of viral levels would appear more appropriate but, in view of the lack of clinical validation and the possibility that blood virus levels may not reflect tissue burden (particularly in bowel, brain and lymph nodes), it is unlikely that viral markers alone will serve as a surrogate end-point.

The search for new immunological markers has focused particularly on tests of functional T cell lymphocyte competence. The most extensively evaluated involves the *in vitro* use of the non-specific activator anti-CD3 to stimulate all T cells and to measure their proliferation by radioisotope incorporation (Miedema *et al.*, 1988). This approach would appear to be particularly suited to the study of children. The alternative approach, using previously encountered environmental stimuli such as extracts of *Candida albicans*, is complicated in neonates by factors which include age and development at testing and differential environmental exposure.

There is increasing interest in the use of post-infection immunisation with genetically engineered fragments of HIV in an attempt to elevate protective anti-HIV immune responses and prolong the period of asymptomatic disease. Assessment of this approach will be particularly challenging in view of the early stages of disease in which such techniques would have to be employed to be effective. CD4 counts will not be suitable for the evaluation of such approaches since levels of the marker will be directly affected by the attempts at vaccine treatment without necessarily influencing the outcome of disease. Such trials will require alternative markers, particularly in children, and a combination of viral quantitation and functional evaluation of immune competence would appear the most appropriate choices at the present time.

Conclusion

Rapid progress has been made in the clinical description of the extent and evolution of the immunodeficiency which follows HIV infection in children. Questions of pathogenesis remain which, when solved, should allow definitive progress towards more effective therapy and preventive immunisation. There is currently much interest in the theoretical possibility that immunisation following infection may slow progression of HIV disease. However, there are no clinical or experimental precedents for this approach and randomised clinical trials will be required using clinical end-points to determine possible efficacy.

Assessment of the extent of immunodeficiency is currently unsatisfactory. Whereas studies of lymphocyte surface markers or immunoglobulin concentrations are useful staging markers for whole patient populations and for defining groups at high risk for progression and clinical trial entry, these markers are less useful in staging individual patients, or for assessing their progression or need for prophylactic antimicrobial therapy. Standardisation of tests of functional immune competence and quantitative virology is required but work in these areas is only in the earliest stages of development and is a high priority for research.

References

Aboulker, J-P. & Swart. A. M. (1993). Preliminary analysis of the Concorde trial. *Lancet*, **341**, 889–90.

Auger, I., Thomas, P., de Gruttola, V., *et al.* (1988). Incubation periods for pediatric AIDS patients. *Nature*, **336**, 575–7.

Bernstein, L. J., Krieger, B. Z., Novick, B., Sicklick, M. J. & Rubinstein, A. (1985a). Bacterial infection in the acquired immuno-deficiency syndrome in children. *Pediatric Infectious Diseases*, **4**, 472–5.

Bernstein, L. J., Ochs., H. D., Wedgwood, R. J. & Rubinstein, A. (1985*b*). Defective humoral immunity in paediatric acquired immunodeficiency syndrome infection. *Journal of Pediatrics*, **107**, 352–7.

Bird, A. G. (1992). Clinical and immunological assessment of HIV infection. *Journal of Clinical Pathology*, **45**, 850–4.

Blanche, S., Le Deist, F., Fischer, A., *et al.* (1986). Longitudinal study of 18 children with perinatal LAV/HTLV III infection: attempt at prognostic evaluation. *Journal of Pediatrics*, **109**, 965–70.

Blanche, S., Rouzioux, C., Moscato, M-L., *et al.* (1989). A prospective study of infants born to women seropositive for human immunodeficiency virus type 1. *New England Journal of Medicine*, **320**, 1643–8.

Blanche, S., Tardieu, M., Duliege A-M. & Rouzioux, C. (1990). Longitudinal study of 94 symptomatic infants with perinatally acquired human immunodeficiency virus infection. *American Journal of Diseases of Children*, **144**, 1210–15.

Bonagura, V. R., Cunningham Rundles, S. L. & Schuval, S. (1992). Dysfunction of natural killer cells in human immunodeficiency virus infected children with or without *pneumocystis carinii* pneumonia. *Journal of Pediatrics*, **121**, 195–201,

Bonavida, B., Katz, J. & Gottlieb, M. (1986). Mechanism of defective NK cell activity in patients with acquired immunodeficiency syndrome (AIDS) and AIDS-related complex. I. Defective trigger on NK cells for NK CF production by larger cells and partial restoration by IL2. *Jounal of Immunology*, **137**, 1157–63.

Borkowsky, W., Rigaud, M., Krasinski, K., Moore, T., Lawrence, L. & Pollack, H. (1992). Cell-mediated and humoral immune responses in children infected with human immunodeficiency virus during the first four years of life. *Journal of Pediatrics*, **120**, 371–5.

Cheynier, R., Langlade-Demoyen, P, Marescot, M-R. (1992). Cytotoxic T lymphocyte responses in the peripheral blood of children born to HIV-1 infected mothers. *European Journal of Immunology*, **22**, 2211–17.

Clerici, M., Stocks, N. I., Zajac, R. A., *et al.* (1989). Detection of three distinct patterns of T helper cell dysfunction in asymptomatic human immunodeficiency virus seropositive patients. *Journal of Clinical Investigation*, **84**, 1892–9.

Clerici, M., Roilides, E., Butler, K. M., *et al.* (1992). Changes in T helper cell function in human immunodeficiency virus-infected children during didanosine therapy as a measure of antiretroviral activity. *Blood*, **80**, 2196–202.

de Martino, M., Tovo P.-A., Galli, C., *et al.* (1991). Prognostic significance of immunologic changes in 675 infants perinatally exposed to human immunodeficiency virus. *Journal of Pediatrics*, **119**, 702–9.

Embretson, J., Zupancic, M., Ribas, J. L., *et al.* (1993). Massive covert infection of helper T lymphocytes and macrophages by HIV during the incubation period of AIDS. *Nature*, **362**, 359–62.

European Collaborative Study (1991). Children born to women with HIV-1 infection: natural history and risk of transmission. *Lancet*, **337**, 253–9.

European Collaborative Study (1992). Age-related standards for T lymphocyte subsets based on uninfected children born to human immunodeficiency virus 1-infected women. *Pediatric Infectious Diseases Journal*, **11**, 1018–26.

Falloon, J., Eddy, J., Wiener, L. & Pizzo, P. A. (1989). Human immunodeficiency virus infection in children. *Journal of Pediatrics*, **114**, 1–30.

Froebel, K. S., Doherty, K. V., Whitelaw, J. A., Hague, R. A., Mok, J. & Bird, A. G. (1991). Increased expression of CD45 RO (memory) antigen on T cells in HIV infected children. *AIDS*, 5, 97–9.

Groenink, M., Fouchier, R. A. M., Broersen, S. *et al.* (1993). Relation of phenotype evolution of HIV-1 to envelope V2 configuration. *Science*, 260, 1513–16.

Johnson, J. P., Nair, P., Hines, S. E., *et al.* (1989). Natural history and serologic diagnosis of infants born to human immunodeficiency virus-infected women. *American Journal of Diseases of Children*, 143, 1147–53.

Krasinski, K., Borkowsky, W., Bonk, S., Lawrence, R. & Chandwani, S. (1988). Bacterial infections in human immunodeficiency virus-infected children. *Pediatric Infectious Diseases*, 7, 323–8.

Lagakos, S. W. & Hoth, D. F. (1992). Surrogate markers in AIDS: where are we? where are we going? *Annals of Internal Medicine*, 116, 599–601.

Learmont, J., Tindall, B., Evans, L., *et al.* (1992). Long-term symptomless HIV-1 infection in recipients of blood products. *Lancet*, 340, 863–8.

Leibovitz, E., Rigaud, M., Pollack, H. *et al.* (1991). *Pneumocystis carinii* pneumonia in infants infected with the human immmunodeficiency virus with more than 450 CD4 T lymphocytes per cubic millimeter. *New England Journal of Medicine*, 323, 531–3.

Leinonen, M., Säkkinen, A., Kalliokoski, R., Luotonen, J., Timonen, M. & Mäkelä, H. (1986). Antibody response to 14 valent pneumococcal capsular polysaccharide vaccine in preschool age children. *Pediatric Infectious Diseases*, 5, 39–44.

Lifson, J. D., Benicke, C. J., Mark, D. F., Koths, K. & Engleman, E. G. (1984). Human recombinant interleukin 2 partially reconstitutes deficient *in vitro* immune responses of lymphocytes from patients with AIDS. *Lancet*, i, 698–702.

Luzuriaga, K. & Sullivan, J. L. (1993). HIV specific CTL in long-term survivors of vertical infection. *Pediatric Research*, 33, 155A.

Maloney, M. J., Guill, M. F., Wray, B. B., Lobel, S. A. & Ebbeling, W. (1987). Pediatric acquired immune deficiency syndrome with panhypogammaglobulinaemia. *Journal of Paediatrics*, 110, 266–67.

Meynard, L., Schuitemaker, H. & Miedema, F. (1993). T-cell dysfunction in HIV infection: anergy due to defective antigen-presenting cell function. *Immunology Today*, 14, 161–4.

Miedema, F., Petit, A. J. C., Terpstra, F. G., *et al.* (1988). Immunological abnormalities in human immunodeficiency virus (HIV)-infected asymptomatic homosexual men. HIV affects the immune system before CD4⁺T helper cell depletion occurs. *Journal of Clinical Investigation*, 82, 1908–14.

Mosier, D. E., Gulizia, R. J., MacIsaac, P. D., Torbett, B. E. & Levy, J. A. (1993). Rapid loss of CD4⁺T cells in human-PBL-SCID mice by non-cytopathic HIV isolates. *Science*, 260, 689–92.

Niven, P, Skuza, C., Chadwick, E., *et al.* (1990). Age-related changes of lymphocyte phenotype in healthy children. *Pediatric Research*, 27, 155A.

Nixon, D. F. & McMichael, A. J., (1991). Cytotoxic T cell recognition of HIV proteins and peptides. *AIDS*, 5, 1049–59.

Oleske, J., Minnefor, A., Cooper, R., *et al.* (1983). Immune deficiency in children. *Journal of the American Medical Association*, 249, 2345–49.

Pahwa, R., Good, R. A. & Pahwa, S. (1987). Prematurity, hypogammaglobulinaemia and neuropathology with human immunodeficiency virus (HIV) infection. *Proceedings of the National Academy of Sciences, USA*, 84, 3826–30.

Panteleo, G., Graziosi, C., Demarest, J. F., *et al.* (1993). HIV infection is active and progressive in lymphoid tissue during the clinically latent stage of disease. *Nature*, **362**, 355–8.

Papiernik, M., Brossard, Y., Mulliez, N., *et al.* (1992). Thymic abnormalities in fetuses aborted from human immunodeficiency virus type 1 seropositive women. *Pediatrics*, **89**, 297–301.

Petersen, J. M., Church, J., Gomperts, E. & Parkman, R. (1989). Lymphocyte phenotype does not predict immune function in pediatric patients infected with human immunodeficiency virus type 1. *Journal of Pediatrics*, **115**, 944–8.

Petersen, J. M., Weinberg, K. I., Annett, G., Church, J., Gomperts, E. & Parkman R. (1992). Correction of antigen-specific T-lymphocyte function by recombinant cytokines in children infected with human immunodeficiency virus type 1. *Journal of Pediatrics*, **121**, 565–8.

Phair, J. P., Munoz, A., Detels, R., Kaslow, R., Rinaldo, C., Saah, A. and the Multicentre AIDS Cohort Study Group (1990). The risk of *Pneumocystis carinii* pneumonia among men infected with human immunodeficiency virus type 1. *New England Journal of Medicine*, **322**, 161–5.

Philips, R. E., Rowland-Jones, S., Nixon, D. F., *et al* (1991). Human immunodeficiency virus genetic variation that can escape cytotoxic T cell recognition. *Nature*, **354**, 453–59.

Roilides, E., Clerici, M., De Palma, L., Rubin, M., Pizzo, P. A. & Shearer, G. M. (1991). Helper T cell response in children infected with human immunodeficiency virus type 1. *Journal of Pediatrics*, **118**, 724–30.

Roilides, E., Holmes, A., Blake, C., Pizzo, P. A. & Walsh, T. J. (1993). Impairment of neutrophil antifungal activity against hyphae of *Aspergillus fumigatus* in children infected with human immunodeficiency virus. *Journal of Infectious Diseases*, **167**, 905–11.

Roilides, E., Mertins, S., Eddy, J., Walsh, T. J., Pizzo, P. A. & Rubin M. (1990). Impairment of neutrophil chemotactic and bacteriocidal function in children infected with human immunodeficiency virus type 1 and partial reversal after *in vitro* exposure to granulocyte-macrophage colony-stimulating factor. *Journal of Pediatrics*, **117**, 531–40.

Rook, A. H., Masur, H., Lane, H. C., *et al.* (1983). Interleukin 2 enhances the depressed natural killer and cytomegalovirus-specific cytotoxic activities of lymphocytes from patients with the acquired immunodeficiency syndrome. *Journal of Clinical Investigation*, **72**, 398–403.

Rowland-Jones, S. L., Nixon, D. F., Aldhous, M. C. *et al.* (1993). HIV-specific cytotoxic T cell activity in an HIV exposed but uninfected infant. *Lancet*, **341**, 860–1.

Rubinstein, A., Sicklick, M., Gupta, A., *et al.* (1983). Acquired immunodeficiency with reversed T4/T8 ratios in infants born to promiscuous and drug-addicted mothers. *Journal of the American Medical Association*, **249**, 2350–56.

Rutstein, R. M. (1991). Predicting risk of *Pneumocystis carinii* pneumonia in human immunodeficiency virus infected children. *American Journal of Diseases of Children*, **145**, 922–4.

Wagasugi, N. & Virelizier, J-L. (1985). Defective IFN$_\gamma$ production in the human neonate. I. Dysregulation rather than intrinsic abnormality. *Journal of Immunology*, **134**, 167–71.

7

The HIV-infected woman

RAYMOND P. BRETTLE

Introduction

Increasing numbers of females are being infected with HIV. In some areas, up to one-third of injection drug users are female and spread to heterosexual partners of HIV-positive individuals, especially females, is occurring with increasing frequency. As vertical transmission is the major mode of acquisition of infection in children it is important to consider the natural history and management of HIV disease in women.

Progression from HIV to AIDS

Extensive data on the time course of progression from HIV infection to AIDS are now emerging from several cohorts with various risk activities and known seroconversion dates. These reports suggest rates of progression to AIDS of 0–2% at 2 years, 5–10% at 4 years, 10–25% at 6 years, 30–40% at 8 years and 48–51% at 10 years (Table 7.1; Moss & Bacchetti, 1989; Rutherford et al., 1990). The median time for progression from infection to AIDS from these studies is 11 years and the annual risk of progression to AIDS is around 8%. The majority of these studies, however, are based on males and there are specific factors relating to women which need to be addressed.

The risk can also be expressed according to CD4 counts, with the risk of progression to AIDS rising as the CD4 count falls (Table 7.2), although even patients with very high CD4 counts can develop AIDS. This is in part explained by the fact that the CD4 count does not measure the individual function of the CD4 cells and the clinical expression of immunodeficiency (AIDS) is dependent on overall function which is determined by both total numbers and individual function.

Pregnancy

Perhaps one of the greatest concerns for both women and their physicians has been the possibility of an interaction between pregnancy and the

124

Table 7.1. *Progression to AIDS*

Time from infection (years)	% progression to AIDS
2	0–2
4	5–10
6	10–25
8	30–40
10	48–51

Table 7.2. *Annual progression according to CD4 counts*

CD4 count (/mm³)	Annual risk of progression to AIDS (%)
>500	1
350–500	3
200–350	10–12
<200	20

From Lau *et al.* (1992).

progression of HIV disease. This concern is hardly surprising when one considers that the median time from infection to the development of AIDS is 10–11 years, and that the majority of infected females are in the reproductive age group and therefore likely to have one or two children during the time they are infected. In Scotland, for instance, 86% of infected females are in the 15–44 year age group and in Europe 76% of women with AIDS are in the 15–49 age group (see Chapter 1). The interaction between HIV disease and pregnancy is discussed later, but to date in Edinburgh there is no evidence that pregnancy in the asymptomatic stage hastens immunological decline.

Gender

There are relatively few cohort studies detailing progression of HIV infection in women compared with men, although studies considering gender are now in progress. Gender has not been reported as a significant factor in HIV progression (Italian Seroconversion Study, 1992; Selwyn *et al.*, 1992). Similarly, results from the Edinburgh study cohort, which contains a substantial number of women and men of comparable age and risk activity, does not show a gender effect for progression measured either from seroconversion or from enrolment to symptomatic disease.

As with drug users, there is concern over whether AIDS accurately reflects the natural history of HIV infection in women since the initial definition was based largely on homosexual men. In Edinburgh there does

Table 7.3. *Survival in AIDS*

Time from diagnosis of AIDS (years)	% survival
1	50
2	25
3–4	5
5	0

not appear to be a separate spectrum of clinical HIV disease for women. In a retrospective survey of 612 HIV-related admissions there was no excess of female admissions except for detoxification, investigation of episodes of loss of consciousness and urinary tract infections (Willocks *et al.* 1991). In addition, the lack of any excess mortality for HIV-infected women compared with men (see below) supports the argument that the AIDS definition (Centers for Disease Control, 1987) as applied in the UK is appropriate for women.

Survival after AIDS diagnosis

Following a diagnosis of AIDS 50% of patients usually survive 1 year (Table 7.3). As with drug users, the initial impression, based on data from the USA, was that women had a poorer survival from AIDS compared with men (Friedland *et al.*, 1991). However, this reduced survival could be related to access to medical services rather than gender, since death at presentation for women was more common in both New York and San Francisco (Rothenberg *et al.*, 1987; Lemp *et al.*, 1990). Further evidence that women generally present late for medical care comes from a study from Minnesota, USA, where two-thirds of women with HIV were detected by neonatal screening rather than via medical care (Danila *et al.*, 1990). Where there is good access to medical care, women have equivalent if not better survival than men (Rothenberg *et al.*, 1987; Batalla *et al.*, 1989; Lemp *et al.*, 1990; Morlat *et al.*, 1992). The most recent San Francisco analysis noted that a significant difference in survival for men and women disappeared when controlled for antiretroviral drug use, which suggests that socioeconomic factors, delays in diagnosis, and poor utilisation of access to medical services are more important than gender (Areneta *et al.*, 1990).

In Edinburgh, unlike the USA or even the rest of the UK, women have tended to present early for treatment. This may be a result of the close integration of obstetric, paediatric and adult HIV services as well as mothers' concerns over their ability to care for their children.

Post-AIDS survival may be influenced by early or late presentation of patients even when good medical care is available. For instance, early presentation to medical services may increase the use of prophylaxis for opportunistic infections (*Candida* and *Pneumocystis carinii* pneumonia (PCP)), thus delaying the diagnosis of AIDS. However, this may paradoxically shorten post-AIDS survival if there is no reduction in immunological decline. Equally, relatively late presentation to medical services may result in an immediate AIDS diagnosis with a relatively well-preserved immunological state (oesophageal candidiasis) as a consequence of a lack of prophylaxis for the common opportunistic infection and thus a paradoxically prolonged post-AIDS survival. The earlier use of prophylaxis may explain the slightly shorter survival in the post-AIDS period for women in Edinburgh.

Clinical problems for HIV-infected women

Problems of drug use

The extent of the injection drug use (IDU)-related HIV epidemic in Edinburgh and elsewhere requires consideration of the clinical features of IDU as well as those of HIV since each may mimic the other. As an example, lymphadenopathy is associated with both HIV and with the injecting of foreign materials. The fatigue, lethargy and excessive sweating which are an early feature of HIV infection can all also be caused by mild withdrawal from opiates. Diarrhoea, a common presentation of early symptomatic HIV (CDC stage IVA), is unfortunately a common problem with opiate withdrawal. A history of diarrhoea for longer than 1 month may be elicited via direct questioning and suggests a possible diagnosis of CDC stage IVA. Such a history would also require a search for specific pathogens such as *Cryptosporidium* which are seen in AIDS. However, early-morning diarrhoea is common for those on methadone and is simply a symptom of early opiate withdrawal. Weight loss and sweating are both key symptoms of constitutional disease (CDC stage IVA) as well as mycobacterial infections, yet both are associated with heavy opiate use or the use of stimulants (amphetamines or cocaine).

Epileptic fits in patients with HIV require consideration of cerebral toxoplasmosis, but the intermittent use of benzodiazepines can also cause seizures. The regular monitoring of CD4 counts and *Toxoplasma* serology helps to identify those patients at-risk of toxoplasmosis and consequently reduces the number of CT scans required. The excessive use of cannabis and benzodiazepines interferes with memory and other cognitive functions in a similar manner to HIV, although in the former, dramatic improvement occurs with reduction or cessation of drugs. Thus early dementia which might be detected in other risk groups by psychometric testing is extremely difficult to diagnose in current drug users, especially since reducing drugs will also help the dementing patient to improve function in activities of daily living. Syncopal attacks in AIDS are often associated with an autonomic neuropathy or a failing adrenal cortex. This problem, however, is associated with the use or misuse of antidepressant tricyclic drugs such as amitriptyline. Lastly shortness of breath and a persistent cough are common early symptoms of PCP but can occur with endocarditis, bacterial pneumonia, excessive smoking, recurrent bronchitis and obstructive airways disease. The medical conditions associated with IDU include asymptomatic abnormalities of pulmonary function tests, life-threatening infections, or immunological problems such as polyarteritis nodosa. The advent of IDU-related HIV has not only widened the spectrum of disease seen in drug users but has also increased the frequency of some existing conditions. As a consequence the differential diagnosis in a patient with IDU-related HIV is extensive. Further examples are detailed in Table 7.4. Because of the difficulties with interpreting the history and the extensive differential diagnosis if there is evidence of current drug use, a short period of admission is often the only way to clarify the situation.

HIV problems

In Edinburgh, other than the fact that women presented earlier in an asymptomatic state, there were no significant gender differences in non-AIDS clinical events.

Non-infective HIV problems

Loss of endocrine function has been reported in patients with AIDS. Overall deficiencies of adrenal or thyroid function were not evident except in association with severe illness (Raffi *et al.*, 1991). As far as sex hormones are concerned most studies have concentrated on testicular function. In the report by Raffi *et al.* (1991), although 25 women were studied, no data were presented with respect to women.

Another common problem with HIV infection is thrombocytopenia, which seems to occur in around 5% of individuals (Peltier *et al.*, 1991). In a cohort of 435 individuals the male to female ratio was 3.8 : 1, whilst for those with platelet counts less than $150\times10^9/1$ the ratio was 13.5 : 1. However, this difference was not statistically significant. It has been reported that women are more likely than men to present with anaemia.

Table 7.4. *Comparison of drug-related and HIV-related problems*

Symptom complex	Drug-related problems	HIV-related problems
Pulmonary		
Recurrent sinusitis	'Snorting' of drugs	Susceptibility to recurrent bacterial infection
Reduced transfer factor for carbon monoxide	Talc granuloma secondary to emboli, cocaine	PCP
Respiratory syndrome (cough, dyspnoea, etc.)	Chronic bronchitis secondary to tobacco and marijuana	Increased susceptibility to bacterial infections
	Emphysema (tobacco)	HIV-related emphysema
	Inhalation or aspiration pneumonia	PCP, TB, other OIs, bacterial pneumonia, KS
	Acute bronchitis Endocarditis 'Heroin asthma' or pulmonary oedema Polyarteritis-nodosa-related pneumonitis	
Pulmonary hypertension (dyspnoea, hypoxaemia, restrictive lung disease)	Talc granuloma secondary to emboli	HIV-related pulmonary hypertension
Constitutional symptoms		
Fever	Endocarditis, septicaemia, etc. 'Bad fix' or endotoxaemia	CDC stage IVA, PCP and OIs such as MAI
Night sweats	Opiate withdrawals	CDC stage III, IVA, or early OI
Weight loss	Heavy addiction, poor diet and use of stimulants such as cocaine or amphetamines	CDC stage IVA, TB or other OI
Gastroenterology		
Diarrhoea	Opiate withdrawals	CDC stage IVA or enteric pathogen
Sore mouth		Thrush, OHL, etc.
Sores around mouth/nose	Poor diet, 'snorting' or sniffing glue or cocaine	HSV
Abdominal pain	Intra-abdominal pathology obscured by opiates, e.g. appendicitis, cholecystitis, pancreatitis	MAI, cryptosporidium, CMV, lymphoma, KS, etc.
Abnormal liver function tests	Acute hepatitis type A, B, C, D Paracetamol overdose	Recurrence of B, C or D hepatitis, drug reactions (e.g. anti-TB drugs) and MAI

Table 7.4 (*contd*)

Symptom complex	Drug-related problems	HIV-related problems
Neurological		
Loss of vision	Endocarditis, ophthalmitis (candidaemia)	CMV/VZV/HSV retinitis, toxoplasmosis, etc.
Toxic confusional state	Drug use or infection	Bacterial infections, OIs, HIV encephalopathy
Epileptic seizures	Withdrawals from benzodiazepines or barbiturates	Toxoplasmosis
Peripheral nerve paralysis	IDU-related traumatic nerve damage	Seroconversion illness of HIV, CDC stage IVB
Hemiparesis	Endocarditis	Toxoplasmosis, cerebral haemorrhage secondary to HIV-related thrombocytopenia
Skin		
Purpura	IDU, endocarditis	HIV-related seborrhoeic dermatitis, scabies, HIV-related papular urticaria
Itching and scratching	Opiates and stimulant use	
Recurrent abscesses	IDU	Susceptibility to bacterial infections, bacillary angiomatosis, lymphoma
Cardiology		
Heart murmurs	Endocarditis	
Cardiomyopathy	Alcohol	HIV
Pulmonary hypertension	Talc granulomas	HIV-related pulmonary hypertension
Endocrinology		
Increased prolactin levels and gynaecomastia	Opiate use	Not recognised
Amenorrhoea (may be secondary to weight loss)		Late-stage disease
Oligospermia, impotence and gynaecomastia	Cannabis	Late-stage disease (not gynaecomastia)

OI, opportunistic infection; HSV, herpes simplex virus; OHL, oral hairy leukoplakia; VZV, varicella zoster virus. For other abbreviations see text.

Infections (non-AIDS)

There is an increased susceptibility to bacterial infections in HIV infection. Encapsulated bacteria such as *Streptococcus pneumoniae* and *Haemophilus influenzae* are frequent respiratory pathogens and causes of bacteraemia in HIV-seropositive individuals (Simberkoff *et al.*, 1984; Polsky *et al.*, 1986; Selwyn *et al.*, 1988). In a study of bacteraemia in Nairobi HIV-seropositive individuals were 5 times more likely to suffer a bacteraemia (26% versus 6%), particularly with *S. pneumoniae* and *Salmonella typhimurium* (Gilks *et al.*, 1990), than HIV-negative controls. In Edinburgh analysis of a cohort of 501 patients with a 3 : 2 male to female ratio showed that admissions for urinary tract infections were increased for females (male to female ratio 4 : 11) whilst admissions for other infections showed no difference in the male to female ratio (Willocks *et al.*, 1991). Only 4 of the 168 female patients required admission with pelvic inflammatory disease. The majority of admissions in both males and females were, as has been reported from drug users in the USA, for respiratory disorders, especially recurrent bacterial infections.

This increased susceptibility to bacterial infections may in part explain the suggestion that genital tract infections are increased in HIV-positive women. The prevalence of lower genital tract infection for HIV-positive drug users is higher than in HIV-negative drug users although many of the infections are in fact genital warts. There is also a significantly higher prevalence of human papilloma virus (HPV) infection. Genital herpes, candidiasis and pelvic inflammatory disease are also of particular concern. These infections were more prevalent, more aggressive and often recurrent in HIV-positive females. In studies of reasonably well HIV-infected women (CDC stage III) there was also an increased prevalence of recurrent vaginal candidiasis. In one study of HIV-infected women, 23% of whom had AIDS, the prevalence of reported genital infections over a 1 year period was 31%. Vaginal yeast infections were reported by 10% (4% with recurrent yeast infections as defined by more than 4 attacks per year), genital herpes infections by 5%, *Trichomonas* infections by 4% and pelvic inflammatory disease by 1% of women (Buehler *et al.*, 1991). In a group of 117 women asymptomatic at the diagnosis of HIV the most common first symptoms were *Candida* vaginitis in 37%, visible lymphadenopathy in 14.5% and bacterial pneumonia in 13% (Carpenter *et al.*, 1991). These infections are likely to be due to a reactivation of previous microbiological exposure. Women with no history of pelvic disease before HIV will probably not develop these problems *de novo*.

Non-AIDS mortality

As with drug users the increased susceptibility to bacterial infections may increase the mortality of non-opportunistic events such that many patients die before the advent of AIDS (Stoneburner *et al.*, 1989). Thus it is important to look at total survival for women rather than just survival after the development of AIDS. In Africa excess mortality of HIV-positive compared with HIV-negative mothers has been noted. For instance after 2 years of follow-up of 460 HIV-infected women and 998 women not infected with HIV the mortality for those women not infected was 0.3% but was 7% for those infected (Lindan *et al.*, 1992). However, in Edinburgh no excess mortality was found for women compared with men, suggesting that in Europe the definition of AIDS is not missing large numbers of deaths in HIV-infected women.

Infections (AIDS-defining events)

In the majority of reports, PCP is the commonest presentation of AIDS and occurs with a frequency varying from 30 to 60%. The frequency of other conditions is variable. A large study of all New York cases revealed that 17% presented with Kaposi's sarcoma (KS) alone, 9% with KS and some other event, 12% with PCP and another event, whilst 4% had two other events (not KS or PCP) as a presenting diagnosis (Rothenberg *et al.*, 1987). In Denmark, KS occurred in 18% of presentations (Smith *et al.*, 1990). The St Mary's group (London) recently reported a frequency of 24% for cutaneous KS, 10% for oesophageal *Candida* and 4% for cerebral toxoplasmosis (Lau *et al.*, 1992). It is important to note that since KS is rare in non-homo/bisexuals the higher percentages for PCP in other risk groups may simply reflect the absence of KS rather than an increased susceptibility to PCP. Similarly other major differences may simply reflect the number exposed to pathogens such as CMV or toxoplasmosis with an established latency.

Tuberculosis (TB) is the opportunistic infection usually associated with a particular risk group (drug users) and is very common in southern Europe where extrapulmonary TB made up 33% of the index diagnoses compared with less than 1% in San Francisco (Batalla *et al.*, 1989; Hessol *et al.*, 1990). In New York a study looking at TB in patients undergoing investigations for PCP revealed that 2.4% had pulmonary TB (Klein & Motyl, 1993). In the UK it has a cumulative rate of only 7% and our experience was that it was a relatively uncommon infection (<2%), presumably because HIV is not common in the populations affected by tuberculosis (Peters *et al.*, 1991).

Further geographical variations are noted in a study from southern France where PCP accounted for only 27% of the initial and 35% of the cumulative events; the second commonest presentation was toxoplasmosis followed by KS and *Candida* oesophagitis (Morlat *et al.*, 1992). The rarer events were extrapulmonary tuberculosis, lymphoma, infections with atypical mycobacteria such as *Mycobacterium avium intracellulare* (MAI), herpes simplex virus (HSV) infections, HIV encephalitis, cryptococcal and cryptosporidial infections, all of which occurred in less than 10% of cases except for cytomegalovirus (CMV) infections which occurred in 13% of cases (Morlat *et al.*, 1992).

Other than genital tract infections and neoplasms there have been few reports to suggest that HIV-infected women have a particular disease spectrum that differs from that seen in men. Women are less likely to present with PCP as the AIDS-defining illness compared with men with AIDS. The most common AIDS indicator diseases in women were *Candida albicans* oesophagitis (34–38%), HIV-related wasting syndrome (25%), PCP (20%) and chronic mucocutaneous herpes simplex (18%). Significantly more women than men suffered from oesophageal candidiasis, atypical mycobacteria and the wasting syndrome (Thompson *et al.*, 1991). However, the majority of these reports come from the USA and clinical presentations may be affected by the time of presentation and access to medical care. For instance, a lack of access to care may mean that candidiasis is the first opportunistic event whereas regular attendance at clinics may provide access to appropriate prophylaxis resulting in delayed or prevented *Candida* infections. As a result other opportunisitic infections may increase in frequency as presenting features. The numbers of patients in all these reports are small and findings need to be confirmed before any definitive conclusions can be drawn.

By comparison the cumulative percentage of AIDS patients ever having particular conditions in Edinburgh were: PCP 91%, disseminated MAI 29%, oesophageal candidiasis 28%, CMV disease 21%, Kaposi's sarcoma 11%, lymphoma 12%, toxoplasmosis 11%, HIV dementia 10%, extra pulmonary tuberculosis 2%. No significant gender differences were noted, however, once homo/bisexuals were removed from the comparison.

Neoplasms

Kaposi's sarcoma

The most common neoplasm associated with AIDS is KS, which occurs in 15% of the reported cases of AIDS. It is more frequent among homosexual AIDS cases than in drug users (Beral *et al.*, 1990). The commonest malignancy associated with drug use appears to be malignant lymphoma, which was reported in 8% of surgical specimens from drug users. In an Italian study of more than 10 000 cases of AIDS of which 6% were due to KS, women were less likely to present with KS than men. The odds ratios for KS amongst drug users (0.6), heterosexuals (0.4) or the undetermined transmission category (0.4) were all more favourable for women (Serraino et al., 1992).

Whilst about 3% of women have developed KS in Europe or the USA there is a suggestion that when it occurs women are more immunodeficient and have a shorter survival. Sixty to seventy per cent of women were dead by 1 year after diagnosis, with a median survival of 3–4 months, whereas 70% of men with KS survived 1 year (Lassoud et al., 1991; Benedetti et al., 1991). However, caution is required because more recent cases of KS in men have been more immunodeficient and had poorer prognostic markers. In Africa, KS seems to affect women fairly frequently, the male to female ratio of epidemic KS being 2 : 1 instead of 5 : 1 for endemic KS, as seen before 1983. In one series of 101 patients, 18% of cases were women and by comparison with the European and US studies only 36% had died by 2 years. It may therefore be that the studies reporting poor prognosis for women are based on small numbers.

It has been suggested that KS is sexually transmitted, as the initial lesions of KS have been found in areas of sexual contact (Lassoud et al., 1991). KS was 4 times more likely in female partners of bisexual men than other risk groups and is more common in Africa (Beral et al., 1990). However, a recent study has failed to confirm this association with bisexual men or partners of patients with KS (Benedetti et al., 1991).

Genital neoplasms

Women with HIV infection have been thought to be at higher risk of developing lower genital tract problems, although well-controlled studies with comparable HIV-negative controls are relatively rare. Since individuals who acquire HIV may be more sexually active and therefore at more risk of becoming infected, simple comparisons of HIV-positive with HIV-negative groups may not be adequately controlled. In a study of HIV-infected women who were clinically well, 18 of 109 had abnormalities of the lower genital tract (Byrne et al., 1989). In general HIV-positive women from a variety of sources have an incidence of cervical intraepithelial neoplasia (CIN) varying between 35% and 80%. A recent review of 21 published studies on the relationship between HIV infection and cervical dysplasia found that only five studies had comparative groups. However, the summary odds ratio indicated that the odds of HIV-infected women having cervical neoplasia was 4.9 times that of HIV-negative women (Mandelblatt et al., 1992). The conclusion of the review was that whilst more work is needed in this area the available data suggest that regular screening of HIV-positive women is necessary and that HIV counselling and testing should be considered in cases of women with cervical neoplasia at-risk of HIV.

From a management point of view it is suggested that HIV-positive women should have two cervical smears within the first 6 months (to reduce the risks of an initial false negative smear) followed by annual smears thereafter. This is mostly to ensure that if cervical dysplasia is present it is detected early prior to invasion and spread.

General management principles

The first general principle of managing women with HIV infection is to engender an awareness in carers of the fact that women are likely to be infected. Services dealing with women such as antenatal, well woman or a gynaecology clinics need to recognise the clinical presentations of HIV infection in women. Secondly some modification of the health care environment is required to cater for the specific needs of infected women. For example many patients are also mothers, and clinics normally caring only for adults need to make provision for children, who may accompany their infected mother to the clinic. In certain circumstances there may be a requirement for single-sex clinics, especially if there is any possibility of victimisation of women by other HIV-positive patients. It may be difficult to attract and retain patients within the health care system and therefore some modification of clinic routines is often necessary, offering more user-friendly clinic times which fit in with a woman's way of life or offering different types of clinics with both male and female doctors to accommodate patients' wishes. Such changes increase the ability of a clinic to attract and retain patients over many years that is necessary with a chronic illness.

Unlike many centres an initial presentation with AIDS was and is unusual for the majority of Edinburgh patients, occurring in only 11% of patients – although it has become more common in recent years. This presumably reflects the effectiveness of the health care system in persuading patients with HIV to enter the system before the onset of ill health. The recent rise may in part be accounted for by referrals of patients with pre-existing AIDS from other centres for access to more difficult treatment schedules.

Specific issues in management for women (Table 7.5)

In an attempt to reduce vertical transmission it makes sense to ensure that all HIV-infected women are aware of effective contraception to enable

Table 7.5. *Management of HIV-infected women*

Problem	Management
Asymptomatic HIV infection	Review 3–6 monthly to establish: baseline CD4 counts, relationship with patient
Symptomatic HIV infection	Review at least 2–4 monthly depending on problems
Vertical transmission	Contraception to ensure only planned pregnancies occur
Horizontal transmission	Encourage barrier contraception if partner is HIV negative
Cervical dysplasia	6 monthly cervical smears or colposcopy for asymptomatic and symptomatic women
Bacterial infections	Reduce smoking, reduce opiate drug use, early use of antibiotics
Antiretroviral therapy	Symptomatic patients: zidovudine with ddc or ddI as second-line agents for patients intolerant of zidovudine

them to avoid unplanned conception. The increased incidence of cervical dysplasia in some populations of HIV-infected women requires an awareness in carers and surveillance for this disorder approximately 6 monthly, via either repeated smears or colposcopy.

An awareness of the increased incidence of severe bacterial infections is required and it is sensible to attempt to reduce this susceptibility further by reducing smoking (tobacco and marijuana) and opiate consumption, both of which increase susceptibility to infections, particularly respiratory infections.

The use of prophylaxis for opportunsitic infections at the required times should be encouraged in women as in men. The only caution is for those women seeking conception. However, co-trimoxazole is contra-indicated in late pregnancy because of the sulphonamide component. The potential risks for the child need to be balanced against the risks for the mother during pregnancy of developing PCP. There is little experience with the use in pregnancy of other agents commonly used in the treatment of AIDS conditions such as CMV or atypical mycobacteria, and again the risks for the pregnancy need to be balanced against the risks for the mother.

The results of the recent Concorde trial of zidovudine in asymptomatic patients with HIV showed no survival advantage for its early use (Aboulker & Swart, 1993). Since there appears to be no clear survival advantage for the patient from early treatment, at present it seems sensible to offer zidovudine only to patients with HIV symptoms. This plan has the benefit that compliance is enhanced by clear improvement in a patient's symptoms. In the event of serious adverse effects from zidovudine two other nucleoside analogues (ddc and ddI) are generally available in Europe, Australia and the USA, either on a named patient basis or via prescription for use as single agent antiretroviral therapy (see Chapter 12). There is some experience of zidovudine in pregnancy suggesting reduction of the risks of vertical transmission (see Chapter 1).

Conclusion

At present there does not appear to be a significant difference in the natural history of women infected with HIV compared with HIV-infected men, although the majority of these studies have concerned patients with early HIV infection and with time other problems may emerge. Of concern for some countries such as the USA is the fact that a different natural history seems to occur because of differential access to medical care. The effect, if any, of pregnancy on the outcome of HIV could be via a variety of pathologies, for instance hormonal, immunosuppression or antigenic stimulation. However, the lack of an overall effect of gender on the progression of HIV would suggest that pregnancy is unlikely to have a significant effect on the natural history of HIV in women. Other than genital tract infections and/or neoplasia there also appears to be little difference in either the clinical presentation or the management issues for women.

Without doubt the increasing number of women infected with HIV and ultimately dying of AIDS will have serious implications for all societies. The psychosocial issues for women with HIV may, or may not, be different from those for homosexual or heterosexual men. However, illness and death of one or both parents, as well as the death of infected children, are important issues that must be considered by society as a consequence of this epidemic.

References

Aboulker, J. P. & Swart, A. M. (1993). Preliminary analysis of the Concorde trial. *Lancet*, **341**, 889–90.

Areneta, M. C. Young, M. A. & Pierce, P. (1990). Natural history of HIV disease in an urban cohort of women (abstract FB 432). San Francisco: VIth International Conference on AIDS.

Batalla, J., Gatell, J., Cayla, J. A., Plasencia, A., Jansa, J. M. & Parellada, N. (1989). Predictors of the survival of AIDS in Barcelona, Spain. *AIDS*, **3**, 355–9.

Benedetti, P., Greco, D., Figoli, F. & Tirelli, U. (1991). Epidemic Kaposi's sarcoma in female AIDS patients – a report of 23 Italian cases. *AIDS*, **5**, 466–7.

Beral, V., Peterman, T. A., Berkelman, R. L. & Jaffe, H. W. (1990). Kaposi's sarcoma among persons with AIDS; a sexually transmitted infection. *Lancet*, **335**, 123–8.

Buehler, J., Farizo, K. & Berkelman, R. (1991). The spectrum of HIV disease in women (abstract MD 4253). Florence: VIIth International Conference on AIDS.

Byrne, M. A., Taylor-Robinson, D., Munday, P. E. & Harris, J. R. W. (1989). The common occurrence of human papillomavirus infection and intraepithelial neoplasia in women infected by HIV. *AIDS*, **3**, 379–82.

Carpenter, C. C. J., Mayer, K. H., Stein, M. D., Leibman, B. D., Fisher, A. & Fiore, T. C. (1991). HIV in North American women: experience with 200 cases and a review of the literature. *Medicine*, **70**, 307–25.

Centers for Disease Control (1987). Revision of the CDC surveillance case definition for AIDS. *Morbidity and Mortality Weekly Report*, **36**, 15–135.

Danila, R., Jones, D., Reier, D., Thomas, J., Osterholm, M. & MacDonald, K. (1990). A comparison of statewide Minnesota HIV/AIDS surveillance data with a population-based HIV seroprevalence study of childbearing women in Minnesota (abstract FC 569). San Francisco: VIth International Conference on AIDS.

Friedland, G. H., Saltzman, B., Vileno, J., Freeman, K., Schrager, L. K. & Klein, R. S. (1991). Survival differences in patients with AIDS. *Journal of Acquired Immune Deficiency Syndromes*, **4**, 144–53.

Gilks, G. F., Brindle, R. J., Otieno, L. S., *et al.* (1990). Life-threatening bacteraemia in HIV-1 seropositive adults admitted to hospital in Nairobi, Kenya. *Lancet*, **336**, 545–9.

Hessol, N. A., Byers, R. H., Lifson, A. R., *et al.* (1990). Relationship between AIDS latency period and AIDS survival time in homosexual and bisexual men. *Journal of Acquired Immune Deficiency Syndromes*, **3**, 1078–85.

The Italian Seroconversion Study (1992). Disease progression and early predictors of AIDS in HIV seroconverted injecting drug users. *AIDS*, **6**, 421–26.

Klein, R. S. & Motyl, M. (1993). Frequency of pulmonary tuberculosis in patients undergoing sputum induction for diagnosis of suspected *Pneumocystis carinii* pneumonia. *AIDS*, **7**, 1351–5.

Lassoud, K., Clauvel, J. P., Fegeux, S., Matheron, S., Gorin, I. & Oksenhendler, E. (1991). AIDS associated Kaposi's sarcoma in female patients. *AIDS*, **5**, 877–80.

Lau, R. K. W., Hill, A., Jenkins, P. *et al.* (1992). Eight year prospective study of HIV infection in a cohort of homosexual men: clinical progression, immunological and virological markers. *International Journal of STD and AIDS*, **3**, 261–6.

Lemp, G. F., Payne, S. F., Neal, D., Temelso, T. & Rutherford, G. W. (1990). Survival trends for patients with AIDS. *Journal of the American Medical Association*, **263**, 402–6.

Lindan, C. P., Allen, S., Serufilira, A., *et al.* (1992). Predictors of mortality among HIV infected women in Kigali, Rwanda. *Annals of Internal Medicine*, **116**, 320–8.

Mandelblatt, J. S., Fahs, M., Garibaldi, K., Senie, R. T. & Peterson, H. B. (1992). Association between HIV infection and cervical neoplasia: implications for clinical care of women at-risk for both conditions. *AIDS*, **6**, 173–8.

Morlat, P., Parneix, P., Douard, D., *et al.* (1992). Women and HIV infection; a cohort study of 483 HIV infected women in Bordeaux, France 1985–91. *AIDS*, **6**, 1187–93.

Moss, A. R. & Bacchetti, P. (1989). Natural history of HIV infection. *AIDS*, **3**, 55–61.

Peltier, J. Y., Lambin, P., Doinel, C., Couroucé, A. M., Rouger, P. & Lefrère, J. J. (1991). Frequency and prognostic importance of thrombocytopenia in symptom-free HIV infected individuals: a 5 year prospective study. *AIDS*, **5**, 381–4.

Peters, B. S., Beck, E. J., Coleman, D. G., *et al.* (1991). Changing disease patterns in patients with AIDS in a referral centre in the United Kingdom: the changing face of AIDS. *British Medical Journal*, **302**, 203–7.

Polsky, B., Gold, J. W., Whimbey, E., *et al.* (1986). Bacterial pneumonia in patients with the acquired immunodeficiency syndrome. *Annals of Internal Medicine*, **104**, 38–41.

Raffi, F., Brisseau, J. M., Planchon Rémi, J. P., Barrier, J. H. & Grolleau, J. Y. (1991). Endocrine function in 98 HIV infected patients: a prospective study. *AIDS*, **5**, 729–33.

Rothenberg, R., Woelfel, M., Stoneburner, R., Milberg, J., Parker, R. & Truman, B. (1987). Survival with the acquired immunodeficiency syndrome. *New England Journal of Medicine*, **317**, 1297–302.

Rutherford, G. W., Lifson, A. R., Hessol, N. A., *et al.* (1990). Course of HIV-1 infection in a cohort of homosexual and bisexual men: an 11 year follow up study. *British Medical Journal*, **301**, 1183–8.

Selwyn, P. A., Feingold, A. R., Hartel, D., *et al.* (1988). Increased risk of bacterial pneumonia in HIV-infected intravenous drug users without AIDS. *AIDS*, **2**, 267–72.

Selwyn, P. A., Alcabes, P., Hartel, D., *et al.* (1992). Clinical manifestations and predictors of disease progression in drug users with HIV infection. *New England Journal of Medicine*, **327**, 1697–703.

Serraino, D., Zaccarelli, M., Franceschi, S. & Greco, D. (1992). The epidemiology of AIDS-associated Kaposi's sarcoma in Italy. *AIDS*, **6**, 1015–19.

Simberkoff, M. S., El-Sadr, W., Schiffman, G. & Rahal, J. J. Jr. (1984). *Streptococcus pneumoniae* infections and bacteremia in patients with acquired immune deficiency syndrome, with report of a pneumococcal vaccine failure. *American Review of Respiratory Disease*, **130**, 1174–6.

Smith, E. & Orholm, M. (1990). Trends and patterns of opportunistic diseases in Danish AIDS patients 1980–90. *Scandinarian Journal of Infectious Diseases*, **22**, 665–72.

Stoneburner, R. L., Des Jarlais, D. C., Benezra, D., *et al.* (1989). A larger spectrum of severe HIV-1 related disease in intravenous drug users in New York City. *Science*, **242**, 916–18.

Thompson, M., Whyte, B., Morris, A., Rimland, D. & Thompson, S. (1991). Gender differences in the spectrum of HIV disease in Atlanta (abstract ME 3115). Florence: VIIth International Conference on AIDS.

Willocks, L., Cowan, F. M., Brettle, R. P., MacCallum, L. R., McHardy, S. & Richardson, A. (1991). Early HIV infection in Scottish women (abstract MB 2433). Florence: VIIth International Conference on AIDS.

8

Issues related to pregnancy

FRANK D. JOHNSTONE

Introduction

HIV infection is now a common medical problem in pregnancy in many parts of the world. There are few purely obstetric issues and pregnancy management is dominated by effective communication, up-to-date knowledge, and expertise in the care of HIV disease (see Addenda, p. 154).

Antenatal HIV testing

Despite greater public awareness, and increased availability of HIV testing, most asymptomatic HIV-infected women probably remain undiagnosed and unaware of their infected status. Thus, in Southeast England only 17% of infected women are identified antenatally (Ades *et al.*, 1993).

There are definite advantages for the infected woman in discovering her infection status. The knowledge allows her to make informed decisions about pregnancy planning; she can take steps to protect a non-infected sexual partner; prophylaxis for *Pneumocystis Carinii* pneumonia (PCP) and antiretroviral treatment can be started at the optimal time; transmission to the baby can be minimised by avoiding breastfeeding; and the knowledge allows her infant to be monitored. However, there are also disadvantages. The knowledge may disrupt her sexual relationship, can result in depression and difficulty in coping, and if her status becomes more widely known discrimination and ostracism can occur. Because the issues are complex, most testing programmes require careful pre-test counselling and fully informed consent.

The balance of advantage/disadvantage in testing is likely to change in future with more effective treatment of established infection in mother and child and the possibility that intervention during pregnancy will substantially reduce the risk of vertical transmission. There will

Table 8.1. *Higher risks in pregnant women indicating the offer of selective testing, and counselling before HIV testing*

The woman herself:
Has a history of drug use, and injected drugs at any time since 1977
Has had sex at any time since 1977 with men from countries with high
   endemic HIV rates (especially sub-Saharan Africa)
Has a history of prostitution
Has particular anxieties about HIV positivity

The woman believes that her current partner, or any previous sexual partner:
Has a history of drug use, and injected drugs at any time since 1977
Is known to have HIV or AIDS
Has had sex with other men at any time since 1977
Is haemophiliac
Has had sex at any time since 1977 with women from countries with high
   endemic HIV rates (especially sub-Saharan Africa)

---

then be a very strong case for universal named testing and the ethical issues surrounding refusal of testing, where perceived needs of mother and child may differ, will be complicated. This scenario emphasises the need for health planners to be sensitive to changing perspectives in the development of the epidemic and in improvements in prevention and treatment.

The main issues to be discussed in pre-test counselling have been well described (Holman, 1992; Sherr, 1993). Although it is sometimes suggested that counselling should not be dependent on assessment of risk, in practice this is unrealistic. Where women are at higher risk (Table 8.1) detailed discussion is required. Some of the issues which may be raised are listed in Table 8.2. Where such a woman does test positive it is important that the main issues have been mentioned beforehand. For the low-risk population, the logistics of time and cost demand a simpler approach to counselling, with written material and a brief interactive discussion (Boyd, 1990; McCarthy *et al.*, 1992; Goldberg & Johnstone, 1992). Topics which should be briefly covered include the risk factors associated with HIV infection, behaviour which protects against transmission of HIV, the advantages and disadvantages of testing for mother and baby, current local prevalence in pregnant women, and the offer of more detailed counselling. The necessity for informed consent remains. Women at higher risk should be reviewed in person, and without delay, specifically to discuss their HIV test result. For women assessed as being at low risk in low-prevalence areas, the arrangement can be made to give the result at their next antenatal appointment, or, if negative, by post.

Table 8.2. *Issues covered in pretest counselling*

Information
Explanation of HIV infection and its relationship to AIDS
Modes of HIV transmission
Sexual and drug-related risk reduction behaviours
The purpose of HIV antibody testing
The meaning of HIV antibody test results
The importance of knowing one's HIV antibody status, particularly with regard
    to treatment, pregnancy and perinatal transmission
The disadvantages of knowing HIV seropositivity, including ineligibility for
    many life insurance schemes
Local prevalence of HIV in pregnant women; if appropriate, within the specific
    risk group

Test results
Arrangements made for giving her the test results (see text)
Equivocal results, and the possible need to repeat the test
Documentation of a test result, confidentiality, and the sharing of information
    with other health professionals

Assessment of the patient
Who are the supportive people in her life?
If HIV positive who would she confide in? Who would be supportive and keep
    her confidence?
How has she generally reacted to stressful situations?
How does she think she might deal with a positive test result?

Partly from Holman (1992).

The effect of pregnancy on maternal HIV disease

Concern has been expressed about possible adverse effects of pregnancy
on the progression of disease in the mother. Some of the reasons for concern are shown in Table 8.3. However, many of the observations could be
explained in alternative ways: a subset of women at particularly high risk
may have been identified, reduction in blood CD4 count may simply represent redistribution to tissues, early reports of fatalities may represent
reporting bias, and the observed gender effect could be attributed to
women's lack of economic power to access health care.

Most studies have methodological limitations. Nevertheless the balance
of evidence from many sources compels the belief that pregnancy at least
does not have a major effect on HIV disease. This area has been well
reviewed (Brettle, 1992; Mandelbrot & Henrion, 1993). Thus, no gender
effect has emerged in several natural history cohort studies (Downs *et al.*,
1990; Dorrucci *et al.*, 1992). Although there are conflicting reports, most
studies have not shown clear differences in clinical outcomes or presence
of adverse prognostic markers; and recent controlled studies directed at

Table 8.3. *Some reasons why pregnancy has been postulated as a possible adverse factor in the progression of HIV*

Follow-up of women who had delivered children who had developed AIDS showed a high progression rate in these women (Scott *et al.*, 1985; Minkoff *et al.*, 1987)
Pregnancy may have an adverse effect on many infectious diseases, viral and non-viral (Weinberg, 1984; Brabin, 1985)
Pregnancy alters cell-mediated immunity; and in particular blood CD4 count falls in early pregnancy (Johnstone *et al.*, 1994)
All early reports of AIDS in pregnancy were of fatalities (reviewed in Johnstone *et al.*, 1992)
Initial reports from the USA suggested a gender effect on survival time, worse for females (Rothenberg *et al.*, 1987)
Pregnancy could result in delay in diagnosis of opportunistic infection or could contribute to less aggressive prophylaxis, investigation or treatment

the rate of fall of CD4 counts in individual women have not shown any long-term effect of pregnancy (Weedon *et al.*, 1993).

However, further research is required, and it remains possible that pregnancy may have some (small) adverse effect. In addition, even if pregnancy does not have a major effect it must be remembered that women with bad prognostic markers or advanced HIV disease are at high risk of short-term deterioration, pregnant or not, and death around pregnancy carries additional consequences for the fetus or child.

Vertical transmission

Transmission from mother to child has been estimated to be 15–20% in Europe, 25–30% in Africa and 16–30% in the USA (see Chapter 1). Much of the variation in transmission rates is related to population differences. The timing of transmission is of key contemporary interest. Whilst there is no doubt that transmission can occur *in utero*, intrapartum or post-natally, the relative contribution of each of these routes remains unknown. However, it has been suggested that much transmission may occur around the time of delivery and this is based largely on two lines of indirect evidence. The first is the demonstration that the number of babies found at birth to be HIV infected is low, with a higher rate weeks or months later (Ehrnst *et al.*, 1991; Krivine *et al.*, 1992). However, this could be due to decreased sensitivity where small volumes of blood are used from newborns, or could relate to the fact that only after birth is the baby subject to antigenic stimulation, and hence only then does significant HIV replication occur. The second line of evidence is based on the International Registry of HIV-exposed twins (Goedert *et al.*, 1991), which

showed a higher rate of infection among first-born twins. This was interpreted as indicating that a substantial proportion of HIV infection occurs
during passage through the birth canal. Increased recruitment of lymphocytes to the cervix as part of the preparation for spontaneous labour could
be a further factor.

Early studies showing transmission apparently due to breastfeeding
involved recent maternal seroconversion and the estimated risk in this
situation was 1 in 3. However, statistical review of the literature has concluded that even where the mother is infected before delivery, breastfeeding imposes an additional 14% risk of transmitting HIV to the baby (Dunn
et al., 1992) and a relationship with duration of breastfeeding has been
suggested (de Martino *et al.* 1992).

Many factors have been shown to relate to vertical transmission. However, few have consistently emerged as risk variables and it seems likely
that multiple factors relating to maternal viral load, viral type, maternal
antibody response, fetal resistance including HLA and other genotype, placental damage including chorioamnionitis, other maternal infections,
interventions around delivery, gestation, length of membrane rupture, and
breastfeeding all inter-relate in a complex fashion (see Chapter 1).

Infectivity is generally believed to relate to viraemia, with high levels of
virus and high infectivity at primary infection (Hague *et al.*, 1993) and in
advanced disease. This may be reflected in immunological and virological
surrogates such as CD4 or p24 antigenaemia. However, the predictive
power of individual clinical and laboratory markers is not high. Studies on
levels of antibody to epitopes on the hypervariable V3 loop of gp120 have
produced conflicting results (Goedert *et al.*, 1989; Parekh *et al.*, 1991)
and infection does seem to have occurred despite high maternal levels of
antibodies. There may be an association with chorioamnionitis (Ryder *et
al.*, 1989). Fetal genotype may be important, with one small study finding
HLA DR3 to be 3 times more common in infected infants (Kilpatrick *et
al.*, 1991) while another reported that susceptibility to HIV infection was
related to genetic variation in HLA immune response genes (Just *et al.*,
1991).

Obstetric factors which could influence transmission are shown in
Table 8.4, though there is little information which allows assessment of
their significance. Interestingly, preterm delivery before 34 weeks was
associated with a doubling of risk in the European Collaborative Study
(1992), possibly because of lower levels of passively transferred maternal
antibodies at early gestations. Length of time between rupture of the membranes and delivery has been related to transmission (Ciraru *et al.*, 1993).

Major current interest surrounds the possible protective effect of elective
caesarean section. In theory, this could be protective by minimising the

Table 8.4. *Obstetric factors which could influence*
vertical transmission

Antenatal
Chorion villus sampling
Amniocentesis
Placental biopsy
Cordocentesis
Antibiotic prophylaxis (e.g. co-trimoxazole)
Antiretroviral drugs[b]
New interventions

Delivery
Premature delivery[a]
Premature spontaneous rupture of the membranes[a]
Duration of labour
Artificial rupture of the membranes[a]
Elective caesarean section[a]
Scalp electrode[a]
Fetal blood sampling[a]
Forceps delivery
Episiotomy
New interventions

After delivery
Early cord clamping
Early washing of the baby
Breastfeeding[b]

[a] Some evidence of an effect or association.
[b] Proven effect or association.

time the baby is exposed to cervical mucus and maternal blood. Prospective studies have generally reported lower rates of infection after a caesarean section delivery (see Chapter 1).

The interim analysis of the zidovudine (AZT) prophylaxis trial (ACTG 076), which shows reduction of vertical transmission from 25% to 8%, appears to open up new scope for prevention (see Chapter 1).

The effect of HIV infection on pregnancy outcome

Studies in the developed world have not shown convincing evidence of important effects of HIV infection on pregnancy outcome. This may be due in part to the small number of cases studied. The much larger studies of outcome from Africa have potential intrinsic problems of bias due to associated adverse factors in cases compared with controls. Nevertheless, several studies attempt to deal with this, and despite different methodological designs, all report reduction in birthweight associated with maternal HIV infection. However, this reduction is relatively modest (around 150 g). Results from a case–control study in Nairobi, Kenya (Temmerman *et al.*, 1992) suggested increased risks of preterm delivery and of intrauterine and intrapartum death, but this has not been found in all African studies. There may be important related factors operating in some areas, such as the load of other infectious disease, especially tuberculosis and malaria, and low nutritional status. On present evidence it seems most plausible that when women are asymptomatic and not significantly immunocompromised, HIV infection *per se* does not have a major effect on pregnancy outcome. It seems inevitable that advancing maternal disease, other infections and deteriorating nutritional status will have a detrimental effect on pregnancy, and there are some data suggesting that this is so (European Collaborative Study, 1994).

Antenatal care

A major interruption of vertical transmission will occur with a reduction in the number of women becoming infected with HIV, or if those infected decide against pregnancy or choose pregnancy termination. For women who continue pregnancy an important principle of antenatal care is a multi-disciplinary approach between the pregnant HIV-infected woman, obstetric and midwifery staff, community care staff and physicians with expertise for both mother and child. Individuals with particular skills can then be involved as required. While this skill mix offers many advantages and opportunities to the pregnant woman it also carries the risk of conveying different, partially confusing messages, and can involve duplication of effort. There is therefore an obligation on such a team to maintain effective communication with each other as well as with the woman.

Investigations which might be done at first contact are shown in Table 8.5. CD4 lymphocyte count is the single most important predictor of HIV disease progression. It should be remembered that in early normal pregnancy there is a fall in blood CD4 count and also that there is a diurnal variation, with a nadir in late morning. In individuals, counts may change suddenly and opportunistic infections can occur at higher than expected counts. Nevertheless, in general practical terms, opportunistic infection is very unlikely with a CD4 count greater than 300 per mm^3. For these women regular detailed physical examination is probably not necessary and medical surveillance may be restricted to retesting of CD4 count and full blood count every 3 months, with prompt investigation of any suspicious symptoms. Where CD4 count is less than 200 per mm^3 opportunistic infection becomes more likely. The count should be confirmed 1 week later. The significance both in terms of her own life expectancy and

Table 8.5 *Investigations which may be appropriate depending on local laboratory facilities and local levels of disease*

Routine
Full blood count
Rubella serology
Syphilis serology
Blood group
Screening for bacteriuria

Assessment of HIV disease
CD4 lymphocyte count (% and absolute)
p24 antigen
p24 antibody titre
β_2-microglobulin
Neopterin

Baseline titres of conditions which may affect the fetus
Hepatitis B or C
Cytomegalovirus
Toxoplasmosis

Screening for other related maternal disease
Mantoux test
Other sexually transmitted disease
Cervical cytology/colposcopy

the likelihood of an increased risk of vertical transmission must be discussed with the woman, who may reconsider her decision to proceed with the pregnancy. She should learn to recognise symptoms which might be important and which might demand investigation (Table 8.6) and she should be recommended to take PCP prophylaxis. Co-trimoxazole 960 mg once daily is probably the prophylaxis of choice. Although there are theoretical concerns about this drug, no adverse effects have been firmly attributed to its use in pregnancy. Dapsone may be a safe second-line drug,

Table 8.6. *Some symptoms which susceptible HIV-infected women should be asked to report, or which may prompt full clinical and laboratory search for HIV disease*

Fever
Night sweats
Difficulty or pain on swallowing
Headache
Cough
Shortness of breath
Visual disturbance
Diarrhoea

judging by experience in leprosy patients, but there is little information relating specifically to pregnant HIV-infected women. For women unable to take these drugs, monthly nebulised pentamidine remains an alternative. It is not routine practice to offer chemoprophylaxis against other opportunistic infection.

The main antiretroviral drug, zidovudine, reaches concentrations in the fetus similar to those in the mother, although its effect on the fetus is not known. In a retrospective series of 43 women who had received zidovudine during pregnancy, Sperling *et al.* (1992) found no association with malformations, premature delivery or fetal distress. However, existing data are insufficient to allow a firm base for recommendations about zidovudine use in pregnancy, and this remains an area for case-by-case individual discussion. This gap in information is being filled by a continuing randomised, placebo-controlled trial (ACTG 076), and the first interim efficacy analysis shows a reduction in vertical transmission in women who were given active treatment (Sperling, 1993; Chapter 1).

Apart from the surveillance of HIV disease, antenatal care for the HIV-infected woman is not greatly different from standard obstetric practice. Where women are current injecting drug users or have particularly disadvantaged social circumstances, attention should be paid to recognition of intrauterine growth retardation. Attempts should be made to prevent preterm labour, especially in view of the apparently higher transmission risk at this time. Apart from infectious complications, pregnancy problems generally do not seem to be more frequent in HIV-infected women. Much attention therefore focuses on communication, and on ensuring that the system of antenatal care is sympathetic and geared to the needs of the individual patient.

The belief that a high proportion of transmission occurs around delivery is encouraging as far as prevention is concerned, and several approaches to interventions have been suggested. The interim analysis of the trial on AZT prophylaxis (ACTG 076) has introduced a new and important subject for discussion (see Chapter 1).

Delivery

There are few substantial differences in obstetric management of the HIV-infected woman. She has the same needs and should have access to the same care as other women. However, a key issue is the suggestion that a high proportion of vertical transmission may occur around delivery. This in turn has raised the possibility that elective caesarean section or antiviral treatment, systemically or vaginally, might be protective. At present, evidence is inconclusive and it is premature to make firm recommendations.

The general belief is that mode of delivery should continue to be indicated by obstetric factors, perhaps with HIV infection as a relative indicator in some circumstances. However, this opinion will have to be reviewed with each patient in the light of accumulating evidence.

Where delivery is by caesarean section, there are possible, largely untested, modifications of technique which could minimise exposure of the baby to maternal blood, such as stapling or suturing large vessels in the lower segment incision and delivering the baby within intact membranes as much as possible. Although there are no conclusive data, it seems appropriate to interfere as little as possible during labour. Thus, it is reasonable to leave the membranes intact and to avoid scalp electrodes or scalp sampling. With modern external monitoring techniques there should be adequate surveillance of the fetus without artificial rupture of the membranes. Furthermore, this technique has not been shown to have clear obstetric advantages (Barrett *et al.*, 1992). This policy in turn has a bearing on any decision to induce labour, which itself can increase other interventions. However, theoretical risks of HIV transmission have to be weighed in the context of standard optimal obstetric management. Thus the theoretical possibility that there might be a small increased risk of transmission with forceps delivery and episiotomy should not be a reason to delay delivery of a baby showing signs of fetal distress.

Other procedures which might be considered are early cord clamping, which conceivably could reduce the risk of maternal cells gaining access to the fetal circulation as the placenta detaches, and early bathing of the baby to minimise the time maternal blood is in contact with the baby's body surface. Although it is unlikely that evidence of the value of early bathing of the baby will emerge, this intuitively seems correct care for the term baby.

Post partum

The postnatal period is another time when further interactive discussion may be helpful. Women in developed countries where bottlefeeding is relatively safe should be advised against breastfeeding (Dunn *et al.*, 1992), but the balance of risk may be different in other situations where breastfeeding should continue to be promoted as offering infants the optimum chances for survival (see Chapter 1). The woman should be encouraged to hug and kiss the baby in the knowledge that this will not transmit HIV infection. She may need to acquire confidence in her ability to care for the infant and knowledge of contact which could and could not be of possible risk to the baby. This is a useful time to review arrangements for follow-up of mother and baby, to answer questions about the baby at-risk of HIV disease and to discuss contraception. Although to the obstetrician the delivery of the baby may seem to be the end of the process, to the woman, her general practitioner and the community carers, it is a beginning. That is why it is so important that care during the pregnancy is supportive, multi-disciplinary, and largely based in the community (see Chapter 9).

Infection control procedures

There is a very small, but not negligible, risk of transmission of infection to staff and potentially to other patients when dissemination of blood-stained body fluid occurs around delivery or postpartum. Therefore, in general terms, no reasonably avoidable personal contact with blood-stained fluid should be allowed to occur. This is the basis for a high level of universally applied infection control standards. Basic precautions to avoid exposure are shown in Table 8.7 and particular issues in obstetrics have been well dealt with in the Royal College of Obstetricians and Gynaecologists report (RCOG, 1990).

Segregation of the HIV-positive woman after delivery is not necessary, but she should be counselled about sensible precautions, including the handling of lochia and pads. Most hospitals do not have personal toilet facilities and meticulous cleaning of any contamination with lochia is essential. She should avoid handling other women's babies.

The debate about whether particular precautions should be universal or selective will continue, though it seems clear that some intermediate position will be adopted by most health care workers (Joint Working Party, 1992). What is often not stressed is that the infected woman should not be subjected to any unnecessary and discriminatory infection control procedures which could isolate her or draw attention to her before other patients or relatives.

The future

There are likely to be important advances in the treatment of HIV infection over the next few years and, in particular, more information will become available about prevention of vertical transmission. Prognostic indicators, for both maternal survival and transmission, should become more precise. Increased identification of infected mothers with improvements in organisation of care, optimal timing of initiation of treatment and advances in treatment should combine to ensure much longer survival with a better quality of life.

Table 8.7. *Ways to avoid exposure to HIV and hepatitis in all departments*

Apply basic hygiene practices with regular handwashing
Cover existing wounds and skin lesions with waterproof dressings
Take simple protective measures to avoid contamination of person and clothing
  with blood
Protect mucous membranes of eyes, mouth and nose from blood splashes
Take care to prevent wounds, cuts and abrasions in the presence of blood
Avoid use of sharps whenever possible
Ensure safe handling and disposal of sharps
Clear spillages of blood promptly and disinfect surfaces
Ensure safe disposal of contaminated water

Precautions recommended for staff performing invasive procedures in all
patients
Have vaccination against hepatitis B
Cover all cuts and abrasions with waterproof dressings
Do not pass sharps hand to hand
Do not use hand needles
Do not guide needles with fingers
Do not resheath needles
Dispose of all sharps safely into approved containers
Put disposables and waste into yellow clinical waste bags for incineration

Additional precautions when caring for known HIV and hepatitis B virus
positive and high-risk patients
Consider non-operative management
Remove unnecessary equipment from theatre
Observe highest level of theatre discipline
Have only experienced surgeons and health care workers in theatre
Use: double glove, high efficiency masks, eye protection, boots, impervious
  gowns, closed wound bandage
Use disposable anaesthetic circuitry or appropriate method of decontamination
Disinfect theatre floor with hypochlorite (refer to local policies)

From Joint Working Party (1992).

Acknowledgements

This chapter has been influenced by many sources but particularly the guidelines for the Management of HIV-positive pregnant women suggested by a working party of the Royal College of Obstetricians and Gynaecologists and Midwives, chaired by Professor C. M. Hudson, and also the Report from Danielle Mercey, Susan Bewley and Peter Brocklehurst. I am grateful to AVERT for research support.

References

Ades, A. E., Davison, C. F., Holland, F. J., *et al.* (1993). Vertically transmitted HIV infection in the British Isles. *British Medical Journal*, **306**; 1296–9.

Barrett, J. F. R., Savage, J, Phillipps, K. & Lilford, R. J. (1992). Randomised trial of amniotomy in labour versus the intention to leave membranes intact until the second stage. *British Journal of Obstetrics and Gynaecology,* **99,** 5–9.

Boyd, K. M., (1990). HIV infection: the ethics of anonymised testing and of testing pregnant women. *Journal of Medical Ethics,* **16;** 173–8.

Brabin, B. J., (1985). Epidemiology of infection in pregnancy. *Reviews of Infectious Diseases,* **7,** 579–603.

Brettle, R. P., (1992). Pregnancy and its effect on HIV/AIDS. In: HIV, infection in obstetrics and gynaecology, ed. F. D. Johnstone. *Baillières Clinical Obstetrics and Gynaecology,* **6,** 125–36.

Ciraru, N., Lefevre, V., Lepage, E. & Ravina, J. H., (1993). Obstetrical risk factors in HIV-I vertical transmission (abstract). *Pediatric AIDS and HIV Infection,* **4,** 304.

de Martino, M., Tovo, P-A., Tozzi, A. E., *et al.* (1992). HIV transmission through breastmilk, appraisal of risk according to duration of feeding. *AIDS,* **6,** 991–7.

Dorrucci, M., Rezza, G., Pezzotti, P., *et al.* (1992). Age accelerates the progression from HIV-seroconversion to AIDS in women (abstract MoC0033). Amsterdam: VIIIth International Conference on AIDS.

Downs, A. M., Ancelle-Park, R. A. & Brunet, J. B. (1990). Surveillance of AIDS in the European Community: recent trends and predictions to 1991. *AIDS,* **4,** 1117–24.

Dunn, D. T., Newell, M. L., Ades, A. E. & Peckham, C. S. (1992). Risk of human immunodeficiency virus type 1 transmission through breastfeeding. *Lancet,* **340,** 585–588.

Ehrnst, A., Lindgren, S., Dictor, M., *et al.* (1991). HIV in pregnant women and their offspring: Evidence for late transmission. *Lancet,* **338,** 203–7.

European Collaborative Study (1992). Risk factors for mother-to-child transmission of HIV-1. *Lancet,* **339,** 1007–12.

European Collaborative Study (1994). Perinatal findings in children born to HIV-infected mothers. *British Journal of Obstetrics and Gynaecology,* **101,** 136–41.

Goedert, J. J., Mendez, H., Drummond, J. E., *et al.* (1989). Mother-to-infant transmission of human immunodeficiency virus type 1: association with prematurity or low anti-gp 120. *Lancet,* **ii,** 1351–4.

Goedert, J. J., Duliege, A. M., Amos, C. I., Felton, S., & Biggar, R. J., (1991). High risk of HIV-1 infection for first-born twins. The International Registry of HIV-exposed twins. *Lancet,* **338:** 1471–5.

Goldberg, D. & Johnstone, F. D. (1992). HIV testing programmes in pregnancy. In: HIV infection in obstetrics and gynaecology, ed. F. D. Johnstone. *Baillières Clinical Obstetrics and Gynaecology,* **3,** 33–51.

Hague, R. A., Mok, J. Y. Q., Johnstone, F. D., *et al.* (1993). Maternal factors in HIV transmission. *International Journal of STD and AIDS,* **4,** 142–6.

Holman, S. (1992). HIV counselling for women of reproductive age, In: HIV infection in obstetrics and gynaecology, ed. F. D. Johnstone. *Baillières Clinical Obstetrics and Gynaecology,* **6,** 53–68.

Joint Working Party of the Hospital Infection Society and the Surgical Infection Study Group (1992). Risks to surgeons and patients from HIV and hepatitis; guidelines on precautions and management of exposure to blood or body fluids. *British Medical Journal,* **305,** 1337–43.

Johnstone, F. D., Willocks, L. & Brettle, R. P. (1992). Survival time after AIDS in pregnancy. *British Journal of Obstetrics and Gynaecology*, **99**, 633–6.

Johnstone, F. D., Thong, K. J., Bird, A. G. & Whitelaw J. (1994). Lymphocyte sub-populations in early human pregnancy. *Obstetrics and Gynecology*, **83**, 941–6.

Just, J., Louie, L., Abrams, E., *et al.* (1991). Genetic risk factors for perinatally acquired HIV infection (abstract MC3044). Florence: VIIth International Conference on AIDS.

Kilpatrick, D. S., Hague, R. A., Yap, P. L. & Mok, J. Y. Q. (1991). HLA antigen frequencies in children born to HIV-infected mothers. *Disease Markers*, **8**, 1–6.

Krivine, A., Firtion, G., Francoval, C., Henrion, R. & Lebon, P. (1992). HIV replication during the first weeks of life. *Lancet*, **339**, 1187–9.

McCarthy, K. H., Johnston, M. A. & Studd J. W. W. (1992). Antenatal HIV testing. *British Journal of Obstetrics and Gynaecology*, **99**, 867–8.

Mandelbrot, L. & Henrion, R. (1993). Does pregnancy accelerate disease progression in HIV-infected women? In *HIV Infection in Women*, ed. M. A. Johnson & F. D. Johnstone, pp. 157–71. Edinburgh: Churchill Livingstone.

Minkoff, H. L., Nanda, D., Menez, R., *et al.* (1987). Follow-up of mothers and children with AIDS. *Obstetrics and Gynecology*, **87**, 288–91.

Parekh, B. S., Shaffer, N., Pau, C. P., *et al.* (1991). Lack of correlation between maternal antibodies to V3 loop peptides of gp 120 and perinatal HIV-1 transmission. *AIDS*, **5**, 1179–84.

Rothenberg, R., Woelfel, M., Stoneburner, R., *et al.* (1987). Survival with the acquired immunodeficiency syndrome. Experience with 5833 cases in New York City. *New England Journal of Medicine*, **317**, 1297–302.

Royal College of Obstetricians and Gynaecologists (1990). HIV infection in maternity care and gynaecology. Revised report of the RCOG sub-committee on problems associated with AIDS in relation to obstetrics and gynaecology. London: RCOG.

Ryder, R. W., Nsa, W., Hassig, S. E., *et al.* (1989). Perinatal transmission of the human immunodeficiency virus type 1 to infants of seropositive women in Zaire. *New England Journal of Medicine*, **320**, 1637–42.

Ryder, R. W., Nsa, W., Hassig, S. E., *et al.* (1992). Intrauterine onset of symptomatic HIV disease (abstract PoC4734). Amsterdam: VIIIth International Conference on AIDS.

Scott, G. B., Fischl, M. A., Klimas, N., *et al.* (1985). Mothers of infants with the acquired immunodeficiency syndrome. Evidence for both symptomatic and asymptomatic carriers. *Journal of the American Medical Association*, **253**, 363–6.

Sherr, L. (1993). Counselling around HIV testing in women of reproductive age. In *HIV Infection Women*, ed. M. A. Johnson & F. D. Johnstone pp. 17–35. Edinburgh: Churchill Livingstone.

Sperling, R. S., Stratton, P., O'Sullivan, M. J., *et al.* (1992). A survey of zidovudine use in pregnant women with human immunodeficiency virus infection. *New England Journal of Medicine*, **326**, 857–61.

Sperling, R. (1993). Prophylaxis and treatment during pregnancy. In *HIV Infection in Women*, ed. F. D. Johnstone & M. A. Johnson, pp. 211–19. Edinburgh: Churchill Livingstone.

Temmermann, M., K'Oduol, T., Plummer, F. A., Ndinya-Achola, J. O. & Piot, P. (1992). Maternal HIV infection as a risk factor for adverse obstetrical outcome (abstract POC 4232 PC283). Amsterdam: VIIIth International Conference on AIDS.

Weedon, J., Machelle, A. & Hutchison, S. (1993). Effect of pregnancy and HIV on CD4 count in women (abstract). *Pediatric AIDS and HIV Infection*, **4**, 312.

Weinberg, E. D. (1984). Pregnancy-associated depression of cell-mediated immunity. *Reviews of Infectious Diseases*, **6**, 814–31.

Addenda

Following the report on the ACTG 076 randomised placebo controlled trial of zidovudine (ZDV), many women are now being offered ZDV to reduce perinatal transmission of HIV (see Chapter 1).

Guidelines on the use of ZDV in pregnancy, specifically to reduce mother-to-child transmission, were issued in the USA after the reports of the 076 trial (see Chapters 1 and 2). This report discusses the limitations of the trial as well (Centers for Disease Control (1994). *Morbidity and Mortality Weekly Report*, **43**, RR11: 1–20).

For the results of the European Collaborative Study on mode of delivery see: European Collaborative Study (1994). Caesarean section and risk of vertical transmission of HIV-1 infection. *Lancet*, **343**, 1464–7.

This report is not based on a randomised trial, but efforts were made to assess confounding factors associated with transmission risk. Preliminary data from some observational prospective studies now show that there may be an association between length of time between rupture of membranes, or duration of labour, and risk of vertical transmission.

Further information is required before caesarean section can be generally recommended for all HIV-infected women. An international randomised trial has started to evaluate the effectiveness of an elective caesarean section in preventing perinatal transmission (for more information contact Dr Marie-Louise Newell at the Institute of Child Health in London, UK).

9

Follow-up of the child born to an HIV-infected woman

JACQUELINE Y. Q. MOK

Introduction

Children born to women with HIV infection usually come from areas of multiple deprivation, where access to health care and other services is limited. The follow-up of the child therefore requires close liaison between professionals working in different agencies. There is also a need for access to laboratory facilities for early diagnosis, preferably in a unit where the needs of the child and parents can be met. For these reasons the follow-up is best done in specialised multidisciplinary units, with the care shared between the specialist paediatrician, adult physician and obstetrician, working closely with general practitioners, general paediatricians and professionals based in the community. In many centres, this is best done in a 'family' clinic (Mok *et al.*, 1989*a*; Gibb & Walters, 1992).

The antenatal period

Pregnant women with HIV infection often want advice about the risk of mother-to-child transmission, the outlook for the infected child, as well as the likelihood of pregnancy affecting their own HIV disease. Follow-up of the baby is facilitated if the responsible paediatrician meets the woman in the antenatal period (see Chapter 8).

During this meeting, individually tailored advice can be given regarding the risk of vertical transmission, based on the mother's clinical status, immune function and laboratory parameters (see Chapter 1). The European Collaborative Study (1992) demonstrated that the risk of transmission is increased with advanced maternal disease, where the mother's CD4 count is below 700 cells/mm^3 and in the presence of p24 antigenaemia. The increased risk due to breastfeeding was also highlighted and, where safe alternatives exist, the woman should be advised against breastfeeding (WHO, 1992).

Table 9.1. *Points to discuss during antenatal counselling*

Transmission of HIV from mother to child: rate and risk factors
Mother's own health, immune function and virological tests
Advise against breastfeeding
Importance of close follow-up of infant
Early diagnosis and difficulties with tests
Outlook for the infected child
Psychosocial support
Coming to terms with the diagnosis
Who needs to know and why
Shortened maternal lifespan
HIV affected children
Liaison with obstetrician

The importance of close follow-up in the first 6 months of life should be emphasised, to allow an early diagnosis of HIV infection in the child to be made. Difficulties with diagnostic tests in a small infant should also be explained to the woman (see Chapter 5). The frequency of and venue for follow-up should be discussed at this stage.

Some women may discover their HIV status for the first time during the antenatal period. A referral should be made for psychosocial support, to help the woman come to terms with the diagnosis. Within the health care team, staff should be clear about which members should be told, and why. Most women recognise the need for the general practitioner to know, as well as the health visitor, so that trivial symptoms in the child can be treated appropriately. The wishes of the woman must be respected, and disclosure of her HIV status should only be done with her consent.

It may also be appropriate to discuss the fact that her own illness is likely to result in a shortened life span, so that although her infant may not be infected, she may not survive to see the child reach an independent age. Many women will already have thought about plans for alternative child care.

Liaison with the obstetrician is also important, to reinforce the message regarding unnecessary exposure to invasive procedures which might put the infant at-risk of HIV infection. Procedures such as amniocentesis, chorionic villus sampling and scalp monitoring should be avoided (see Chapter 8). Table 9.1 summarises the discussion points during antenatal counselling.

The neonatal period

It is unusual for AIDS to present in the newborn period. In the developed world, prospective studies of all infants born to HIV-infected women have documented that newborns who are subsequently found to be infected do not differ at birth from those who are not infected (Johnstone *et al.*, 1988; Selwyn *et al.*, 1989; Semprini *et al.*, 1990; European Collaborative Study, 1994). However, the infant should be seen in the first week of life to obtain baseline measurements of growth, clinical signs, immunological and virological parameters. The infant should be nursed in the newborn nursery with no special precautions unless medically indicated. Drug withdrawal symptoms, prematurity or intrauterine growth retardation may require special care facilities. It is important that infection control guidelines are not limited to those women and infants known to be HIV seropositive. All health care staff in the delivery room and newborn nursery should adopt a one-tier system of universal precautions, to protect themselves against untested, infected patients as well as other blood-borne infections.

The advice against breastfeeding should be reinforced. The paediatrician should be responsible for checking for mother's hepatitis B status and organise passive and active immunisation against hepatitis B for the infant if necessary. Other congenital infections, such as cytomegalovirus, should also be sought for.

The follow-up schedule for the infant should be planned with the mother, taking into account her wishes as to where she might like her infant to be seen. In some centres, home visits are offered and this increases compliance (Mok *et al.*, 1989a). If the child is seen in a specialist centre, the mother must be given clear guidelines as to whom to contact should the child become unwell. Good communication with the general practitioner or local paediatrician ensures that they are informed of the follow-up plans.

Table 9.2 summarises the action required in the neonatal period. The paediatrician must be receptive to the emotional state of the mother at all times, and refer her for counselling and support if necessary.

Immunisations and prophylaxis

Infants born to HIV-infected women should be offered the same immunisations as all children, at the usual ages and the same intervals. Theoretical arguments prevail as to why live vaccines should not be administered to individuals with HIV infection, but have not withstood results of retrospective reviews (McLaughlin *et al.*, 1988). With the exception of BCG, all other childhood live vaccines (polio, measles, mumps, rubella) are considered safe for HIV-infected children. BCG may be given to infants irrespective of their mother's HIV status, but should be withheld from children known to be HIV infected (Lallemant-Le Coeur *et al.*, 1991). BCG

Table 9.2. *Action required in the neonatal period*

Clinical examination of newborn
Venesection for:
   Full and differential blood count
   Hepatitis B serology
   HIV serology
   Virus culture
   p24 antigen   } If available
   Polymerase chain reaction in lymphocytes or plasma
   Immunoglobulin levels
Urine for cytomegalovirus isolation
Reinforce advice against breastfeeding
Offer passive and active immunisation against hepatitis B, if appropriate
Plan follow-up programme with mother, with clear lines of referral if baby
   becomes unwell
Refer for counselling and support if necessary

vaccination has resulted in disseminated infection in up to 30% of cases of primary immune T cell deficiency (Stephan *et al.*, 1993) and in some cases of HIV-infected children (CDC, 1986).

There have been no reports of increased adverse reactions to other live vaccines in children with HIV infection. In certain circumstances, inactivated polio vaccine should be administered because of the theoretical risk of transmission of the vaccine virus to other family members who may be immune deficient due to HIV infection. Experience from primary immune deficiency states suggests that oral attenuated poliovirus vaccination can lead to paralytic disease in contacts (Wyatt, 1973). Even if the parents are immune competent, it is prudent to advise stringent hand-washing after changing the baby's nappy, to minimise faeco-oral transmission of the vaccine virus.

In most countries in the developed world, children are also offered immunisation against *Haemophilus influenzae* type B (Hib), a major cause of meningitis. Children who are known to be HIV infected should receive the Hib vaccine at the usual times; also pneumococcal vaccine at 2 years, as they are particularly prone to recurrent respiratory infections with these organisms. Influenza vaccine should be offered at annual intervals in the autumn.

There is evidence in adults with HIV infection that immunisation with both protein and polysaccharide vaccines results in suboptimal responses, especially to new immunogens in the later stages of the disease (Amman *et al.*, 1984). There are strong arguments for completing the course of primary immunisations as early as is feasible, prior to the onset of immune dysfunction (Bernstein *et al.*, 1985; Borkowsky *et al.*, 1987). Even in early disease there is a failure to prime memory cell responses (Adamson *et al.*, 1989), especially to polysaccharide and protein antigens (Huang *et al.*, 1987). Despite documented immunisations, many infected children fail to mount an adequate antibody response, especially with the onset of immune deficiency. Minor bacterial and viral infections also contribute to significant morbidity, and immune modulatory therapy with intravenous immunoglobulins has been shown to have a beneficial effect in reducing viral infections as well as minor bacterial infections in children with CD4 counts of greater than 200 cells/mm³ (Mofenson *et al.*, 1992; Hague *et al.*, 1992; Molyneaux *et al.*, 1993).

Most argument has centred on the risks and benefits of the measles vaccine or the measles, mumps and rubella (MMR) vaccine. Initial recommendations were that these should be avoided in symptomatic children, along with other live vaccines (Immunisation Practices Advisory Committee, 1986). However, primary measles infection has been associated with severe or fatal disease in children infected with HIV (Krasinski & Borkowsky, 1989; Embree *et al.*, 1992). Subsequently, a retrospective review of HIV-infected children who had received measles immunisation identified no adverse reactions (McLaughlin *et al.*, 1988). Where there is a high prevalence of both HIV and measles infection, immunisation should continue. This is especially so for many parts of Africa, where the benefits outweigh the risks (Lepage *et al.*, 1992). United States guidelines have also been amended to take these considerations into account, and now recommend routine MMR immunisation in all children with HIV infection (Immunisation Practices Advisory Committee, 1988). Since immunisation will not be effective in all children, exposure to measles should also be followed by intramuscular administration of immunoglobulin, in the following doses: <1 year, 250 mg; 1–2 years, 500 mg; >3 years, 750 mg. Children who are symptomatic should receive zoster immunoglobulin (ZIg) following close contact with chickenpox. If varicella or zoster develops despite ZIg, then intravenous acyclovir should be commenced immediately (500 mg/m² per dose, three times a day).

PCP prophylaxis

Pneumocystis carinii pneumonia (PCP) is the most common AIDS indicator disease in HIV-infected children (see Chapters 3 and 4). It occurs most frequently in infants under 6 months of age, and has a high mortality (Bernstein *et al.*, 1989; Tovo *et al.*, 1992; Gibb *et al.*, 1994, European Collaborative Study, 1994). In many cases, the child presenting with an acute respiratory illness subsequently diagnosed to be PCP may be the first indication of AIDS in the family.

For these reasons, current recommendations are that children with HIV infection should be started on primary prophylaxis against PCP, based on the age-appropriate CD4 count (Centers for Disease Control, 1991). These recommendations rest on the strong association between low CD4 counts and the risk of PCP in homosexual men (Phair *et al.*, 1990). PCP has also been reported in children with CD4 counts well above that recommended for initiation of prophylaxis (Leibovitz *et al.*, 1990), which has prompted many paediatricians to commence prophylaxis as soon as a diagnosis of HIV infection is made, regardless of CD4 counts. Others would suggest that the high mortality of PCP in young infants justifies the regime of starting prophylaxis from three weeks of age, irrespective of the infection status, especially if the frequency of follow-up is likely to be suboptimal (Gibb & Walters, 1992).

The risk of PCP in children born to HIV-infected mothers depends on the probability of vertical transmission as well as the incidence of PCP in those infected children. The European Collaborative Study (1994) has examined data on 924 children followed prospectively, and found the cumulative incidence of PCP by 6 years of age to be only 2%. The limitations of monitoring CD4 counts was also highlighted, as only three of 14 children with PCP fulfilled the criteria for prophylaxis. With the low cumulative incidence of PCP found in this large cohort, it would be difficult to justify giving prophylaxis to all children born to HIV-infected mothers irrespective of the child's status of infection.

At present, data are lacking to guide clinical practice regarding primary prophylaxis against PCP. The risks and benefits of initiating early PCP prophylaxis have to be considered on an individual basis, along with the impact of the disease on the family. Fig. 9.1 sets out a flow diagram which might help in the decision to commence prophylaxis. Suggested drugs and dosages are outlined in Chapter 10.

The follow-up schedule

Prior to discharge of the baby from the newborn nursery, the responsible paediatrician should discuss with the family the frequency, content and venue for follow-up. The mother should have the name of a paediatrician and a telephone number to call, in case of need. This is especially important if the centre of follow-up is not the local paediatric unit, so that no confusion should exist about lines of communication and referral. Most specialist centres have community nurses who will liaise with the infant's generic health visitor on the follow-up programme.

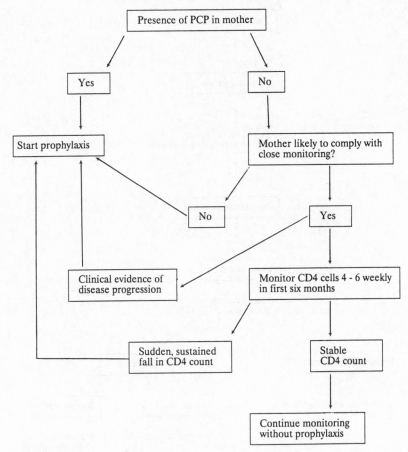

Fig. 9.1. When to start PCP prophylaxis in the infant born to an HIV-infected mother.

Fig. 9.2 summarises the follow-up schedule. After discharge from the maternity unit, intensive monitoring is recommended in the first six months of life to enable an early diagnosis to be made and also to allow detection of immunological deterioration which might necessitate intervention such as prophylaxis against PCP. Follow-up can be relaxed to three monthly from the age of six months until 18 months. Thereafter, the frequency of follow-up depends on the manifestation of HIV disease in infected children. Children who are not infected should also be monitored, albeit less intensively, as these affected children are likely to exhibit behavioural and emotional disorders when their parents' health fails.

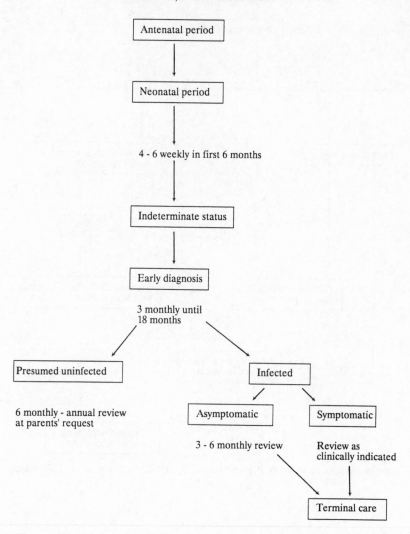

Fig. 9.2. Follow-up schedule for an infant born to an HIV-infected mother.

Indeterminate status/early diagnosis

The Centers for Disease Control (1987) has classified children born to HIV-infected mothers who are less than 15 months old as 'indeterminate status', because of the possible persistence of maternal HIV antibodies until that age. The European Collaborative Study (1988) has shown that although the median age of antibody loss is 10 months, antibodies may persist until 18 months of age. For these reasons, the first 18 months of life is usually considered the time during which the infant's infection status is not known.

With advances in diagnostic tests, many children with HIV infection can be detected in the first few weeks or months of life (see Chapter 5). A positive result should be confirmed with blood taken on a separate occasion, and the mother then informed that her child is infected. Early knowledge of the infant's infection status allows the mother and health care professionals to be particularly vigilant in responding to clinical symptoms and laboratory markers which might herald more serious disease (see Chapter 10). However, it remains difficult to exclude infection.

For the above reasons, the infant should be seen 4–6 weekly in the first 6 months of life. During each visit, a thorough examination should include growth monitoring and developmental assessment. Non-specific clinical signs which predict HIV infection include persistent lymphadenopathy (especially axillary and post-occipital), splenomegaly and hepatomegaly, recurrent oral candidiasis, frequent respiratory infections, protracted diarrhoea and failure to thrive (European Collaborative Study, 1991). Physical findings are significant if present for more than 2 months. Laboratory evidence of infection which can be detected early include non-specific hypergammaglobulinaemia (Mok *et al.*, 1989*b*; European Collaborative Study, 1991). As with physical signs, laboratory parameters must also be persistently abnormal, on two or more occasions, to allow a definitive diagnosis to be made.

The procedure at each visit is outlined in Table 9.3. Table 9.4 summarises the clinical and laboratory markers which are useful in making an early diagnosis.

The infected child

The diagnosis of HIV infection must be disclosed to the parents or care givers by a doctor experienced in the management of paediatric HIV infection, so that the carers have an opportunity to ask questions about the clinical outcome and therapeutic options for the child. The need for close follow-up should again be stressed; the frequency of follow-up depends on the medical condition of the child and the psychosocial support required for the family, as well as the network of other professionals involved with the family. Children who are in good health need be seen only 3 to 6 monthly, with the frequency of visits increased according to clinical needs (Fig. 9.2). For asymptomatic and symptomatic children, the procedure at each visit is as described in Table 9.3. Classifying the child's signs and symptoms enables the paediatrician to stage the disease process, as well as to offer the carers a prognostic value for disease patterns (Tovo *et al.*, 1992) (see

Table 9.3. *Procedure at follow-up*

History
HIV-related symptoms
Dietary intake
Child care issues
Immunisation status
Examination
Height, weight, head circumference
Developmental progress
Evidence of HIV infection
Laboratory tests
Haematology
Full blood count
White cell count with differential
Immunology
Immunoglobulin levels
T lymphocyte subsets
Others (e.g. cytotoxic T cell activity, β_2-microglobulin)
Virology
p24 antigen (this might predict disease progression)
Biochemistry
Liver function tests 6–12 monthly
Radiology
Chest X-ray annually
Liaison with, and referral to, other professions if necessary

Table 9.4. *Early clinical and laboratory markers of
HIV infection*

Clinical
Persistent lymphadenopathy
Recurrent candidiasis
Frequent respiratory infections
Protracted diarrhoea
Failure to thrive
Laboratory
Polymerase chain reaction
Virus culture
Hypergammaglobulinaemia

Clinical signs must be present for at least 2 months, and
laboratory tests positive on two or more occasions, to allow
a definitive diagnosis of HIV infection.

Chapter 3). Specific care for the infected child with symptoms is outlined in Chapter 10.

The uninfected child

Loss of HIV-antibody, which has been confirmed on more than two occasions, usually implies lack of HIV infection. If the child has been commenced on PCP prophylaxis, this should be discontinued. The presumed uninfected child is usually older than 18 months, is clinically well, has tested negative for HIV-antibody, antigen, culture and polymerase chain reaction (PCR), and has normal immune function. Current knowledge is that seroconversion following seroreversion is rare. As the long-term outlook for children born to HIV-infected women is not yet known, it is prudent at present to continue to review these uninfected children on an annual basis. However, experience suggests that the stigma of the disease, as well as the implications of follow-up for the mother's own illness, mean that many families opt out of follow-up at this stage (see Chapter 15).

The affected child

The added benefits of continued contact with the families include the ability to identify and manage emotional and behavioural difficulties in children that arise with the onset of parental ill-health and death. Over the past decade, the organisation and provision of health care has focused primarily on infected individuals. Parents who are HIV infected may fail to provide for their child due to circumstances such as chaotic drug use, ill health, HIV-related dementia or death. Although many members of the extended family may take on the care of children bereaved by AIDS, the extra pressures brought on by orphaned children should be addressed. Studies in Europe and North America have identified the scale of the problem, although the needs of children living with HIV and AIDS have not yet been defined (Giaquinto *et al.*, 1992; Principi *et al.*, 1992; Michaels & Levine, 1992; Ronald *et al.*, 1993).

Where contact has been maintained with the families, it is likely that the carers will turn to the paediatrician for help and support when the child exhibits behavioural problems which might be associated with parental illness or death. Physical complaints may be the presenting feature, and the paediatrician must be sensitive and responsive to the emotional needs of the child, making referrals to the appropriate professionals as necessary.

Chronic illness and terminal care

Paediatric HIV disease has been recognised as the most recent chronic illness of childhood (Meyers & Weitzman, 1991). With increasing numbers of children infected with HIV but surviving into later childhood, the impact will be felt in all areas of health care. The complex medical and social needs of HIV-infected children and their families demand a multi-disciplinary team approach, which can be drawn from existing models provided for children with chronic illness. In providing for the medical needs, the paediatrician must always remember the association of mental health problems and chronic illness. A survey of primary care providers revealed increased prevalence rates of behavioural and emotional disorders in children with a serious chronic illness, with a negative effect of having more than one handicap. Despite these findings, there were few referrals to mental health services for these children (Weiland *et al.*, 1992).

Children with HIV infection represent a wide clinical spectrum, but are usually characterised by poverty and multiple deprivation, with poor access to health care. Although poverty encompasses a heterogeneous group of people, it is a predominant social precursor to poor health (Kliegman, 1992). In many communities, large numbers of infected children are born to parents who have emigrated from countries with endemic heterosexual spread of HIV. Immigrant families may have uncertain legal status and little concept of health care, including that required for their child. The services provided must therefore be appropriate to the family's culture, beliefs and language, as well as taking into account the needs of the mother who is also likely to be infected (see Chapter 17). This approach requires commitment and financial support from professionals in public health, medicine, social work and education, as well as the voluntary agencies (Van Dyke, 1991).

Although there is no cure for AIDS, the goals for treatment are to achieve a long-term disease-free survival and to improve the quality of life for children infected with HIV. Throughout the course of the illness, the primary focus should be on helping the family come to terms with HIV infection in the child. When all treatments have failed, families become aware of a terminal illness. Feelings of guilt, anger and denial will re-emerge, together with the added pain of the secrecy of AIDS.

The stigma of AIDS in the family usually prevents many parents from discussing the child's illness. The lack of communication and the lack of explanation for frequent painful procedures result in a wall being built up. Children usually have a greater awareness of their illness than their carers believe. Disclosure and discussion usually help to reduce the sense of isolation and fear experienced by families facing death (Lewert, 1990). However, the decision to involve the child lies entirely with the family, and must be respected. If the carers decide to tell the child, this must be done on a developmentally appropriate level, with help from professional counsellors trained in child development (see Chapter 17).

The carers may wish to take the child home for terminal care. In such circumstances, support must be available from home care nurses as well as social workers to manage the practical aspects of care. A primary concern of parents and carers is that their child is free from pain. It behoves all doctors caring for children to ensure that the final stages of the child's life are comfortable and dignified. The effects on other family members, especially children, also have to be considered when a terminally ill child is nursed at home. When the child dies, bereavement counselling must be offered to the family; although some families may wish to seek alternative sources of support.

HIV testing in paediatric practice

The General Medical Council (1988) in the UK has laid down specific guidelines on testing for HIV infection, because of the unique social and financial consequences which follow a positive diagnosis. In all circumstances, doctors must ensure that the patient's consent has been obtained. Consent can be implicit, as when blood is drawn for multiple investigations; or explicit when blood is tested for a specific condition.

In the case of the majority of children, testing the child implicitly tests the mother's HIV status. Often, the mother may be unavailable for consent, or the parents may withhold consent. The paediatrician must judge whether some children are competent to consent or withhold consent on their own behalf – including consent to disclose information on the test to their parents. When the child is unable or unfit to consent, the paediatrician must decide whether the interests of the child override the wishes of the parents and justify performing HIV testing without parental consent (see Chapter 11). HIV testing usually arises in the following circumstances:

Diagnostic purposes

This process is part of the consultation for which a diagnosis is expected, and consent is implied. Good practice dictates that the parents are informed of the need for HIV testing, and consent obtained before any investigations are undertaken.

Children who have been sexually abused

Although there is a theoretical risk of HIV infection following child sexual abuse, the frequency of HIV transmission by this route is not known. In a recent report, 64% of 28 children had sexual abuse as the sole risk factor for HIV infection. The perpetrators were either known to be HIV infected at the time of assessment for the abuse (67%) or had behavioural risk factors for, or signs of, HIV infection (58%). Penile vaginal and/or rectal penetration occurred in only 50% of cases (Gellert *et al.*, 1993). For these reasons, children who have suffered sexual abuse should be evaluated for the risk of HIV infection. Clinical indications which justify testing for HIV infection include the following:

Perpetrator known to be HIV infected
Perpetrator known to engage in high-risk behaviour
Abuse occurred in an area of high HIV prevalence
Child has another proven sexually transmitted disease
Child has clinical evidence of HIV infection

Every effort should be made to discover the HIV status and risk activities of the abuser. As part of the specialist paediatric examination, blood can be taken and stored for HIV testing, with a repeat specimen sent 6 months later. The parents and child should be offered counselling, and if they decline HIV testing, their wishes must be respected. Storage of serum samples allows for retrospective testing should clinical indications arise; and most parents readily agree to this.

Placement in foster care

There are no indications for testing children who are received into foster care, as HIV transmission does not occur during casual household contact. In the case of young infants, the presence of maternal HIV antibodies will complicate rather than resolve the issue, and testing is therefore not recommended.

Older children may present a dilemma with testing, especially if they are sexually active or are injecting drug users. The young person, as well as the person named *in loco parentis*, must be involved in the discussions around testing, and the young person's wishes taken into account (see Chapter 15).

Adoption

With the spread of HIV infection into the heterosexual population, and the availability of children from Eastern Europe, medical advisers to adoption panels are increasingly being asked to consider HIV testing. Adoption agencies are required to compile comprehensive medical reports on the child, as well as on each birth parent, to be made available to all prospective adopters. Therefore, careful enquiry must be made into the mother's past history to elicit activities which might have put her at risk of HIV infection. If necessary, the birth mother must be counselled with a view to testing, although a positive HIV test in the mother does not resolve the issue for a young infant. The adoptive parents may wish to pursue further investigations on assumption of parental rights; and advice should be made available to adoptive parents who wish to discuss the implications of HIV testing (see Chapter 15).

Before testing a child for HIV, the following guidelines should be considered:

Counselling must be available on the implications of a positive test
Informed consent must be obtained from the parent, or from the child if of the age of consent
A definite appointment must be made when the results can be discussed. Results should never be given over the telephone or on a Friday
Further counselling will be required if the result is positive. Ensure that a referral is made to a paediatrician experienced in the management of HIV disease in children
Where parental consent is withheld, the paediatrician must decide whether the child's interests overrides the wishes of the parents, and be prepared to justify his or her action in a court of law

School placement

The extensive media coverage on a few cases of children with AIDS attending school generated fear and anxiety among the general public, concerned that their children may be attending the same school as children with HIV. In reality, school-aged children infected with the virus are still few in number, but with increased survival of infected children it is likely that the numbers will rise. In many communities children affected by HIV have also encountered discrimination, because of the stigma of AIDS in the family.

There have been no documented reports of HIV transmission amongst family members during household contact, or between children in playgroup or school settings (Rogers *et al.*, 1990; Simonds & Rogers, 1993). National guidelines have been recommended but local policies and

Table 9.5. *Guidelines for school attendance of children infected with HIV*

In general, children infected with HIV should be allowed to attend school in an unrestricted setting

Some children with neurodevelopmental delay, behavioural difficulties or with open skin lesions may require special educational placements

An individual review of each child should be conducted prior to school placement, involving a multidisciplinary team

Disclosure of the child's HIV status should be based on the 'need to know', and with the parents' consent

Universal hygiene precautions should be adopted by schools

HIV/AIDS awareness programmes should be in place for all parents, students and staff at school

procedures must be developed, based on cooperation between professionals in health, education and social work. The emphasis for local procedures should be on the following:

Respect for the child and family's right to privacy

Lack of casual transmission at school

Protection of the child who is immune compromised

Practice of universal hygiene by all staff

Raising awareness of HIV/AIDS at school

The guidelines for school attendance of children with HIV infection are summarised in Table 9.5, from the American Academy of Pediatrics (1991) and the Department of Education at the Scottish Office (1992).

On a practical level, a successful placement hinges on the presentation to the school staff of a new child. Experience has shown that if a knowledgeable professional accompanies the parent, the placement passes without difficulties. This provides a chance for the teachers to ask questions, and allays fears. Protection of confidentiality in schools is a major concern, as in most schools there is a professional expectation that all information disclosed to the class teacher must be relayed to the head teacher. Sharing of educational reports among teachers is a common part of education, and parents worry about the passing on of medical information. A good working relationship between the paediatrician in charge of the child's health care, professionals from the School Health Service and educational staff will optimise the school placement. The appointment of teaching staff with the specific remit to raise awareness about HIV, AIDS, healthy lifestyles, sexual health and harm avoidance is an important component of the strategy.

Prior to enrolling the child at school, the paediatrician must review the clinical condition, neurodevelopmental status and immune function of

Table 9.6. *Infection control in day care and schools*

Children and staff should have cuts covered with waterproof dressings
Bleeding should be controlled by covering abrasions, lacerations or other lesions
Gloves or other protection should be used when attending to wounds
Sponges, water or other first aid items used to care for injuries involving blood should not be reused
Contact of blood on skin or mucous membranes should be washed immediately with soap and water
Blood-stained surfaces should be cleansed with bleach solution (diluted 1:10)
Dressings and other material used to dress wounds should be placed in a bag and disposed of carefully

the child. A meeting with the parents or carers should then be arranged, to discuss whether or not it is in the best interest of the child to inform the school of his or her HIV status. Advantages of disclosure include the need to advise the parents of outbreaks of communicable diseases (especially measles and chickenpox); the ability of teachers to identify educational deterioration which may be related to HIV brain involvement; and the relief, for the parents, of the burden of secrecy or the fear of inadvertent disclosure. Most parents can see the advantages but still fear the adverse effects, and their wishes should be respected. The paediatrician must then ensure that the universal guidelines for handling blood and body fluids are practised in the school. Infection control procedures are outlined in Table 9.6.

A school placement policy for children infected with or affected by HIV must also include support for the other children as well as staff at school, who will have to cope with chronic ill health, death and bereavement in the HIV-affected family. Fig. 9.3 outlines the procedure for the school placement of children living with HIV and AIDS.

Multidisciplinary working

Paediatric HIV infection is like many other chronic childhood illnesses in the following ways:

Life-long illness with acute exacerbations
Repeated hospitalisations with painful procedures
Need for early intervention and possible special educational placement
Psychosocial dysfunction of child and family
Multisystem disease requiring coordination of medical and non-medical care givers

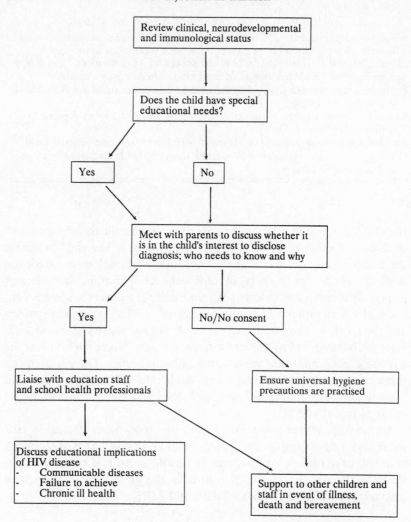

Fig. 9.3. Procedure for school placement for children living with HIV.

All too often, the care of children with chronic illnesses is focused on medical interventions, with many doctors regarding the social and psychological aspects of the disease as 'second rate'.

In Europe, inequalities of care are seen in many countries, where there is little link between primary and secondary health care and no integration between hospital and community-based services. Often, the system works well for those with legal status. In many European countries a high proportion of children with HIV are born to immigrant women from Africa, who have no legal status and therefore no access to health or social services.

Many specialist centres have been set up to coordinate the medical management of the child and family. However, hospital-based specialists usually have little understanding of the set up of services in the community. As with other chronic childhood illnesses, families affected by HIV could be faced with either a famine or a feast of professionals, who hinder rather than help the family. Inter-professional suspicion or jealousy further jeopardises working with the family. In the planning of any care to the child with HIV infection, it is important to remember that services must be coordinated, child-centred, family focused and involve professionals in the community, as well as being culturally appropriate and sensitive to the psychosocial dimensions of the illness.

Conclusion

HIV disease has emerged as a major chronic illness affecting children and their families. The challenges raised by a child with HIV infection are immense, but it is important to draw on models of good practice which have existed for children with other chronic illnesses rather than to 're-invent the wheel'. Substantial progress has been made in understanding the natural history of the disease, as well as in therapeutic interventions. These advances can only benefit the child if the care provided is comprehensive, seamless, multidisciplinary and coordinated, and includes the psychosocial needs of the whole family.

References

Adamson, P. C., Wu, T. C., Meade, B. D., Rubin, M., Manclark, C. R. & and Pizzo, P. A. (1989). Pertussis in a previously immunised child with human immunodeficiency virus infection. *Journal of Pediatrics*, **115**, 589–92.

American Academy of Pediatrics (1991). Task Force on Pediatric AIDS. Education of children with HIV infection. *American Academy of Pediatrics News*, June, 21–2.

Amman, A. J., Schiffman, G. & Abrams, D. (1984). B cell immunodeficiency in acquired immune deficiency syndrome. *Journal of the American Medical Association*, **251**, 1447–9.

Bernstein, L. J., Ochs, H. D., Wedgwood, R. J., *et al.* (1985). Defective humoral immunity in pediatric acquired immune deficiency syndrome. *Journal of Pediatrics*, **107**, 352–7.

Bernstein, L. J., Bye, M. R. & Rubinstein, A. (1989). Prognostic factors and life expectancy in children with acquired immunodeficiency syndrome and *Pneumocystis carinii* pneumonia. *American Journal of Diseases of Children*, **143**, 775–8.

Borkowsky, W., Steele, C. J., Grubman, S., et al. (1987). Antibody responses to bacterial toxoids in children infected with human immunodeficiency virus. Journal of Pediatrics, 110, 563–6.

Centers for Disease Control (1986). Disseminated Mycobacterium bovis infection from BCG vaccination of a patient with acquired immunodeficiency syndrome. Morbidity and Mortality Weekly Report, 34, 227–8.

Centers for Disease Control (1987). Classification system for human immunodeficiency virus (HIV) infection in children under 13 years of age. Morbidity and Mortality Weekly Report, 36, 225–30, 235–6.

Centers for Disease Control (1991). Guidelines for prophylaxis against Pneumocystis carinii pneumonia for children infected with human immunodeficiency virus. Morbidity and Mortality Weekly Report, 40, 1–13.

Embree, J. E., Datta, P., Stackiw, W., et al. (1992). Increased risk of early measles in infants of HIV type 1-seropositive mothers. Journal of Infectious Diseases, 165, 262–7.

European Collaborative Study (1988). Mother-to-child transmission of HIV infection. Lancet, ii, 1039–43.

European Collaborative Study (1991). Children born to women with HIV-1 infection: natural history and risk of transmission. Lancet, 337, 253–60.

European Collaborative Study (1992). Risk factors for mother-to-child transmission of HIV-1. Lancet, 339, 1007–12.

European Collaborative Study (1994). CD4 T cell count as a predictor of Pneumocystis carinii pneumonia in children of mothers infected with HIV. British Medical Journal, 308, 437–40.

European Collaborative Study (1994). Perinatal findings in children born to HIV infected mothers. British Journal of Obstetrics and Gynaecology, 101, 136–41.

Gellert, G. A., Durfee, M. J., Berkowitz, C. D., Higgins, K. V. & Tubiolo, V. C. (1993). Situational and sociodemographic characteristics of children infected with human immunodeficiency virus from pediatric sexual abuse. Pediatrics, 91, 39–44.

General Medical Council (1988). HIV infection and AIDS: the ethical considerations. London: General Medical Council.

Giaquinto, C., Giacomet, V., Pagliaro, A., et al. (1992). Social care of children born to HIV infected parents. Lancet, 339, 189–90.

Gibb, D. & Walters, S. (1992). Guidelines for Management of Children with HIV Infection. Horsham, West Sussex. AIDS Virus Education and Research Trust (AVERT),

Gibb, D. M., Davison, C. F., Holland, F. J. et al. (1994). Pneumocystis carinii pneumonia in vertically acquired HIV infection in the British Isles. Archives of Disease in Childhood, 70, 241–4.

Hague, R. A., Burns, S. E., Hargreaves, F. D. et al. (1992). Virus infections of the respiratory tract in HIV-infected children. Journal of Infection, 24, 31–6.

Huang, K. L., Ruben, F. L., Rinaldo, C. R., Kingsley, L., Lyter, D. W. & Ho, M. (1987). Antibody responses after influenza and pneumococcal immunisation in HIV-1 infected men. Journal of the American Medical Association, 257, 2047–50.

Immunisation Practices Advisory Committee (1986). Immunisation of children infected with HTLV III/LAV. Morbidity and Mortality Weekly Report, 35, 595–8; 603–6.

Immunisation Practices Advisory Committee (1988). Immunisation of children infected with human immunodeficiency virus. Supplementary ACIP Statement, Morbidity and Mortality Weekly Report, 37, 181.

Johnstone, F. D., MacCallum, L., Brettle, R., *et al*. (1988). Does infection with HIV affect the outcome of pregnancy? *British Medical Journal*, **296**, 467.

Kliegman, R. M. (1992). Perpetual poverty: Child health and the underclass. *Pediatrics*, **89**, 710–13.

Krasinski, K. & Borkowsky, W. (1989). Measles and measles immunity in children infected with human immunodeficiency virus. *Journal of the American Medical Association*, **261**, 2512–16.

Lallemant-Le Coeur, S., Lallemant, M., Cheynier, D., Nzingoula, S., Drucker, J. & Larouze, B. (1991). Bacillus Calmette-Guerin immunization in infants born to HIV-1-seropositive mothers. *AIDS*, **5**, 195–9.

Leibovitz, E., Rigaud, M., Pollack, H., *et al*. (1990). *Pneumocystis carinii* pneumonia in infants infected with the human immunodeficiency virus with more than 450 CD4 T lymphocytes per cubic millimeter. *New England Journal of Medicine*, **323**, 531–3.

Lepage, P., Dabis, F., Msellat, P., *et al*. (1992). Safety and immunogenicity of high dose Edmonston-Zagreb measles vaccine in children with HIV1 infection. *American Journal of Diseases of Children*, **146**, 550–5.

Lewert, G. (1990). Psychosocial needs of HIV infected children and their families. *Pediatric AIDS and HIV Infection. Fetus to Adolescent*, **1**, 141–4.

McLaughlin, M., Thomas, P., Onorato, I., *et al*. (1988). Live virus vaccines in human immunodeficiency virus-infected children: a retrospective survey. *Pediatrics*, **82**, 229–33.

Meyers, A. & Weitzman, M. (1991). Pediatric HIV disease. The newest chronic illness of childhood. *Pediatric Clinics of North America*, **38**, 169–94.

Michaels, D. & Levine, C. (1992). Estimates of the number of motherless youths orphaned by AIDS in the United States. *Journal of the American Medical Association*, **268**, 3456–61.

Mofenson, L. M., Moye, J. Jr., Bethel, J., Hirschhorn, R., Jordan, C. & Nugent, R. (1992). Prophylactic intravenous immunoglobulin in HIV-infected children with CD4+ counts of $0.20 \times 10(9)$/L or more. Effect on viral, opportunistic, and bacterial infections. *Journal of the American Medical Association*, **268**, 483–8.

Mok, J. Y. Q., Hague, R. A., Taylor, R. F., *et al*. (1989*a*). The management of children born to human immunodeficiency virus seropositive women. *Journal of Infection*, **18**, 119–24.

Mok, J. Y. Q., Hague, R. A., Yap, P. L., *et al*. (1989*b*). Vertical transmission of HIV: a prospective study. *Archives of Disease in Childhood*, **64**, 1140–45.

Molyneaux, P. J., Mok, J. Y. Q., Burns, S. M. & Yap, P. L. (1993). Measles, mumps and rubella immunisation in children at-risk of infection with human immunodeficiency virus. *Journal of Infection*, **29**, 251–3.

Phair, J., Munoz, A., Detels, R., *et al*. (1990). The risk of *Pneumocystis carinii* pneumonia among men infected with human immunodeficiency virus type 1. *New England Journal of Medicine*, **322**, 161–5.

Principi, M. D., Fontana, M., Marchisio, P., Picco, P., Massironi, E. & Tornaghi R. (1992). Changes in family structure of children born to HIV-infected mothers. *Pediatric AIDS and HIV Infection*, **3**, 15–18.

Rogers, M. F., White, C. R., Sanders, R., *et al*. (1990). Lack of transmission of human immunodeficiency virus from infected children to their household contacts. *Pediatrics*, **85**, 210–14.

Ronald, P. J. M., Robertson, J. R., Duncan, B. M. & Thomson, A. S. (1993). Children of parents infected with HIV in Lothian. *British Medical Journal*, **306**, 649–50.

Scottish Office Education Department (1992). A guide for the Education Services in Scotland. HIV and AIDS. Facts for teachers, lecturers and youth workers. Edinburgh: Scottish Office Education Department.

Selwyn, P. A., Schoenbaum, E. E., Davenny, K., *et al.* (1989). Prospective study of human immunodeficiency virus infection and pregnancy outcomes in intravenous drug users. *Journal of the American Medical Association*, **261**, 1289–94.

Semprini, A. E., Ravizza, M., Bucceri, A., Vucetich, A. & Pardi, G. (1990). Perinatal outcome in HIV-infected pregnant women. *Gynecologic and Obstetric Investigation*, **30**, 15–18.

Simonds, R. J. & Rogers, M. F. (1993). HIV prevention – bringing the message home. *New England Journal of Medicine*, **329**, 1883–5.

Stephan, J. L., Vlekova, V., Le Deist, F., *et al.* (1993). Severe combined immunodeficiency: a retrospective clinical study of clinical presentation and outcome of 117 patients. *Journal of Pediatrics*, **123**, 564–72.

Tovo, P. A., De Martino, M., Gabiano, C., *et al.* (1992). Prognostic factors and survival in children with perinatal HIV-1 infection. The Italian Register for HIV Infections in Children. *Lancet*, **339**, 1249–53.

Van Dyke, R. B. (1991). Pediatric human immunodeficiency virus infection and the acquired immunodeficiency syndrome. A health care crisis of children and families. *American Journal of Diseases in Children*, **145**, 529–32.

Weiland, S. K., Pless, I. B. & Roghmann, K. J. (1992). Chronic illness and mental health problems in pediatric practice: Results from a survey of primary care providers. *Pediatrics*, **89**, 445–9.

WHO Global programme on AIDS (1992). Consensus statement from the WHO/ UNICEF consultation on HIV transmission and breastfeeding. *Weekly Epidemiological Record*, **67**, 177–9.

Wyatt, H. V. (1973). Poliovirus in hypogammaglobulinaemia. *Journal of Infectious Diseases*, **124**, 802–6.

10

The infected child with HIV-related symptoms

CARLO GIAQUINTO and JACK LEVY

Introduction

HIV infection is a multi-system disease causing a wide spectrum of manifestations. After an acute non-specific illness, HIV-infected adults or children who acquire the virus by transfusion may remain symptom free for a long period. In contrast, most vertically infected children show HIV-related manifestations in early infancy. At birth neonates born to HIV-infected mothers and who will eventually prove to be infected have no clinical or immunological signs of disease and are indistinguishable from those who will be found to be uninfected. However, on a population basis, the birthweight (Lepage *et al.*, 1992) and the CD4 counts (Blanche *et al.*, 1989) of infected neonates tend to be lower than those of uninfected infants. By 1 year of age, 90% of infected children will have shown some clinical and immunological manifestations (European Collaborative Study, 1991) and 17% will have died from AIDS. The evolution of these children towards disease is bimodal (Blanche *et al.*, 1990): some present with severe symptoms in the first months of life, whereas others have milder manifestations that become apparent later (see Chapter 4). The former group has a high rate of opportunistic infections and central nervous system manifestations, with a very poor prognosis, whereas the latter may develop lymphoid tissue hyperplasia and bacterial infections and usually survive beyond infancy (Italian Register for HIV Infection in Children, 1994).

Recurrent infections

Infection by HIV leads progressively to profound immune dysfunction, the pathogenesis of which is not yet fully understood. The primary targets of HIV in the immune system are CD4-positive helper-inducer T lymphocytes (see Chapter 6). The invasion of these cells results in a progressive decrease in their numbers, as well as in qualitative defects in T cell function. HIV-infected children also appear to develop defects in B cell function early in the course of the disease. Hypergammaglobulinaemia is the earliest immunological marker of infection in vertically infected infants (European Collaborative Study, 1991) and is the result of polyclonal activation of B lymphocytes. In contrast, antibody production after specific antigen stimulation is diminished (Borkowsky *et al.*, 1987).

The major consequence of this immune dysfunction is an increased susceptibility to infection by a number of fungi, bacteria, viruses or parasites. Oral candidiasis, recurring or persisting despite therapy, is one of the earliest signs of this increased susceptibility (European Collaborative Study, 1991) and, when associated with lymphadenopathy and/or hepatosplenomegaly, is highly suggestive of HIV infection in children born to infected mothers. Bacterial infections have been identified as a major complication of HIV infection in earlier retrospective studies (Bernstein *et al.*, 1985; Krasinski *et al.*, 1988). A number of prospective cohort studies and case–control comparisons have confirmed these findings and found bacterial infections to be more frequent in HIV-infected than in uninfected children born to infected mothers (Lepage *et al.*, 1989; European Collaborative Study, 1991). The organisms most frequently isolated are encapsulated bacteria and are not different from those isolated from the general paediatric population in the same epidemiological setting: *Streptococcus pneumoniae* and *Haemophilus influenzae*, enterobacteria, staphylococci, *Pseudomonas* spp. in industrialised countries, and non-typhoid *Salmonella* in Central Africa (Bernstein *et al.*, 1985; Krasinski *et al.*, 1988; Lepage *et al.*, 1989). The clinical spectrum associated with bacterial infections is wide, extending from minor and localised infections such as otitis media, chronic purulent rhinitis, conjunctivitis, soft tissue infection and gastroenteritis to more severe or generalised manifestations such as pneumonia, bacteraemia and meningitis. With the increasing use of central venous catheters in these children, infections of these devices, frequently accompanied by bacteraemia, are now a common problem. Recurrent viral infections are due mainly to herpes viruses, with recurrent stomatitis and zoster as the main clinical manifestations.

Although they are responsible for significant morbidity, recurrent infections are usually readily treatable and are not associated with a high rate of immediate mortality. The medical management of these infections requires prompt aetiological diagnosis and administration of appropriate antimicrobial agents. Prophylactic interventions include general measures such as adequate nutritional support and immunisations. Post-exposure prophylaxis after measles or varicella contact is indicated. Administration of intravenous immunoglobulins (IVIG) to children with recurrent bacterial infections is widely recommended although criteria for initiation of this prophylaxis are not clearly established. At the dose of 400 mg/kg every 28 days, IVIG has been shown to increase the time free from serious bacterial infections and to reduce the frequency of acute hospitalisations compared with placebo in symptomatic children. However, this benefit was limited to children with >200 CD4+ lymphocytes per mm^3 and was not accompanied by improvement in survival (National Institute of Child Health and Human Development, 1991). In a further study performed in patients treated with zidovudine (AZT), IVIG provided protection against serious bacterial infections in children not receiving *Pneumocystis carinii* pneumonia (PCP) prophylaxis with trimethoprim-sulphamethoxazole (TMP-SMX). In those receiving TMP-SMX, there was no additional benefit of IVIG (see Chapter 12).

Central nervous system manifestations

Although the incidence is not established with certainty, central nervous system (CNS) manifestations of HIV in children are among the most severe complications of the disease and the least amenable to treatment. Studies of symptomatic children have provided estimates of neurological involvement in 24–29% of HIV-infected children in Europe (Tardieu *et al.*, 1987) and in 50–88% in the USA (Belman *et al.*, 1985, 1988; Epstein *et al.*, 1986). More recent prospective follow-up studies of infants born to HIV-infected mothers from Europe have found encephalopathy to occur in less than 2% of infected children (Blanche *et al.*, 1990; European Collaborative Study, 1990). The discrepancy between these numbers might be due to selection bias in the retrospective studies, insufficient length of follow-up in the prospective studies, or might reflect differences in populations or in the level of social and health care.

Severe encephalopathy occurs mainly in younger children, with the onset of symptoms before 15 months in most patients, and is associated with a poor prognosis (see Chapter 4). A variety of clinical manifestations have been described including developmental delay or loss of acquired developmental milestones, cognitive impairment, axial hypotonia and abnormal reflexes in infants, pyramidal signs evolving towards spastic quadriplegia and severe pain in older children, often associated with bucco-lingual dyspraxia. Microcephaly has been observed in about one-third of the patients and cortical atrophy is documented by cerebral imaging in 50–85%. Other characteristic neuroradiological findings include calcifications of the basal ganglia and frontal white matter, and attenuation of periventricular white matter. The encephalopathy is progressive, with periods of rapid deterioration alternating with plateaus of stable neurological status (Tardieu *et al.*, 1987; Epstein *et al.*, 1986).

In most patients, the motor impairment remains more severe than the intellectual involvement throughout the evolution (Tardieu et al., 1987). At the onset of encephalopathy, affected children usually already have other severe clinical manifestations and profound immune deficiency.

In a recent prospective evaluation of their cognitive and motor development, HIV-infected infants scored significantly lower than controls in the absence of other significant non-neurological manifestations (Aylward et al., 1992). Whether the subtle neurodevelopmental alterations detected in this study are early manifestations of the major disorders remains to be established. Therapy of encephalopathy attributed to HIV rests mainly on the use of antiretroviral agents (Working Group on Antiretroviral Therapy: National Pediatric HIV Resource Center, 1993) (see Chapter 12).

CNS manifestations can also be due to infections by pathogens other than HIV. Bacterial meningitis occurred in 3% and 11% of patients in two reviews of bacterial infections in children with HIV infection (Bernstein et al., 1985; Krasinski et al., 1988). S. pneumoniae, H. influenzae, enterobacteria and Staphylococcus aureus are the main pathogens. Congenital transmission of cytomegalovirus and Toxoplasma gondii can occur in infants born to mothers with dual infection with HIV and either of these two pathogens. In these circumstances, CNS involvement is a poor prognostic sign (Mitchell et al., 1990). Opportunistic infections of the CNS are seen much less frequently in children than in adults. Cerebral Toxoplasma abscesses, among the most frequent opportunistic infections in adults, fungal (Candida and cryptococcal) meningitis and progressive multifocal leucoencephalopathy (PML), a chronic demyelinating disease caused by Jakob–Creutzfeldt virus, have all been described in children, but remain rare (Civitello, 1991). PML initially manifests by cognitive impairment, followed by focal signs such as hemiparesis, cerebellar dysfunction or hemianopia. The only method of diagnosis of PML is histopathological examination of a brain biopsy associated with viral genome detection, although neuroradiological imaging associated with the clinical picture is usually highly indicative of this disease.

Primary CNS B cell lymphoma has been reported in HIV-infected children and, in one large series, was the most common cause of CNS mass lesions (Epstein et al., 1988). Systemic lymphoma metastatic to the brain and leukaemia with epidural infiltration (Civitello, 1991) are other possible causes of malignant CNS complication.

Vascular accidents due to thrombocytopenia or other coagulation disorders are rarely seen in children.

Haematological manifestations

Anaemia and thrombocytopenia are frequent complications of HIV infection in children: 16% of those in the Italian Register for HIV infection in children had a haemoglobin level <8 g/dl before the introduction of zidovudine and the same proportion had <10^{11} platelets/l (Tovo *et al.*, 1992). Neutropenia (<10^9/l) occurred in 3.7% of these children.

As in adults, thrombocytopenia and neutropenia are mediated by immune mechanisms. Thrombocytopenia is frequently accompanied by haemorrhagic signs which can be life threatening (Ellaurie *et al.*, 1988). High-dose IVIG (0.5–1 g/kg per dose for 3–5 days followed by maintenance therapy) is currently accepted as the treatment of choice (Working Group on Antiretroviral Therapy: National Pediatric HIV Resource Center, 1993). Immune thrombocytopenia in children seems to be less responsive to zidovudine treatment than that in adults. Steroids are effective in some patients and can be recommended if IVIG is ineffective.

Anaemia is usually of multifactorial aetiology, and chronic inflammation and nutritional deficiencies are common in these patients. Coombs-positive autoimmune anaemia has also been observed. Bone marrow suppression is associated with the use of potentially toxic drugs such as zidovudine, TMP-SMX or ganciclovir, which can cause or exacerbate anaemia and neutropenia (Working Group on Antiretroviral Therapy: National Pediatric HIV Resource Center, 1993). In these circumstances, erythropoietin and granulocyte-colony stimulating factor may be beneficial. Aplastic anaemia caused by persisting or secondary (reinfection or reactivation) parvovirus B19 is increasingly recognised among children with HIV infection (Griffin *et al.*, 1991) and responds to therapy with IVIG (400 mg/kg per day for 5 days, with monthly IVIG maintenance necessary in patients with severely depressed CD4 counts).

Respiratory manifestations

Pulmonary disease and respiratory manifestations play a major role in the morbidity and mortality of HIV-infected children. More than 80% of children develop lung diseases during the course of their illness, including infections (PCP, viral or bacterial pneumonia) and chronic pulmonary disease (European Collaborative Study, 1991; Tovo *et al.*, 1992).

Pneumocystis carinii *pneumonia (PCP)*

PCP has consistently been the most common AIDS indicator disease in children infected with HIV (Hughes, 1991; Centers for Disease Control, 1991; Tovo *et al.*, 1992) and the most common cause of death in the first year of life. Although PCP can occur at any age, the incidence is highest between 3 and 6 months (Simonds *et al.*, 1993; European Collaborative Study, 1994*a*). Data from the European Collaborative Study (1994*a*) showed that the cumulative incidence of PCP by 6 years of age was 16% (95% confidence interval 7.3–24%) in infected children, and 2% in all children born to infected mothers.

PCP is characterised by four main clinical signs: tachypnoea, dyspnoea, cough and often fever, which, however, are not specific and common to many other lung diseases. Whereas in adults the development of PCP becomes increasingly likely with decreasing CD4 count, in children the value of the CD4 lymphocyte count as a predictor of PCP is limited, especially during the first year of life (European Collaborative Study, 1994*a*). The chest X-ray may reveal bilateral diffuse alveolar disease. The earliest findings are usually perihilar, and a typical X-ray pattern often appears after the clinical manifestations. A definitive diagnosis of PCP requires the demonstration of the organism in the pulmonary parenchyma or in broncho-alveolar secretions. If there is clinical and radiographic suspicion of the infection, bronchoalveolar lavage (BAL) should be performed. If the organism cannot be identified using this procedure a lung biopsy may be considered. Other diagnostic approaches such as the presence of *Pneumocystis carinii* antigen in nasopharyngeal secretions, are under evaluation (Hague *et al.*, 1990).

Once PCP has been identified, or if there is a strong suspicion of its presence, therapy must be started immediately. The drug of choice is TMP-SMX (20 mg/kg per day trimethoprim intravenously) rather than pentamidine because TMP-SMX has fewer adverse effects. Side-effects of both drugs are less severe in paediatric patients with HIV infection than in adults. Children who cannot tolerate TMP-SMX (10% of children with AIDS) or who fail to respond to this therapy should be treated with intravenous pentamidine (4 mg/kg per day). Two to three weeks of treatment are usually needed with both drugs, after which the child should be put on prophylactic treatment (Table 10.1).

Considering the frequency of PCP among HIV-infected children, the high mortality of the disease and the demonstrated efficacy of prophylaxis in adults with HIV infection, prevention is a high priority. Although both TMP-SMX and aerosolised pentamidine have been recommended for prophylaxis in children (Centers for Disease Control, 1991), TMP-SMX is preferred to pentamidine, especially in infants.

The Centers for Disease Control (CDC) guidelines recommend that PCP prophylaxis is started on the basis of age-adjusted CD4 cell count. However, the predictive value of the CD4 cell count for PCP has not been

Table 10.1. *Drugs used for PCP prophylaxis*

Trimethoprim-sulphamethoxazole	150 mg/m² and 750 mg/m² By mouth daily or ×3 per week
Pentamidine	300 mg By inhalation, via Respigard II nebuliser ×3–4 weekly
Dapsone	1 mg/kg By mouth daily

assessed in prospective studies. A recent study shows that PCP may occur in young children with a CD4 count above these thresholds (European Collaborative Study, 1994*a*). These observations suggest that monitoring the CD4 cell count is of limited value in deciding when to initiate PCP prophylaxis, but stress the importance of an early diagnosis of HIV infection in order to start prophylaxis in all infected infants. An alternative approach would be to give prophylaxis to all children born to HIV-infected mothers; however, this would be very difficult to justify since the cumulative incidence of PCP by 6 years is only 2.% (see Chapter 9).

Lymphoid pulmonary lesions

Children with perinatal HIV infection may develop chronic pulmonary disease characterised by peribronchiolar lymphoid hyperplasia (PLH) or by diffuse infiltration of the alveolar septa by both mature and immature lymphoid cells (lymphoid interstitial pneumonitis, LIP) (Joshi *et al.*, 1989; Connor *et al.*, 1991).

PLH/LIP has been attributed to an abnormal immunological response to inhaled antigen and primary pulmonary infection with HIV, Epstein–Barr virus (EBV) or some other antigen not yet identified (Andiman *et al.*, 1985). Prospective studies have shown that the incidence of PLH/LIP is about 13–15% in children with vertically acquired HIV infection (Tovo *et al.*, 1992), which is lower than previously reported. The introduction of antiretroviral therapy that will reduce the lymphoid proliferation may account for these differences.

PLH/LIP is seldom present before 2 years of age and has a better prognosis for survival than other AIDS indicator diseases (European Collaborative Study, 1991; Tovo *et al.*, 1992). Usually PLH/LIP is asymptomatic or mildly symptomatic and only the chest X-ray may suggest the diagnosis. Generalised lymphadenopathy and splenomegaly are often present. During the course of the disease dyspnoea, cough and hypoxia may appear and are exacerbated when superinfections occur. Sometimes PLH/LIP may result in bronchial dysplasia.

The diagnosis of PLH/LIP can be difficult because of other overlapping cardiac and respiratory problems. Often the chest X-ray is the only available diagnostic procedure. Bilateral reticulonodular interstitial pulmonary infiltrates persisting for more than 2 months in the absence of pathogen identified and no response to antibiotic treatment have been shown to correlate with the pathological diagnosis of PLH/LIP.

The differentiation of this disease from other causes of pulmonary infiltrates often cannot reliably be made using chest radiography. However, lung biopsy is seldom indicated due to the lack of severe respiratory distress. Once the diagnosis of PLH/LIP is established or strongly suspected, regular follow-up should be planned. If the PaO$_2$ drops below 8 kPa (60 mmHg) a 4–12 week course of steroid therapy may be indicated.

Viral infections

Respiratory viruses (respiratory syncytial virus (RSV), influenza virus, adenovirus, etc.) or herpes viruses frequently cause lung infections. Infections with common respiratory viruses rarely have a severe prognosis and only few cases have been reported in which RSV infection was associated with respiratory distress (Chandwani *et al.*, 1990). Disseminated cytomegalovirus (CMV) infection is one of the most common AIDS indicator diseases in developed countries. Although most HIV-positive adults and children shed CMV in urine, the infection is usually asymptomatic. However, between 20% and 40% of children with AIDS have been reported to have disseminated infection. As with other herpes viruses, these infections may be due either to a reactivation of endogenous latent CMV in immunocompromised patients or to reinfection with exogenous viral strain.

The lung is one of the main targets of CMV, and interstitial pneumonitis with severe hypoxia and respiratory failure is often present. The diagnosis of CMV pneumonitis is difficult and differential diagnosis with PCP, PLH/LIP and other infections must be considered. The diagnosis can be made by demonstrating the CMV antigen in bronchoalveolar lavage fluid by immunofluorecence or by *in situ* hybridisation techniques. Therapy includes the use of ganciclovir alone or in association with acyclovir (less effective on CMV) and specific immunoglobulins. However, despite therapy, the mortality of CMV pneumonia remains high.

Fig. 10.1 outlines a management protocol for an HIV infected child presenting with respiratory symptoms.

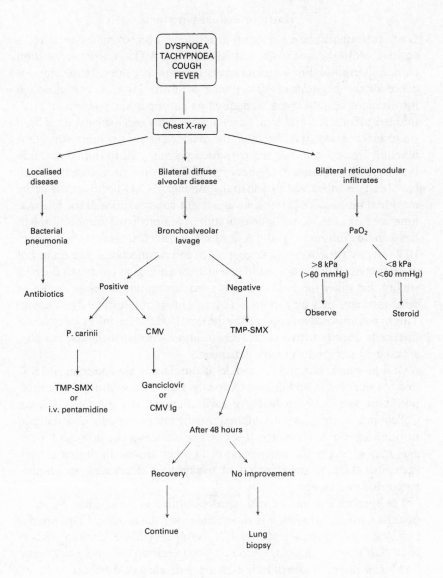

Fig. 10.1. Management of the child with respiratory symptoms.

Gastrointestinal symptoms

Gastrointestinal disease is a common and debilitating complication in HIV-positive adults; between 50% and 90% of adult AIDS patients suffer from chronic diarrhoeal illness and its presence is now considered sufficient evidence for the diagnosis of AIDS (Janoff & Smith, 1988). Gastrointestinal involvement has also been recognised as an important problem in HIV-infected infants and children. Several pathogenic mechanisms have been suggested; however, it is likely that the major causes of gastrointestinal dysfunction are opportunistic and parasitic infections. Significant abnormalities in the distribution of lymphocyte subsets in the gastrointestinal wall have been described. A decrease in the number of CD4-positive cells in the intestinal mucosa could result in significant abnormalities in the mucosal immune function, including defects both in cell-mediated immunity and in the secretory immunoglobulin A (IgA) system. Such alterations may render HIV-infected patients more susceptible to enteric infections. The finding of gastrointestinal pathology without evidence of infection has raised the possibility that other mechanisms such as malabsorption of disaccharides or other nutrients may play an important role in gastrointestinal dysfunction. This hypothesis is also supported by the fact that HIV can infect gastrointestinal cells directly with a subsequent immune-mediated cellular atrophy, which may account for chronic diarrhoea.

Oral lesions and especially recurrent candidiasis are common in HIV-infected children. Candidiasis is strongly associated with the HIV infection status and highly predictive of the imminent onset of AIDS (European Collaborative Study, 1991). Children usually respond rapidly to oral nystatin administered for few days. If severe immunodeficency is present, *Candida* may spread to the oesophagus or to other organs. In this case more aggressive therapy, such as oral or intravenous fluconazole or amphotericin B, is warranted.

The spectrum of enteric pathogens identified as aetiological agents of gastrointestinal dysfunction is wide. Some are parasites (e.g. *Cryptosporidium, Microsporidium, Giardia lamblia, Isospora belli*) while others are bacteria (*Salmonella, Shigella, E. coli*). *Mycobacterium avium-intracellulare* (MAI) has also been identified in children with chronic diarrhoea and malabsorption. Viruses such as rotavirus, adenovirus and CMV may also play a role; CMV may cause severe gastrointestinal dysfunction with or without other organ involvement. CMV, *Cryptosporidium*, MAI, hepatitis virus and HIV itself may infect the hepatobiliary system causing mild to severe forms of hepatitis. Whenever gastrointestinal symptoms are present, a careful microbiological evaluation considering rare pathogens and viruses must be performed before initiating a specific therapy.

Enteric infections in immunocompromised patients are not self limiting and appropriate antimicrobial therapy is often necessary. However, specific therapy is not always available, and alternative supportive measures must be considered. Some patients with CMV colitis benefit from the treatment with ganciclovir; however, symptoms often recur shortly after termination of therapy.

Failure to thrive

Failure to thrive (FTT) is among the most commonly observed symptoms in children with HIV infection. A wasting syndrome without underlying cause is considered an AIDS-defining event (Centers for Disease Control, 1987). It may appear at any age and is especially common in children with advanced disease.

A child is classified as having severe FTT when the weight/height curve crosses at least two centile lines on the growth chart or is below the third centile and continues to deviate downwards from it over a 3 month period, or if there is more than 10% loss of body weight in children over 5 years of age.

Children born to seropositive mothers often have a low birthweight or are small for gestational age. However, it has been shown that injecting drug use during pregnancy had the most marked effect on birthweight and gestational age (European Collaborative Study, 1994b). Multivariate analysis demonstrated a weak association between the birthweight and the child's HIV infection status, but this could partly be explained by the confounding effect of maternal immunological status. HIV infection in the infant is not associated with gestational age (European Collaborative Study, 1994b). Postnatal growth retardation has been observed in up to 50% of infants with perinatally acquired HIV infection and is associated with a relative risk of death fourfold that of normal children (Tovo et al., 1992).

The pathogenesis of FTT in children with HIV infection is unclear but is likely to be multifactorial, including effects of malnutrition, malabsorption (probably due to HIV enteropathy), psychosocial deprivation, recurrent infections and decreased production of growth factors.

The manifestations of HIV disease that influence the development of malnutrition in adults (anorexia, oral lesions, diarrhoea, malabsorption and chronic infections) also affect children. Likewise, the synergism between the malnutrition associated with chronic disease and the immunological deficit caused by the HIV infection and probably enhanced by malnutrition will further predispose patients to infection and malabsorption.

It has been suggested that nutritional deficits may contribute to the cerebro-cortical degeneration seen in children with AIDS (Lane & Certler,

Table 10.2. *Management of failure to thrive*

Nutritional assessment
Evaluation of nutritional status (anthropometric measures, plasma protein determination, evaluation of appetite and food intake)
Psychosocial evaluation
Clinical and immunological evaluation
Hypercaloric formula or/and food supplements
Tube feeding
Transcutaneous gastrostomy
Total parenteral nutrition
Social and psychological support

1991). Furthermore, neurological complications may affect feeding behaviours. Adequate nutrition is an obvious prerequisite for normal growth and development; however, in children with AIDS a diet with sufficient protein and caloric intake or parenteral hyperalimentation may not alter the degree of growth failure. Normal growth is a complex process that includes many interacting factors. During HIV infection both the production of hormonal and non-hormonal factors and the response of target organs may be affected (Janoff & Smith, 1988).

Treatment of growth retardation includes adequate nutritional support, prompt treatment of intercurrent infections and antiretroviral therapy. Results from open studies in children have shown that zidovudine may increase the weight gain; however, this effect is less evident in children with full-blown AIDS and severe failure to thrive. Table 10.2 outlines the management of children who fail to thrive.

Nutritional support

Nutritional assessments should be performed routinely in children with HIV infection (Table 10.2). Evaluation of the nutritional status must be performed in combination with an overall 'psychosocial', clinical and immunological evaluation for the described interaction between environment, growth, immunity and infections. Nutritional assessment should include anthropometric measures, evaluation of appetite and food intake and complete blood counts. Plasma proteins such as albumin, transferrin, prealbumin or retinol binding protein may be used as markers of the nutritional status of the child. Eating ability should be determined and the social situation evaluated. In many cases the child's home environment may be inadequate; the parents may be intravenous drug users, or have AIDS and could be unable to care for their children.

Providing sufficient calories and protein to maintain normal growth is often difficult. Every effort should be made to ensure social and psychological support when needed. The use of hypercaloric formula or food supplements may have to be considered. Sometimes adjustments of diet, consistency and temperature according to the needs of the infant or child have been effective in overcoming feeding difficulties associated with disease complications. If oral intake is inadequate to maintain normal growth, tube feeding may be used to provide total or partial nutritional support in the presence of a functioning gastrointestinal tract. In some cases transcutaneous gastrostomy may be used, but special care is needed to minimise the risk of infections with this procedure.

In symptomatic children the presence of malabsorption, chronic diarrhoea or severe oesophageal candidiasis reduces the effectiveness of oral feeding. In these cases total parenteral nutrition is indicated. However, before starting these procedures the potential nutritional benefit must be balanced against the risk of infection and the results of prolonged hospitalisation. In order to maintain the sucking and swallowing abilities it is always advisable to encourage oral alimentation, regardless of method of feeding.

With longer survival of paediatric patients and to slow disease progression, early and preventive nutritional support is becoming one of the main issues in the management of children with HIV at an early stage of the disease.

Conclusion

In children, HIV infection has a wide spectrum of clinical manifestations that often differ from those found in adults. PLH/LIP and serious bacterial infections are common whereas Kaposi's sarcoma and other tumours are rare. Moreover the opportunistic pathogens responsible for infections in the paediatric population are different, as are the course of the diseases.

The natural history of vertically acquired HIV infection is only partially known. Many HIV-infected children are now more than 10 years of age and are still asymptomatic or mildly symptomatic. It is likely that some of these children will survive longer, but it is possible that some will develop symptoms similar to those found in adults. Only a careful follow-up of these children will allow an exact definition of the natural history and clinical spectrum of the disease in children born to HIV-infected mothers.

References

Andiman, W., Eastman, R., Martin, K. *et al.* (1985). Opportunistic lymphoproliferations associated with Epstein–Barr viral DNA in infants and children with AIDS. *Lancet*, **ii**, 1390–3.

Aylward, E. H., Butza, M., Hutton, N., et al. (1992). Cognitive and motor development in infants at-risk for human immunodeficiency virus. American Journal of Diseases of Children, 146, 218–22.

Belman, A. S., Ultmann, M. H., Horonpian, D., et al. (1985). Neurological complications in infants and children with AIDS. Annals of Neurology, 18, 560–6.

Belman, A. S., Diamond, G. & Dickson, D. (1988). Pediatric acquired immunodeficiency syndrome – Neurologic syndromes. American Journal of Diseases of Children, 142, 29–55.

Bernstein, L. J., Krieger, B. Z. & Novick, B. (1985). Bacterial infections in the acquired immunodeficiency syndrome of children. Pediatric Infectious Disease Journal, 4, 472–5.

Blanche, S., Rouzioux, C., Guihard Moscato, M. F., et al. (1989). A prospective study of infants born to women seropositive for Human Immunodeficiency Virus type I. New England Journal of Medicine, 320, 1643–8.

Blanche, S., Tardieu, M., Duliège, A. M., et al. (1990). Longitudinal study of 94 symptomatic infants with perinatally acquired human immunodeficiency virus Infection. American Journal of Diseases of Children, 144, 1210–5.

Borkowsky, W., Steele, C. J., Grulman, S., et al. (1987). Antibody responses to bacterial toxoids in children infected with human immunodeficiency virus. Journal of Pediatrics, 110, 563–6.

Centers for Disease Control (1987). Classification system for human immunodeficiency virus (HIV) infection in children under 13 years of age. Morbidity Mortality Weekly Report, 15, 225–36.

Centers for Disease Control (1991). Guidelines for prophylaxis against Pneumocystis carinii pneumonia for children infected with human immunodeficiency virus. Journal of the American Medical Association, 265, 1637–44.

Chandwani, S., Borkowsky, W. B., Krasinki, K., Lawrence, R. & Welliver, R. (1990). Respiratory syncytial virus infection in HIV infected children. Journal of Pediatrics, 117, 251–4.

Civitello, L. A. (1991). Neurologic complications of HIV infection in children. Pediatric Neurosurgery, 17, 104–12.

Connor, E. M., Marquis, J. & Oleske, J. M. (1991). Lymphoid interstitial pneumonitis. In: Pediatric AIDS, ed. P. Pizzo & M. Wilfert, pp. 343–5. Baltimore: Williams and Wilkins.

Ellaurie, M., Burns, E. R., Bernstein, L. J., et al. (1988). Thrombocytopenia and human immunodeficiency virus in children. Pediatrics, 82, 905–8.

Epstein, L. G., Di Carlo, F. J., Joshi, W., et al. (1988). Primary lymphoma of the central nervous system in children with acquired immunodeficiency syndrome. Pediatrics, 82, 355–63.

Epstein, L. G., Scharer, L. R. & Oleski, J. M. (1986). Neurologic manifestations of HIV infection in children. Pediatrics, 78, 678–87.

European Collaborative Study (1990). Neurologic signs in young children with human immunodeficiency virus infection. Pediatric Infectious Disease Journal, 9, 402–6.

European Collaborative Study (1991). Children born to women with HIV-1 infection: natural history and risk of transmission. Lancet, 337, 253–60.

European Collaborative Study (1994a). Does CD4+ T-cell count predict Pneumocystis carinii pneumonia in children born to HIV infected mothers? British Medical Journal, 308, 437–40

European Collaborative Study (1994*b*). Perinatal findings in children born to HIV-infected mothers. *British Journal of Obstetrics and Gynaecology*, **101**, 136–41

Griffin, T. C., Squires, J. E., Timmons, C. F. & Buchanan, G. R. (1991). Chronic human parvovirus B19- induced erythroid hypoplasia as the initial manifestation of human immunodeficiency virus infection. *Journal of Pediatrics*, **118**, 899–901.

Hague, R. A., Burns, S. M., Mok, J. Y. R. & Yap, P. L. (1990). Diagnosis of *Pneumocystis carinii* pneumonia from non-invasive sampling of respiratory secretions. *Archives of Disease in Childhood*, **65**, 1364–5.

Hughes, W. T. (1991). *Pneumocystis carinii* pneumonia: new approaches to diagnosis, treatment and prevention. *Pediatric Infectious Disease Journal*, **10**, 391–9.

Italian Register for HIV Infection in Children (1994). Features of children perinatally infected with HIV-1 surviving longer than 5 years. *Lancet*, **343**, 191–5

Janoff, E. N. & Smith, P. (1988). Perspectives on gastrointestinal infections in AIDS. *Gastroenterology Clinics of North America*, **17**, 451–63.

Joshi, V. V., Morrison, S., Connor, E. M., Marquis, J. & Oleske, J. M. (1989). Pulmonary pathology of AIDS in children. In: *Pediatric Pulmonary Disease*, ed. J. T. Stocke, pp.187–206. New York: Hemisphere Publishing Corporation.

Krasinski, K., Borkowski, W. & Bonk, S. (1988). Bacterial infections in human immunodeficiency virus infected children. *Pediatric Infectious Disease Journal*, **7**, 323–328.

Lane, L. & Certler, G. (1991). Neuroendocrine and growth dysfunction. In: *Pediatric AIDS*, ed. P. Pizzo & K. Wilfert, pp. 343–54. Baltimore: Williams and Wilkins.

Lepage, P., Msellati, P., van de Perre, P., Hitmana, D. G. & Dabis, F. (1992). Newborn characteristics and HIV infection in Rwanda. *AIDS*, **6**, 882–3.

Lepage, P., van de Perre, P., Nsengumuremyi, F., *et al.* (1989). Bacteremia as predictor of HIV infection in African children. *Acta Paediatrica Scandinavica*, **78**, 763–6.

Mitchell, C. D., Erlich, S. S., Mastrucci, M. T., *et al.* (1990). Congenital toxoplasmosis occurring in infants perinatally infected with human immunodeficiency virus I. *Pediatric Infectious Disease Journal*, **9**, 512–18.

National Institute of Child Health and Human Development Intravenous Immunoglobulin Study Group (1991). Intravenous immunoglobulin for the prevention of bacterial infections in children with symptomatic HIV infection. *New England Journal of Medicine*, **325**, 73–80.

Simonds, R. J., Oxtoby, M., Blake Caldwell, M., Gwinn, M. & Rogers, M. (1993). *Pneumocystis carinii* pneumonia among U.S. children with perinatally acquired HIV infection. *Journal of the American Medical Association*, **270**, 470–3.

Tardieu, M., Blanche, S., Rouzioux, C. *et al.*. (1987). Atteinte du système nerveux au cours des infections à HIV 1 chez le nourrisson. *Archive Français Pediatrie*, **44**, 495–9.

Tovo, P. A., De Martino, M., Gabiano, C. *et al.* (1992). Prognostic factors and survival in children with perinatal HIV-1 infection. *Lancet*, **339**, 1249–53.

Working Group on Antiretroviral Therapy: National Pediatric HIV Resource Center (1993). Antiretroviral therapy and medical management of the HIV-infected child. *Pediatric Infectious Disease Journal*, **12**, 513–22.

11

Haemophilia and HIV infection: some lessons learned

PETER JONES

Introduction

In 1973 the British government licensed the first imports of clotting factor concentrates for the treatment of haemophilia. This decision recognised that inadequately treated severe haemophilia resulted in early arthropathy with crippling and sometimes in premature death (Birch, 1937). The answer was the provision of rapid treatment, preferably given at home by patients or by their relatives. The decision was followed by a remarkable change in the health of people with haemophilia. The incidence of painful arthritis and muscle contractures fell. Patients were no longer confined to bed for long periods of time. School and work attendance records improved. Days in hospital for out-patient or in-patient investigation and treatment were dramatically reduced. The long-term quality of life of the most severely affected children and adults improved to the extent that haemophilia became a secondary factor in most of their lives. Easy treatment was assured; this was one of the success stories of modern medicine. Then, in July 1982, the Centers for Disease Control (CDC) reported that three men with haemophilia had died in the USA (CDC, 1982). Other than their bleeding disorder their deaths were linked by *Pneumocystis carinii* pneumonia (PCP). The dream had ended.

It took time for proof of the link between blood products and AIDS to emerge. There were several reasons for this, including the lack of an identifiable pathogen, the initial paucity of cases of overt disease in the haemophilic population and the suspicion that the emerging immune deficiency in haemophilia had a different aetiology from that affecting other groups. The real dilemma for doctors responsible for the health of people with haemophilia was if, and how, treatment should be modified to reduce a risk which by 1983 was perceived as being only 1 case of AIDS per 1000 infected patients. Given the magnitude of the change in people's lives following the introduction of lyophilised factor VIII and IX concentrates, their withdrawal from the market and a return to hospital-based

Table 11.1. *HIV infection, including AIDS, in children aged 14 years or under at time of diagnosis in the UK*

Probable aetiology	Total	Death
Clotting factor product	250	38
Blood transfusion	28	6
Total infected children (all causes)	483	94

Cummulative total to 31 July 1993. Figures from the Public Health Laboratory Service Communicable Diseases Surveillance Centre. *Communicable Disease Report* (1993), vol. 3, p. 43.

therapy with fresh frozen plasma and cryoprecipitate seemed unthinkable. In retrospect (always the easiest part of a story such as this) it was probably too late for the majority of patients. Some lives might have been saved at the expense of haemophilic complications, but it was soon evident that people treated only with the single donor products (which are pooled prior to transfusion in order to provide the correct dose of clotting factor) had been infected too. Of all the subsequent answers to the question of how to ensure a safe blood supply to the haemophilic population the most effective proved to be the virucidal treatment of blood products. Coupled with the exclusion of people most likely to be infected and the HIV-antibody testing of individual donors, the changes in manufacture of the clotting factor concentrates have ensured that no further cases of HIV infection have occurred in the haemophilic population treated with reputable products since 1984.

The extent of the problem

Haemophilia is rare. Factor VIII deficiency, known as haemophilia A, affects 1 in 10 000 people. Factor IX deficiency, known as haemophilia B or Christmas disease, is 5 times less common. The rationale of therapy in both the disorders is simple. Those affected know they are bleeding into their major joints or muscles before there are any physical signs. Replacement transfusion with a product containing sufficient factor VIII or IX at this time aborts the bleed. Nowadays, more patients are being treated with regular prophylaxis in order to prevent bleeding altogether. Children started on prophylaxis before the first haemarthrosis at around the age of 2 years, and maintained on the regimen until the cessation of growth at around 18 years, have normal joints. We are back to the very long-term advantages of adequate therapy signalled before the advent of HIV infection.

Table 11.1 shows the numbers of children with HIV infection as a result of haemophilia therapy or blood transfusion in the UK. Transmission of infection by blood is comparatively rare, and should now be confined to sporadic cases where patients have been recipients of blood donated in the 'window' period of a few weeks between infection and seroconversion to HIV-antibody positivity which can then be picked up on individual donor testing. The testing of individual donations is vital because the test used may not be sensitive enough to register infectivity in plasma pools from multiple donors. In countries unable to test donors the risk will, of course, be directly proportional to the prevalence of HIV infection in the donor population.

Within Europe as a whole 149 cases of AIDS in children with haemophilia or a related disorder were known by 30 June 1993 (European Centre for the Epidemiological Monitoring of AIDS, 1993). These children represented 3.6% of the total cases of paediatric AIDS reported; for many (40%) the aetiology of their infection was unknown. Figures for individual countries reflect the nature of the therapeutic products in use for haemophilia in the early 1980s. France, Italy, Spain and the UK each notified more than 10 cases of paediatric AIDS.

Progression of disease and comparison with other groups

Jason and her colleagues (1988) compared HIV-infected haemophilic children and adolescents with a group of infected paediatric patients without haemophilia. Not unexpectedly the haemophilic group was older and lymphocytic interstitial pneumonitis was less common. The incidence of PCP and case-to-fatality ratios were virtually identical. The study supported the later findings of Darby *et al.* (1989), in that an older group of infected men with haemophilia fared less well than a paediatric group.

Goedert *et al.* (1989) reported a prospective study of 1219 people with haemophilia in the USA, of whom 319 were HIV-1 infected. Adults aged between 35 and 70 years who were HIV-antibody positive had a significantly higher incidence of low CD4 counts than young subjects. Adolescents had a low rate of p24 antibody loss, and children aged between 1 and 17 years a lower incidence of AIDS following p24 antibody loss than older people. The authors suggested that viral replication rates in adolescents may be low, and that the slower progression of HIV disease in the paediatric group might be linked to some as yet unspecified immune alteration in late infection in adults. In this study 44% of those infected after the age of 34 years, 27% of those infected between the ages of 18 and 34, and 13% of those infected under the age of 18 years, had developed AIDS in an 8 year period. The figures were comparable with other groups at risk of AIDS. There was no correlation between progression of disease and either severity of the haemophilia or the overall use of clotting factor concentrate.

Progression rates of haemophilic patients and homosexual men were also found to be similar in studies by Lee *et al.* (1989) and Rutherford *et al.* (1990), and the results from a follow-up investigation (Lee *et al.*, 1991) continued to support this finding. However, the authors wondered whether the higher average age of the haemophilic patients compared with that in other groups might mask a more favourable progression rate in younger people with haemophilia. The effect of age in this cohort was striking and it was projected that 15 years from seroconversion 25% of patients would still not have developed AIDS. In the words of the authors 'some younger patients clearly have the prospect of a slow, indolent disease'.

Cuthbert *et al.* (1990) reported their results from the Edinburgh haemophilic cohort. Eighteen of 32 patients exposed to the same infected batch of factor VIII had seroconverted. Those infected had received significantly more of the batch than those who did not seroconvert but otherwise there were no pre-exposure differences. The ages of the HIV-infected group ranged from 14 to 42.5 years (mean 31 years). In this study there was no correlation between age and disease progression.

Wagner *et al.* (1990) plotted the course of HIV-1 infection in 53 children and adolescents with haemophilia, with ages of between 2 and 20 years. Over a median follow-up period of 30 months, 32 (60%) of the youngsters showed evidence of deterioration. They had been infected between 7 and 9 years before the study. Two patients died of AIDS during follow-up. The authors thought that their findings were comparable with the development of HIV infection in other groups. There was no difference between those with haemophilia A and a small number of haemophilia B patients. The range of symptoms were those expected in any paediatric HIV-infected cohort, although the authors specifically noted a remarkable number (8) of cases of herpes zoster, in accord with the results of Aronstam *et al.* (1993).

As mentioned earlier, Lee *et al.* (1991) reported the progression of HIV disease in 111 people with haemophilia followed over an 11 year period. Median age at seroconversion had been 24 years with a range of 2 to 77 years. PCP prophylaxis with pentamidine had been used by 35 patients. Eleven years from seroconversion, progression to AIDS was 42%, to symptoms 85% and to death 41%. Again, progression was linked to age. Patients under 25 years progressed at a significantly slower rate than those over 25 years of age. One conclusion from the survey was that intervention with prophylaxis, zidovudine and early treatment of infection was slowing progression of the underlying HIV disease.

Aledort *et al.* (1992) studied the relationship between CD4 counts and progression to AIDS in haemophilic patients. A total of 555 HIV-infected people were studied over 30 months between 1986 and 1989. Both low

CD4 counts and increasing age at recruitment were independently and significantly related to progression to AIDS. Progression measured in 149 patients showed an 11% decline in CD4 counts each 6 months regardless of the preliminary count. However, overall counts provided a poor index for identifying people likely to progress rapidly to overt disease, and therefore possibly the last target group for active therapy with zidovudine.

Aronstam and his colleagues (1993) studied the progress of 202 HIV-infected haemophilic children attending centres in northern Europe. In common with adults with haemophilia most children had been infected in the early 1980s with a range between 1979 and 1986. By July 1991, 37 (18%) had developed AIDS and 15 of these boys were dead. During the course of the study treatment patterns had changed and PCP prophylaxis was being used widely. As a result the incidence of PCP as an indicator disease for AIDS fell from 56% in 1989 to 20% in 1991. Other findings were that whilst persistent generalised lymphadenopathy was of no prognostic significance, a history of herpes zoster correlated with an earlier diagnosis of AIDS. Overall it was felt that outcome for the cohort was gloomy because CD4 counts continued to fall despite antiviral therapy, prophylaxis and the earlier treatment of opportunistic infection.

Although there have been suggestions that the progression of disease may differ according to the mode of infection, there is no convincing evidence of this in the haemophilic population. Here the only factor shown to be significant is age, older HIV-infected patients developing overt disease and dying earlier than younger infected patients (Darby *et al.*, 1989). In addition there is some evidence, much publicised by the manufacturers of the relevant blood products, that the more pure a clotting factor concentrate is, the less the decline in a recipient's immune status over time (Brettler & Levine, 1989; Rocino *et al.*, 1990; di Biasi *et al.*, 1991; Seremites *et al.*, 1993).

One of the difficulties with this argument is that there is no rational definition of purity. The term is intended to relate to the ratio between factor VIII or IX protein and all other proteins present after plasma fractionation. However, factor VIII is very labile and needs stabilising in the final vial if it is not to lose its efficacy. Most manufacturers use albumin as a stabiliser and, of course, albumin contains extraneous proteins. So we are in the paradoxical situation of being able to manufacture very pure factor VIII concentrates, including recombinant genetically engineered products, which then have to be adulterated by the addition of a multi-donor human blood product.

The evidence is, however, sufficiently valid to give patients the benefit of the doubt, and all HIV-positive people with haemophilia should now have the option of therapy with a high purity factor VIII or IX concentrate.

The argument for high purity factor IX is more compelling because the less pure products are associated with a risk of thromboembolism (Lusher, 1991). To date there is no evidence that the newer products are associated with undue clotting, but only prolonged surveillance will confirm this.

HIV-infected youngsters with haemophilia

In the early years of the epidemic the haemophilic population contained a unique cohort of boys in late childhood and adolescence. In contrast, within the general population most infected people were adult males who had become infected as a result of anal intercourse with an infected partner, and men or women infected in the practice of intravenous drug abuse. There was a small number of perinatally infected infants. Understandably, the thrust of the early government programmes of public education was to alert the population to the risks of unprotected intercourse and unsafe drug use. Equally understandably haemophilic families felt increasingly threatened by the avalanche of publicity that followed, much of it ill informed and hurtful to them (Jones, 1989).

This was reflected in the decision of most parents not to tell anyone outside their haemophilia centre about their child's infection. Thus siblings, relatives, teachers and even family doctors were unaware of the truth. Predictably, the result was isolation. From the paediatrician's viewpoint the stigma and secrecy of HIV infection cut across all the usual practices of professional work and communication. The friendly telephoned enquiry about progress at school, and the free exchange of information between hospital and family practice ceased. Parents were terrified that knowledge of their son's HIV status would attract media attention, expulsion from school or work, and the loss of friends and neighbours. Sometimes they were right, but experience showed that the only vindictive incidents involving destruction of property or the daubing of slogans on walls were associated more with longstanding underlying social problems than with AIDS.

When to tell

Most parents decided not to tell their younger children with haemophilia that they were HIV-antibody positive, at least initially. The majority were secure in the knowledge that there was no risk to themselves or to siblings in their everyday lives. They wanted to enjoy the time left to the family without constant recognition of the underlying infection and, in general, they succeeded. In contrast a small minority, usually represented by an individual parent, became obsessive. Constant rumination fuelled by the fact that their children had an iatrogenic disease, and later by the searching for some form of compensation that culminated in long months of litigation, disrupted family life sometimes irretrievably. Families usually work better when knowledge is shared. Once the infected child knows the diagnosis, his siblings and close relatives should also know, preferably with his permission.

Occasionally, parents asked a member of staff to break the news for them. This was as painful as the breaking of any bad news to a patient; it was made more comfortable through having known the boy over the years because of his haemophilia. Interestingly when boys were told the diagnosis late, either by their parents or by their doctor, they said, matter of factly, that they already knew. One youngster said that he had not wanted to tell his parents for fear of worrying them!

Adolescence brings its own problems. Boys with haemophilia are routinely counselled about the inheritance of their disorder and, as they become sexually active, know that they can rely on haemophilia centre staff for information about sex and contraception. This background practice probably made it easier for both patients and staff when it came to discussing protected sex in order to reduce the risk of HIV transmission. However, it also added the burden of having to talk through fears about not being able to form meaningful relationships, and not being able to marry or have children. Not surprisingly for this age group, these concerns were far more relevant and real than fears about premature death.

Others had different experiences. Evans (1987) sent a questionnaire to the parents of haemophilic boys over the age of 10 years who were attending his centre. Staff had previously told the parents, but not the boys, the individual results of HIV testing. All 22 questionnaires were returned. Of the 15 HIV infected boys, only 5 had been told. All 7 remaining uninfected boys had been told they were seronegative. No parent of an uninformed infected boy wanted a member of staff to disclose the diagnosis, even after a meeting called to discuss why it was considered to be important. Subsequently, only one further boy was told his diagnosis, and that was only after he asked himself.

Evans pointed out that this enforced failure to impart information to teenagers, despite a longstanding professional relationship with them and their families, created difficulties both for the boys and for any sexual partners. Given the negative attitude of many teenagers to the 'safer sex' message he wondered whether knowledge of HIV infection would really help to prevent its spread, or simply 'placate our own consciences'.

Subsequent experience suggests that the attitude of many schools towards education about HIV infection is indeed more to do with the easing of conscience than with any thought of epidemiological control.

This attitude has not been helped by the early, inflated predictions on the size of the epidemic in the UK, or by the recent government decision to drop HIV education from the National Curriculum.

A template for care

Early in the epidemic it seemed that the haemophilia comprehensive care model could be useful in the management of AIDS. Haemophilia and HIV infection have much in common. Both are chronic disorders with acute exacerbations of ill health. Both are transmitted sexually. Both at some stage require hospital-based therapy. Both are expensive to manage properly. Both have profound long-term effects on families. Both require interdisciplinary specialist care.

The haemophilia model is based on teamwork, and ease of communication. It works best without the usual barriers of conventional medical practice, individuals adding their expertise freely and sometimes doing tasks usually reserved by other disciplines. For instance, nurses are trained to diagnose bleeds and treat bleeding episodes by giving intravenous blood product therapy, and some doctors even become skilled in aspects of social work. The requirements for comprehensive haemophilia care have recently been set out in a health circular (NHS Management Executive, 1993). In the following amended form some may be helpful to those setting up a resource to help people with HIV infection. Briefly, what people need are:

1. A clinical service provided by experienced staff and available at short notice at any time of the day or night
2. Laboratory services capable of providing fast HIV-antibody testing, and all the other investigations required for HIV-positive patients
3. Ease of access to specialist advice on all matters relating to HIV infection
4. Counselling in privacy of patients and their relatives
5. Provision of regular follow-up
6. Access to all relevant information on the treatment of HIV infection and associated disease including, when appropriate, the provision of prophylactic therapy
7. Immediate access to in-patient facilities staffed by people experienced in caring for those with HIV infection

To these should be added home visiting by nurses and social workers, the provision of group therapy and access to other support groups, and the reassurance that people who are terminally ill will be nursed in privacy by staff they know.

The difficulty in using this approach in the average hospital is that it does not fit the usual pattern of medical consultation. Typically people attending a genitourinary medicine clinic are referred when sick to a specialist in infectious diseases, with their social and other needs being addressed by further, unrelated departments. Whilst this fragmentation of care works well in acute medicine, when the majority of hospital referrals need short-term help, it does not commend itself to the needs of the person with a chronic disorder such as HIV infection, or to the needs of his or her family.

As far as paediatrics is concerned the difficulties are not so apparent as with adult patients because of the psychosocial and family approach of most paediatric staff. It is clearly much better to nurse HIV-infected children who need in-patient care in bright and colourful paediatric wards rather than in the isolation of an infectious diseases unit catering for all age groups. The need for barrier nursing these children rarely arises. In addition haemophilic boys frequently require factor VIII or IX therapy, and are used to receiving this from haemophilia centre staff. As these staff work with patients with haematological disorders, including leukaemia and lymphoma, they are also used to treating the opportunistic diseases of AIDS. Further, over the years an emotional link develops between staff and patients with a chronic disorder. Doctors, nurses and other staff enjoy watching children grow and thrive despite the problems posed by their underlying diagnosis. Nurses in particular have felt strongly that this bond with staff can be crucial to the wellbeing of youngsters struggling with a diagnosis of HIV infection. They need to feel safe and valued, that people are not frightened of them, and that when sick they will be nursed by people they know. Naturally, counselling about AIDS involves work both with sexual problems and with death. It is to the nurses that young people turn to talk about their misery and to ask questions about how to cope.

In order to undertake this role the nursing staff have to be tough, and to know they have the support of managers and colleagues. Often they feel guilt or remorse about the fate of their haemophilic patients. Although they did not prescribe the blood products responsible for the infection, it was they who either gave the transfusions or taught the patients or the parents to do so.

If it is bad for the nurses it does not take too much imagination to appreciate how difficult it must be for the mothers of haemophilic boys. They already feel 'responsible', because of their carrier status, for their son's haemophilia. Now they are also 'responsible' for his HIV infection, most poignantly because they must have injected the virus when they gave him treatment in the home.

It has been salutary to watch the courage of parents and children faced with this catastrophe, and humbling to realise how few have felt the need for anger or recrimination directed at the medical profession. The situation in France is not typical, but was recently the subject of a paper by Alain Abelhauser (personal communication 1993), who wondered why the question of contaminated blood should give rise to a blanket condemnation of the medical profession in that country. He thought that the answers lay on an emotional and on a political level. Emotionally, there were all the ties between care givers and patients which cannot remain neutral. Abelhauser is a psychoanalyst and in professional terminology says the French story is one of 'transfer' and 'counter transfer', a subconscious drive by patients to be freed from the emotional cage of the underlying haemophilia. Politically, the answer lies in the public impression of medicine as a power system, easiest to attack at points of perceived weakness. One such area, paradoxically designed to free people from disease, is haemophilia comprehensive care.

The safety of others

Throughout the epidemic health educators and advisory bodies have stressed the fact that HIV causes an infectious but not a contagious disease. The infection can only be transmitted from an infected to an uninfected person in specific ways, predominantly by unprotected penetrative sex or the sharing of equipment when injecting drugs. The infection is not transmitted through ordinary, everyday contact.

This view continues to be supported by the epidemiological evidence. To date, only four cases of probable child-to-child transmission in the home have been reported (Centers for Disease Control, 1993; Fitzgibbon *et al.*, 1993; Simonds & Chanock, 1993). In their paper Simonds & Chanock remarked that none of the cases of AIDS reported to CDC had been attributed to casual contact; by June 1993 CDC knew of 339 250 cases of AIDS in the USA (Centers for Disease Control, 1994). Within the UK none of 20 543 HIV infections reported implicated casual contact, and only 3 cases may have occurred as a result of blood contact involving broken skin (Public Health Laboratory Service, 1993). This small number of cases underlines the need for people to avoid exposure to blood through common sense measures such as not sharing wet razors, and covering open wounds with waterproof dressings.

These observations are crucial to the wellbeing of families with an infected child, especially when that child goes to school. For instance, they form the basis of the guidelines for local and education authorities in the

UK (Department of Education and Science, 1991; Department of Health, 1992). These guidelines recognise the right to privacy of the infected child in the context of the need for overall, general hygiene in the prevention of HIV transmission in community activities.

Children of HIV-infected haemophilic fathers

Despite the risks, couples with a haemophilic partner known to be HIV infected still opt for pregnancy. To date 20 babies have been born to the partners of men with haemophilia attending our centre. Three of the mothers were seropositive at the time of their pregnancies. Fourteen of the babies have been tested and shown to be seronegative after the age of 18 months. Goldman and her colleagues (1993) reported on 14 children born to the partners of 12 HIV-infected haemophilic fathers. All were HIV-antibody negative and physically and mentally healthy. All but one of the mothers were seronegative.

When intended conception is discussed, couples have been advised to have unprotected intercourse only at the time of ovulation, measured using either a prediction test or natural family planning techniques. At all other times abstention or protected sex is suggested to lessen fetal risk from an infected father. It is clear that more research is needed in order to help couples desiring pregnancy to achieve this, despite the risk of HIV infection and the ominous long-term problems associated with the premature loss of one or both parents (Jones, 1994).

Conclusions

Children and adolescents infected with HIV have special needs resulting from the stigma and isolation that have become synonymous with AIDS. Their care may be made more difficult because of the need to preserve confidentiality which, in turn, may prevent exposure to some of those agencies used to helping young people cope. Although there do not appear to be differences in terms of disease progression between those with haemophilia and others infected with HIV, there are differences in perspective. Families with haemophilia face two life-threatening diseases which, in the public mind, are linked. Disclosure of the underlying bleeding disorder may be very difficult for them.

Of the several elements that make up an effective and practical approach to the care of affected families, one of the most important is continuity. This means regular follow-up by experienced staff used to coping sensitively with the myriad problems posed by HIV infection. As the epidemic has developed it has become clear that not everyone dies early from an

AIDS-related disease. For the foreseeable future management therefore needs to address the care of long-term survivors, as well as the provision of help for increasing numbers of HIV-infected children and adolescents.

References

Aledort, L. M., Hilgartner, M. W., Pike, M. C., *et al.* (1992). Variability in serial CD4 counts and relation to progression of HIV-1 infection to AIDS in haemophilic patients. *British Medical Journal*, **304**, 212–16.

Aronstam, A, Congard, B, Evans, DIK, *et al.* (1993) HIV infection in haemophilia in a European cohort. *Archives of Disease in Childhood*, **68**, 521–4.

Birch, C. LaF. (1937). Hemophilia: clinical and genetic aspects. University of Illinois, Urbana; cited in Lee, C. A. (1992). Coagulation factor replacement therapy. In *Recent Advances in Haematology*, vol. 4, ed. A. V. Hoffbrand & M. K. Brenner, pp. 73–88. Edinburgh: Churchill Livingstone.

Brettler, D. B. & Levine, P. H. (1989). Factor concentrates for treatment of haemophilia: which one to choose? *Blood*, **73**, 2067–73.

Centers for Disease Control (1982). *Pneumocystis carinii* pneumonia among persons with haemophilia A. *Morbidity and Mortality Weekly Report*, **31**, 365–7.

Centers for Disease Control (1993). HIV transmission between two adolescent brothers with hemophilia. *Morbidity and Mortality Weekly Report*, **42**, 948–51.

Centers for Disease Control (1994). Statistics. *AIDS*, **8**, 399.

Cuthbert, R. J. G., Ludlam, C. A., Tucher, J., *et al.* (1990). Five year prospective study of HIV infection in the Edinburgh haemophilic cohort. *British Medical Journal*, **301**, 956–61.

Darby, S. C., Rizza, C. R., Doll, R., *et al.* (1989). Incidence of AIDS and excess of mortality associated with HIV in haemophiliacs in the UK. Report on behalf of the directors of haemophilia centres in the UK. *British Medical Journal*, **298**, 1064–8.

de Biasi, R., Rocino, A., Miraglia, E., *et al.* (1991). The impact of a very high purity factor VIII concentrate on the immune system of human immunodeficiency virus infected haemophiliacs: a randomised, prospective, two-year comparison with an intermediate purity product. *Blood*, **78**, 1919–22.

Department of Education and Science (1991). *HIV and AIDS. A Guide for the Education Service. Facts for Teachers, Lecturers and Youth Workers.* London: Department of Education and Science.

Department of Health (1992). *Children and HIV: Guidance for Local Authorities.* London: Department of Health.

European Centre for Epidemiological Monitoring of AIDS (1993). Quarterly Report 38, tables 5 and 6.

Evans, D. I. K., (1987). Human immunodeficiency virus and the law. *Lancet*, **ii**, 574–5.

Fitzgibbon, J. E., Gaur, S., Frenkel, L. D., *et al.* (1993). Transmission from one child to another of human immunodeficiency virus type 1 with a zidovudine-resistance mutation. *New England Journal of Medicine*, **329**, 1835–41.

Goedert, J. J., Kessler, C. M., Aledort, L. M., *et al.* (1989). A prospective study of human immunodeficiency virus type 1 infection and the development of AIDS in subjects with haemophilia. *New England Journal of Medicine,* **321,** 1143–8.

Goldman, E., Lee, C., Miller, R., *et al.* (1993). Children of HIV positive haemophilic men. *Archives of Disease in Childhood,* **68,** 133–4.

Jason, J. M., Stehr-Green, J., Holman, R. C. & Evatt, B. L. (1988). Human immunodeficiency virus infection in haemophilic children. *Pediatrics,* **82,** 565–70.

Jones, P. (1989). The counselling of HIV-antibody positive haemophiliacs. In *Counselling in HIV Infection and AIDS,* ed. J. Green & A. McCreaner, pp. 108–20. Oxford: Blackwell Scientific Publications.

Jones, P. (1994). HIV in childhood. *British Medical Journal,* **308,** 425–6.

Lusher, J. M. (1991). Thrombogenicity associated with factor IX complex concentrates. *Seminars in Hematology* (Suppl 6), 3–5.

Lee, C. A., Phillips, A. N., Elford, J., *et al.* (1989). The natural history of human immunodeficiency virus infection in a haemophilic cohort. *British Journal of Hematology,* **73,** 228–34.

Lee, C. A., Phillips, A. N., Elford, J., *et al.* (1991). Progression of HIV disease in a haemophilic cohort followed for 11 years and effect of treatment. *British Medical Journal,* **303,** 1093–6.

National Health Service Management Executive UK (1993). Provision of haemophilia treatment and care. Health Service Guidelines (93) 30. London: HMSO.

Public Health Laboratory Service (1993). HIV transmission between children at home. Communicable Disease Report 3;52:1. London: PHLS.

Rocino, A., Miraglia, E., Mastrullo, L. *et al.* (1990). Prospective controlled trial of an ultra-pure factor VIII concentrate to evaluate the effects on the immune status of HIV-antibody positive haemophilia patients. *Acta Toxicologica et Therapeutica,* **XI,** 49–58.

Rutherford, G. W., Lifson, A. R., Hessal, N. A., *et al.* (1990). Course of HIV-1 infection in a cohort of homosexual and bisexual men: an 11-year follow-up study. *British Medical Journal,* **301,** 1183–9.

Seremetis, S. V., Aledort, L. M., Bergman, G. E., *et al.* (1993). Three-year randomised study of high purity or intermediate purity factor VIII concentrates in symptom-free HIV seropositive haemophiliacs: effects on immune status. *Lancet,* **342,** 700–3.

Simonds, R. J. & Chanock, S. (1993). Medical issues related to caring for human immunodeficiency virus-infected children in and out of the home. *Pediatric Infectious Disease Journal,* **12,** 845–52.

Wagner, N., Bialek, R., Radinger, H., *et al.* (1990). HIV-1 infection in a cohort of haemophilic patients. *Archives of Disease in Childhood,* **65,** 1301–4.

12

Antiretroviral therapy for disease progression

DIANA M. GIBB

Introduction

Antiretroviral therapy for children with HIV infection and AIDS is a rapidly changing field and one where efficacy data are frequently unavailable. Many aspects of HIV infection in children are similar to those in adults and therefore it is often possible to extrapolate from the results of adult trials, where the number of available participants far exceeds the numbers which can be recruited into paediatric trials.

There are, however, aspects of the disease which are specific to children which may result in different responses to therapy. Not only does the natural history of the disease in vertically infected children differ from that in adults, but interaction between the virus and the developing immune system in the very young child may mean that early intervention could play a more important role in children than in adults. Issues of tolerance and acceptability of paediatric formulations are of importance, particularly if drug combinations become more widely used. The bioavailability and pharmacokinetics of antiretroviral drugs in children, particularly infants, need to be studied separately because of differences in the metabolism and excretion of drugs in this age group. Finally, if in the future it becomes possible to identify accurately those children at-risk of rapidly progressive HIV disease, then this group might help to accelerate knowledge about the efficacy of drugs and multi-drug combinations. Table 12.1 lists the main areas of antiretroviral therapy which require separate paediatric studies. With the rapid developments in this area, it is important that wherever possible children should have the opportunity to be enrolled into clinical trials. This is happening in the USA through the AIDS clinical trials group (ACTG), and a network is also being developed in Europe where, because of the large numbers required, trials organised through the Paediatric European Network for Treatment of AIDS (PENTA) are both multicentre and multinational.

Table 12.1. *Trials of antiretroviral therapy in children*

Cannot extrapolate from adult data alone because of differences in:
Natural history of the disease
Developing immune system
Pharmacokinetics/bioavailability
Tolerance/acceptability
Areas of evaluation to concentrate on:
Pharmacokinetics
Toxicity/tolerance
Timing of initiation of antiretroviral therapy
Identification of, and trials in, rapid progressors
Prevention of vertical transmission

This chapter will concentrate on the use of currently available antiretroviral agents, and will also allude to antiretroviral agents under development. The use of both antiretrovirals and immunotherapeutic agents to attempt to reduce the transmission of HIV infection from mother to child is discussed in Chapter 1.

Zidovudine (ZDV, 3'-azido-3'deoxythymidine) has been used in children for over 5 years and is the only antiretroviral drug licensed for children in all European countries. Dideoxyinosine (ddI) has been licensed in many countries following its release for children in 1992 in the USA. Dideoxycytidine (ddC), while available as a salvage therapy for children intolerant to ZDV in the USA, has not been licensed for paediatric use in Europe. Non-nucleoside reverse transcriptase inhibitors have been little used in children but may have potential as agents for use in combination therapies. New drugs under evaluation include other nucleoside reverse transcriptase inhibitors (stavudine (d4T) and 2'-deoxy-3'-thiacytidine (3TC)), the proteinase inhibitors and immune-based therapies. The main sites of action of antiretroviral drugs are shown in Table 12.2.

Zidovudine (ZDV, 3'-azido-3'-deoxythymidine, AZT, retrovir)

Zidovudine (ZDV) is a nucleoside analogue which inhibits viral reverse transcriptase activity (see Chapter 5). The half-life of the drug in plasma is approximately 1 hour (Furman *et al.*, 1986), although that of the active intracellular triphosphate is about 3 hours (Yarchoan *et al.*, 1989). The cerebrospinal fluid to plasma ratio is 0.6. It is available in 250 mg and 100 mg capsules and as a paediatric syrup at a concentration of 10 mg/ml. It was initially developed as an anticancer agent in 1964, and found to have activity against HIV in 1985.

Table 12.2 *Potential targets for antiretroviral therapy in the HIV life cycle*

Stage of life cycle	Process/enzyme involved	Antiretroviral agents
Cell membrane binding	CD4 receptor	Monoclonal anti-CD4 antibodies; soluble CD4
	gp 120	Monoclonal anti-envelope antibodies; sulphated polysaccharides
Membrane fusion and cell entry	gp41	
DNA provirus synthesis	Reverse transcriptase	Dideoxynucleosides (ZDV, ddI, ddC, 3TC, d4T); non-nucleosides (nevirapine, pyridinone, TIBO, BHAP)
Host DNA integration	DNA polymerase Integrase	
Transcription	RNA polymerase Regulatory and suppressor proteins mRNA translation Viral mRNA	Anti-sense phosphorothioate oligomers
	Ribosomes Regulatory proteins	
Viral assembly	Glycosylation Proteinase Regulatory proteins	Proteinase inhibitors
Budding		Interferon alpha

In 1987 the first clinical trial of 282 adults with AIDS or severe AIDS-related complex (ARC) demonstrated that survival was significantly prolonged in those taking ZDV compared with placebo (19 deaths in the placebo group, 1 death in the ZDV group after 16 weeks) (Fishl et al., 1987). In addition, there were fewer opportunistic infections, greater weight gain, more normal neuropsychological tests of cognition, and increased CD4 counts in the treated group. However, at a dose of 1500 mg per day there was also significant haematological toxicity, mainly anaemia and granulocytopenia. In subsequent trials it was shown that lower doses of ZDV (600 mg/day) were as efficacious as the high dose in patients with advanced disease and caused less toxicity (Degrattola, 1993). Current recommended doses in adults are 500–600 mg daily, often given three or four times daily, although the best dose interval is not known.

The use of ZDV monotherapy in asymptomatic adults with HIV infection has been evaluated in five clinical trials (Volberding, 1990; Fishl *et al.*, 1990; Hamilton *et al.*, 1992; Cooper *et al.*, 1993; Aboulker & Swart, 1993). Two trials reported that the progression to AIDS in those with CD4 counts less than $500 \times 10^6/1$ was reduced by up to 50% in the short term (about 1 year) (Volberding, 1990; Fishl, 1990). Although this finding was confirmed in the US Veterans Affairs Co-operative Study of 338 patients with early symptomatic disease and CD4 counts between 200 and $500 \times 10^6/1$ (Hamilton *et al.*, 1992), no survival advantage was demonstrated in this study in those receiving 'early' treatment. In a study by Cooper *et al.* (1993) which lasted 3 years, benefit was reported from early therapy in asymptomatic patients with CD4 counts above $400 \times 10^6/1$. However, in this study the number of clinical endpoints was small (22 AIDS events in the placebo versus 11 in the ZDV group at 2 years) and those stopping the trial drug were censored at the time of stopping, which limited the true 'early versus deferred therapy' comparison and could have led to bias in favour of ZDV.

The largest trial in asymptomatic HIV-infected adults with the longest follow-up (started 1988, median follow-up 3 years) has been the Anglo-French Concorde trial (Concorde Coordinating Committee, 1994). The number of clinical endpoints in this trial exceeds those of all previous trials put together. Preliminary results of the Concorde trial released in April 1993 (Aboulker & Swart, 1993) showed that although there was a suggestion of benefit in the early treated group at 1 year, comparable to previous trials, this was not sustained. After a median of 3 years follow-up there was no significant difference in progression to AIDS or death in those receiving ZDV early compared with those receiving it only when they developed symptoms. CD4 counts were not evaluated as endpoints in this trial, but analysis of this variable showed that despite the lack of significant difference in clinical endpoints in the two groups there was a highly statistically significant difference of an average of $30 \times 10^6/1$ cells in the CD4 count between those receiving early compared with deferred ZDV; this effect was sustained throughout the trial. This finding has implications for future efficacy trials of antiretrovirals as it suggests that although the CD4 count may be a good marker of progression of HIV disease in adults, it cannot be used as a surrogate endpoint in the evaluation of response to antiretroviral drugs. In children, in whom normal CD4 counts vary with age, the role of the CD4 count even as a marker of disease progression has been less well studied.

ZDV in children

In general, the pharmacokinetics of ZDV in children (5 months to 12 years of age) are similar to those in adults; it has higher oral bioavailability than other nucleoside analogues but a short half-life of about 1 hour (Balis *et al.*, 1989; Barry *et al.*, 1994). A greater variation in clearance, which was on average higher than in adults and older children, has been observed in younger children 2–3 years of age (Balis *et al.*, 1989). A dose of 150–180 mg/m^2 6 hourly has been recommended for paediatric use because of concerns about encephalopathy in children (Pizzo *et al.*, 1988). A paediatric study (ACTG 128) is fully recruited and in progress in the USA comparing 360 with 720 mg/m^2 per day, administered four times daily, the principal endpoint being a change in neurodevelopmental score. This study is discussed in Chapter 13.

No placebo-controlled efficacy studies of ZDV have been performed in children, although data from studies of open ZDV (i.e. with no placebo) suggest benefit in children with symptomatic HIV disease, particularly those with encephalopathy (Pizzo *et al.*, 1988; McKinney *et al.*, 1990, 1991). Other positive effects observed in these studies include an increase in weight and well-being and decreases in total immunoglobulin G and M (IgG and IgM) concentrations. Italian and French phase I studies have reported similar results, the former also reporting good tolerance when the drug was taken twice daily as opposed to 6 hourly. This was felt to increase compliance greatly, especially amongst families where injecting drug use was a problem (Giaquinto *et al.*, in press). Preliminary pharmacokinetic data on the twice-daily regimen suggest that there is a dose-related peak in plasma levels but that the drug then rapidly disappears from plasma. How this relates to tissue levels is unknown.

Even more so than in adults, the optimum timing of initiation of ZDV in children remains unclear. HIV disease in children differs from that in adults as regards both the incubation period and the illnesses associated with the disease (see Chapters 3, 4 and 5). It is also possible that early therapy could play a greater role in children because of the interaction between the virus and the developing immune system (see Chapter 6.)

The PENTA I trial is comparing the efficacy and acceptability of ZDV treatment started early in the disease with treatment started only at the onset of HIV-related symptoms. The design is similar to that of the Concorde trial of early ZDV in asymptomatic adults. The trial commenced in autumn 1992, and is open to recruitment (Gibb *et al.*, 1993). It is a multicentre, multinational trial aiming for an intake of 400 children.

Impact of the results of the ZDV in pregnancy trial

The ACTG 076 trial was a phase III trial comparing ZDV with placebo in antiretroviral-naive pregnant women (see Chapter 1). Trial drug was started orally between 14 and 34 weeks of pregnancy, given intravenously intrapartum, and to the neonate for 6 weeks. Results from the first interim efficacy analysis on 364 mother–baby pairs showed a decrease in transmission rate from mother to child from 25.5% in the placebo group to 8.3% in the ZDV-treated group (Medical News, *Journal of the American Medical Association*, 1994). There was minimal short-term toxicity reported in the babies.

The trial has been discontinued and is likely to have a major impact on clinical practice in USA and Europe. However, it remains unknown which of the times of ZDV administration contributed most to the reduced transmission rate, and many other questions remain unanswered. Of particular importance is the possibility of long-term toxicity in babies who would in any case be uninfected (about 80%). Other issues include the possibility of transmission of resistant virus and questions about how implementation of the results of this trial may affect the natural history of disease in children who are infected despite their mothers having received ZDV in pregnancy. Infected children may also develop resistance more quickly when given ZDV later in childhood. These questions can only be answered by careful follow-up of *all* children whose mothers have received ZDV in pregnancy, both in cohort studies and future trials of antiretroviral therapy.

Adverse effects of ZDV

ZDV can cause a reduction in neutrophil count and haemoglobin concentration, particularly in the first weeks of therapy (Fishl *et al.*, 1987; Richman *et al.*, 1987). These side-effects are, however, reversible. Non-haematological side-effects include nausea and headaches and, very rarely, myositis (Fishl *et al.*, 1987, 1990; Volberding *et al.*, 1990; Hamilton *et al.*, 1992, Cooper *et al.* 1993; Aboulker & Swart, 1993). In trials in asymptomatic adults, including the Concorde trial, the incidence of toxicity was low. In children, ZDV has generally been well tolerated, especially in those in whom treatment is given early in the course of disease. This has been the case so far in the PENTA 1 trial and was an additional factor taken into consideration when the decision was made to continue the trial after the preliminary results of the Concorde trial became available.

ZDV resistance

There is concern that the efficacy of ZDV decreases with time if the drug is given as monotherapy. In 1989, Larder *et al.* demonstrated that *in vitro* resistance to ZDV appears in adults with advanced HIV disease treated for more than 1 year. The relationship between clinical resistance to ZDV and laboratory evidence of ZDV-resistant HIV strains is as yet unclear, but the laboratory findings are disconcerting. In children receiving ZDV monotherapy, decreased *in vitro* ZDV susceptibility has been reported to be associated with poor clinical response to the drug (Tudor-Williams *et al.*, 1992); however, the numbers in this study were small. Further results on the relationship between resistance and disease progression are awaited from virology performed in trials of asymptomatic adults (ACTG 019; Volberding *et al.*, 1990; Aboulker & Swart, 1993).

Dideoxyinosine (2′,3′-dideoxyinosine, didanosine, ddI)

Didanosine (ddI) is another nucleoside analogue which is active *in vitro* against HIV (Mitsuya & Broder, 1986). It has a plasma half-life of only 30 minutes but the intracellular half-life is 12 hours, which allows twice-daily administration. The drug is inactivated by gastric acid and must therefore be taken on an empty stomach, with an antacid. Oral bioavailablity is variable, and the cerebrospinal fluid to plasma ratio is only 0.2 (Yarchoan *et al.*, 1989). The toxicities of ddI are different from those of ZDV and consist of peripheral neuropathy, pancreatitis (in about 5% of children) and occasionally hepatic problems. Toxicities are dose related, occurring especially at doses above 360 mg/m^2 per day (Connoll *et al.*, 1991).

There have been no placebo-controlled efficacy trials of ddI but in adults who have already received ZDV, switching to ddI was reported to be at least as effective in the short term as remaining on ZDV alone (Kahn *et al.*, 1992). In a sister study (ACTG 116A), ZDV appeared to be superior to ddI as first-line monotherapy (AIDS Clinical Trials Group, 1992). In two adult trials (ALPHA trial and ACTG 118), preliminary results reported no clinical or survival benefit in those taking ddI 750 mg/day compared with 500 mg/day or 200 mg/day for late-stage disease, although there was a significantly greater rise in CD4 count in those taking the higher dose (Darbyshire & Aboulker, 1992).

Fewer data are available on the use of ddI in children. In a dose ranging study in which children received between 60 and 540 mg/m^2 per day, the bioavailability was variable and low, being 21% compared with 35% in adults (Butler *et al.*, 1991). Improvements in CD4 counts, decreased p24 antigenaemia and weight gain were reported. In a dose comparison study in 34 French children receiving 120 or 270 mg/m^2 per day for 6 months, the decrease in viraemia and increase in CD4 was similar for both doses and pancreatitis was not observed (Blanche *et al.*, 1994). However, 5 children in the French study developed abnormalities of liver function, and 1 child died of hepatic failure. As 3 of these children had pre-existing liver disease, the possibility that the liver failure was secondary to HIV itself cannot be ruled out.

ddI is now licenced in the USA, and in many European countries including the United Kingdom, France, Italy, Spain and Germany, as monotherapy for children with HIV infection who are intolerant of ZDV or where disease progression is occurring despite ZDV therapy. The available formulations are either a powder with buffer (100 mg) for older children or buffered tablets (to be crushed or dissolved in water: 25 mg, 50 mg, 100 mg). Specific ddI-selected amino acid substitutions on the HIV reverse transcriptase enzyme have been observed after prolonged therapy with ddI. It is of interest, but requires further study, that one of the ddI-selected substitutions can reduce resistance induced by some of the ZDV-selected substitutions (St Clair *et al.*, 1991).

Dideoxcytidine (ddC)

Dideoxycytidine (ddC, zalcitabine) is a third nucleoside analogue with potent *in vitro* activity against HIV (Broder, 1990). Pharmacokinetics of ddC have been studied mainly in adults. The mean oral bioavailability is 87% (ZDV, 63%); plasma half-life and intracellular half-life of ddC are 1.2 and 2.6 hours respectively (Yarchoan *et al.*, 1989; Broder, 1990). ddC is cleared mainly by the kidneys and 75% of the parent drug is recovered in the urine. The cerebrospinal fluid penetration of ddC is about a third of that obtained with ZDV (Yarchoan *et al.*, 1989).

There have been no placebo-controlled efficacy studies of ddC. As monotherapy, in advanced disease in antiretroviral-naive adults, it appears to be inferior to ZDV (Follansbee *et al.*, 1993). The American study CPCRA002 compared ddI and ddC in an open label study of 467 adults with advanced disease previously treated with (but either intolerant of, or progressing despite) ZDV (Abrams *et al.*, 1994). Rates of disease progression and death were slightly better in the ddC-treated group and suggested that ddC is at least as effective as ddI in delaying disease progression and death. More patients suffered from peripheral neuropathy and stomatitis on ddC, while there were more cases of pancreatitis and gastrointestinal disturbances with ddI. The total number of adverse reactions was similar in both groups.

The major dose-limiting toxicity of ddC is a painful sensorimotor peripheral neuropathy; this toxic effect occurs at doses >0.06 mg/kg per day in adults 8–14 weeks after initiation of treatment (Merrigan *et al.*, 1989). Other common side-effects which may occur at any dose level include skin rashes and stomatitis. In most adults, doses of 0.03 mg/kg per day given on an 8 hourly dosing schedule have been tolerated for 6 months or more, although reversible peripheral neuropathy may occasionally develop.

Pharmacokinetic data on ddC in children are limited. In a study conducted by Pizzo and colleagues (1990) the pharmacokinetics in children were similar to those in adults at ddC doses of 0.03–0.04 mg/kg. There is a paucity of cerebrospinal fluid pharmacokinetic data in children. In the above study, an 8 week course of ddC was followed by alternating ZDV and ddC in cycles consisting of ZDV 720 mg/m² per day for 3 weeks followed by 1 week of ddC. This regimen was reported to sustain the reduction in viral burden (observed after 8 weeks of ddC) and to result in some observable clinical benefit in the majority of cases. Psychometric test results did not change, although improved behaviour was reported in all 4 children who presented with encephalopathy. No neutropenia, anaemia or neuropathy were observed at ddC doses of 0.06, 0.08, 0.12 and 0.16 mg/kg per day for 8 weeks. Mouth ulcers occurred in some children at all doses, with onset 2–3 weeks after initiation of treatment. ddC is not yet licensed for children in Europe or the USA, but may be available on a compassionate basis.

Combination therapies

As in the treatment of other infectious diseases, combination therapy for HIV infection may not only result in synergism between different drugs (both those acting on similar and on differing sites of the viral replication cycle), but may limit the emergence of drug resistance. In addition, if lower doses of drugs with different toxicity profiles are combined, this may reduce the overall toxicity. Drugs may be used concurrently, in alternating fashion or sequentially. Clinical trials of combination therapy are only just beginning, and at present there are few data available to favour any of these approaches. Many would argue, however, that concurrent therapy might have the greatest success in preventing the emergence of resistance and delaying disease progression (Yarchoan, *et al*. 1992).

Combination trials in adults are in progress in antiretroviral-naive patients as well as those who have already received ZDV. Two major phase III efficacy trials of ZDV monotherapy versus combination therapy with ZDV+ddI and ZDV+ddC are in progress (ACTG 175 in the USA, DELTA trial in Europe) in antiretroviral-naive adults, as is a phase III trial in children comparing ZDV with ddI with ZDV+ddI in children in USA (ACTG 152). While it will not be necessary to repeat all efficacy studies of drug combinations, it will be important to perform phase I and II studies of pharmacokinetics, toxicity and tolerability in children. Phase I/II studies of ZDV with ddI in children reported no evidence of new or enhanced toxicity (Husson *et al.*, 1994). A US phase II study comparing ZDV+ddC with ZDV+ddC placebo in children who had previously received ZDV is under way (ACTG 190) and a complementary study in ZDV-naive children is in progress in Europe (PENTA 3).

Other antiretroviral drugs under evaluation

Other nucleoside reverse transcriptase inhibitors are under investigation in both adults and children, including 3-thiacytidine (3TC) and stavudine (D4T). To date 3TC has shown little toxicity up to a dose of 20 mg/m^2 per day, but also little effect on surrogate marker response (van Leeuwen *et al.*, 1992). D4T has serious toxicity, particularly pancreatitis.

Non-nucleoside reverse transcriptase inhibitors

The non-nucleoside reverse transcriptase inhibitors include nevirapine, pyridinone (L-697, 66), TIBO and the BHAP compounds such as U-87201E and U-90152S. They bind directly to the enzyme complex and prevent DNA polymerisation, instead of being incorporated into viral DNA to produce 'corrupt DNA' as is the case with the nucleoside analogues. They are HIV-1 specific, but high-level resistance develops rapidly, limiting their use as monotherapeutic agents (Nunberg *et al.*, 1991). They are being evaluated at higher doses and in combination with other antiretrovirals, in both adults and children in the USA. The toxicity of nevirapine, which has been most studied, consists mainly of rashes when used at high doses. The frequency of this adverse effect may be diminished by slowly increasing the dose at the introduction of therapy. One short-term use for these compounds may be in the prevention of intrapartum transmission of HIV from mother to child (see Chapter 1).

Proteinase inhibitors

The HIV proteinase is essential for manufacturing viral core and polymerase proteins in order that infectious virions are produced. Thus far, phase I/II trials in Europe show that proteinase inhibitors are well-tolerated as monotherapy and in combination with ZDV, with very few side-effects. Increases in CD4 counts were observed in all studies; these were dose related and higher with combination therapy (Delfraissy *et al.*, 1993; Danner *et al.*, 1993). Further phase II and III studies of monotherapy and combination therapy with these drugs are planned and the production of preparations for children is being researched. Lack of oral bioavailability has been a difficulty in the development of this group of compounds. Unfortunately the development of resistance to proteinase inhibitors has already been documented.

Immune-based therapies

The elucidation of the immunopathogenesis of HIV-1 infection and development of immune-based therapies are only in the investigational stages. Strategies aimed at general immune enhancement have included use of putative cytokines such as interleukin-2 (IL-2), interferon alpha and interferon gamma as well as inhibitors of cytokines (with potentially deleterious effects) such as tumour necrosis factor (TNF). None of these approaches has yet demonstrated more than minor effects on surrogate markers, but they may prove useful in combination with antiretroviral therapies. At present, the administration by the intramuscular or intravenous routes is a disadvantage for their use, especially in children.

HIV-specific immune enhancement aims to increase responses to neutralising antibodies, antibody-dependent cellular toxicity and cytotoxic T cells. Enhancement of antibody protection has been either by passive immunisation or by active vaccination in an attempt to enhance virus-specific immune responses. Neither of these approaches has yet shown any convincing evidence of clinical efficacy in HIV-infected adults. However, the fact that the majority of mothers do not transmit HIV to their offspring provides an opportunity to examine the mechanisms of protective immune responses. Immunisation of the mother and/or infant remains an attractive strategy to prevent transmission from mother to child (see Chapters 1 and 13).

Passive immunisation

Production of polyclonal antibody from a number of HIV-infected donors is one approach to passive immunisation (Jackson *et al.*, 1988). The advantage of pooling of donors is that the product will contain many component antibodies against several viral variants present in the donors, and donors could be selected from the same population as the prospective recipients. However, this therapy is expensive, and difficult to standardise. In addition, it is possible that such an approach could result in immune activation and actually do harm by increasing HIV replication. A second approach is to use synthesised monoclonal antibodies (Gowland *et al.*, 1992). However, it is likely that a combination of monoclonal antibodies will be required to achieve neutralisation. The most promising role for passive immunisation is in attempting to prevent perinatal transmission; two phase II trials using polycloncal antibody are under way in the USA and Africa (see Chapter 1).

Vaccine therapy

Active immunisation can produce both humoral and cellular immune responses (Redfield *et al.*, 1991) and might be used both as therapy and to prevent mother-to-child transmission. Initial studies of recombinant envelope vaccines given to mothers in early pregnancy, to newborns (as post-exposure prophylaxis) and to HIV-infected children (therapeutic model) are under way in the USA (see Chapters 1 and 13).

Guidelines for antiretroviral management

Treatment guidelines for antiretroviral therapy are continuously evolving over time as results from trials in both adults and children become available. In the USA the National Pediatric HIV Resource Center produced the most recent guidelines in June 1993 (Pizzo & Wilfert, 1993).

ZDV is licensed for children with symptomatic disease and 'significant' immunological compromise, although this is not defined specifically. The initiation of antiretroviral therapy (at present ZDV monotherapy) in the USA guidelines is based on age-related CD4 counts. However, in Europe, especially following the results of the Concorde trial, these CD4-based guidelines are rarely followed. Wherever possible parents and children should be given the opportunity to enrol in the PENTA I trial when there is uncertainty about when to start therapy. Within this trial, clinical guidelines were defined for transfer of children from trial drug (ZDV or placebo) to open label ZDV. These were devised after consultation with European paediatricians and include the development of AIDS or the presence of specific clinical conditions (Table 12.3). Some paediatricians will commence ZDV in children with rapidly falling CD4 counts or p24 antigenaemia, particularly if this occurs early in life.

The optimum dose of ZDV is also unclear and results of ACTG 128 are awaited. The licensed dose is 600–720 mg/m² per day in four divided doses. In the USA the higher dose has been recommended because of concerns about HIV encephalopathy. In Europe the lower dose, often given three times daily, is more frequently used.

For children intolerant to ZDV, ddI is the main second-line treatment and has been licensed or is available on a compassionate basis in most European countries. For children who are progressing but are able to tolerate ZDV, another option would be to add ddI or ddC to ZDV therapy, although ddC syrup is not yet available in Europe. In USA it is recommended that changing antiretroviral therapy should be based on either growth failure (decline over 2 centile lines) or neurodevelopmental deterioration (Pizzo & Wilfert, 1993).

Table 12.3. *Clinical guidelines for initiation of antiretroviral therapy*

AIDS
AIDS-defining opportunistic infection
Severe failure to thrive (crossing 2 centiles or below the 5th centile and deviating from it)
HIV encephalopathy
Recurrent severe bacterial infection (septicaemia or meningitis)
HIV-associated malignancy
Other clinical conditions which may warrant initiating antiretroviral therapy
Symptomatic LIP with/without parotitis
Persistent oral candidiasis
Recurrent unexplained diarrhoea
Cardiomyopathy
HIV nephropathy
Symptomatic thrombocytopenia
Chronic/recurrent severe bacterial infections
Recurrent herpes simplex/varicella zoster infections
Moderate failure to thrive
Developmental delay thought to be HIV-related

LIP, lymphoid interstitial pneumonia.

Conclusion

In the immediate future, it can be hoped that trials of combination therapy in antiretroviral naive adults may show better clinical efficacy than ZDV monotherapy. Phase I and II paediatric studies to evaluate toxicity and tolerability should continue to be set up in parallel so that children can benefit immediately from the results of adult trials. In the long term better antiretroviral agents are needed, to which HIV remains sensitive over time to enable effective early use of these drugs to prevent viral replication and destruction of the immune system in HIV infection. Approaches to affect HIV at different sites of its life-cycle combined with strategies to enhance immune defence against it may be of value. Finally, the most important strategy will come from approaches to prevent vertical transmission. With the results of the ACTG 076 trial, there are clearly future challenges to be met in the use of ZDV, combination antiretroviral and immune based agents in pregnancy and the newborn.

References

Abrams, D. I., Goldman, A. I., Launer, C., *et al.* (1994). A comparative trial of Didanosine or Zalcitabine after treatment with Zidovudine in patients with human immunodeficiency virus infection. *New England Journal of Medicine*, **330**, 657–62.

Aboulker, J. P., Swart, A. M., (1993). Preliminary analysis of the Concorde trial. *Lancet*, **341**, 889–90.

Aids Clinical Trials Group (1992). Executive summary for the final analysis of ACTG 116A. December 22 1992. Bethesda, Maryland:

Balis, F. M., Pizzo, P. A., Eddy J., *et al.* (1989). Pharmacokinetics of Zidovudine administered intravenously and orally in children with human immunodeficiency virus infection. *Journal of Pediatrics*, **114**, 880–4.

Barry M., Howe J. L., Back, D. J., Han, I & Gibb D. M. (1994). Zidovudine pharmacokinetics in children with symptomatic HIV infection. *Drug Investigation*, **7**, 143–7.

Blanche, S., Calvez, T., Rouzioux, C., *et al.* (1994). A randomised study of two doses of didanosine in HIV-infected children (in press).

Broder, S. (1990) 2',3'-Dideoxcytidine: an inhibitor of human immunodeficiency virus. *American Journal of Medicine*, **88** (Suppl 5B), 2S–7S, 27.

Butler, K. M., Husson, R. N., Balis, F. M., *et al.* (1991). Dideoxyinosine in children with symptomatic human immunodeficiency virus infection. *New England Journal of Medicine*, **324**, 137–44.

Concorde Coordinating Committee. (1994). Concorde: MRC/ANRS randomised double blind controlled trial of immediate and deferred zidovudine in symptom-free HIV infection. *Lancet*, **343**, 871–81.

Connoll, K. J., Allan, J. D., Fitch H, *et al.* (1991). Dideoxyinosine administered orally twice daily to patients with AIDS or AIDS-related complex and hemotological intolerance to zidovudine. *American Journal Medecine*, **91**, 471–8.

Cooper, D. A., Gatell, J. M., Kroon, S., *et al*, and the European-Australian Collaborative Group (1993). Zidovudine in persons with asymptomatic HIV infection and CD4⁺ cell counts greater than 400 per cubic millimeter. *New England Journal of Medicine*, **329**, 297–303.

Danner, S. A. Reedijk, M., Boucher, CAB, *et al.* (1993) Phase-I study of A-77003, a HIV proteinase inhibitor in man (abstract WS-B26–6) Berlin: IXth International Conference on AIDS.

Darbyshire, J. H., Aboulker, J. P. (1992) Didanosine for zidovudine-intolerant patients with HIV disease (letter). *Lancet*, **340**, 1346–7.

Degrattola, V. (1993) Modelling the relationship between survival and CD4 lymphocytes in patients with AIDS and AIDS-related complex. *Journal of AIDS*, **6**, 359–365.

Delfraissy, J. F., Sereni, D., Brun-Vezinet, F., *et al.* (1993) A phase I/II dose ranging study of the safety of Ro31–8959 (HIV proteinase inhibitor) in previously zidovudine treated HIV-infcted individuals abstract WS-B26–3. Berlin: IXth International Conference on AIDS.

Fishl, M. A., Richman, D. D., Grieco, M. H., *et al.* (1987) The efficacy of azidothymidine (AZT) in the treatment of patients with AIDS and AIDS-related complex: a double-blind, placebo-controlled trial. *New England Journal of Medicine*, **317**, 185–91.

Fishl, M. A., Richman, D. D., Hansen, N., *et al.* (1990) The safety and efficacy of zidovudine (AZT) in the treatment of subjects with mildly symptomatic human immunodeficiency virus type I (HIV) infection: a double-blind, placebo controlled trial. *Annals of Internal Medicine*, **112**, 727–37.

Follansbee, S., Lalezari, J., Olson, R., *et al.* (1993). The efficacy of zalcatabine (ddC,HIVID) versus zidovudine (ZDV) as monotherapy in naive patients with advanced HIV disease: a randomised, double blind, comparative trial (ACTG 144:N3300) PO-B26–2113. Berlin: IXth International Conference on AIDS.

Furman, P. A., Fyfe, J. A., St Clair, M. H., *et al.* (1986). Phosphorylation of 3'-azido-3'-deoxythymidine and selective interaction of the 5'-triphosphate with human immunodeficiency virus reverse transcriptase. *Proceedings of the National Academy of Sciences, USA,* **83**, 8333–7.

Giaquinto, C., Cozzini, S., Plebani, A., *et al.* (1994). Pharmacokinetic and long-term tolerance of twice daily zidovudine administration in children with mildly symptomatic HIV infection. *Journal of Paediatrics* (in press).

Gibb, D. M., Debre, M., for the Paediatric European Network for Treatment of AIDS (PENTA) Steering committee (1993). The PENTA I Trial (abstract PO-B26-2117). Berlin: IXth International Conference on AIDS.

Gowland, P., Gunthard, H., Schupbach, J., *et al.* (1992). Phase I/IIA clinical studies of a chimeric mouse–human monoclonal antibody to HIV-1 gp120 (abstract PoB3445). Amsterdam: VIII International Conference on AIDS.

Hamilton, J. D., Hartigan, P. M., Simberkoff, M. S., *et al.* (1992). A controlled trial of early versus late treatment with zidovudine in symptomatic human immunodeficiency virus infection: results of the Veterans Affairs Cooperative Study. *New England Journal of Medicine,* **326**, 437–43.

Husson, R., Mueller, B., Farley, M., *et al.* (1994). Zidovudine and Didanosins combination therapy in children with human immunodeficiency virus infection. *Pediatrics,* **93**, 316–322.

Jackson, G. G., Rubenis, M., Knigge, M., *et al.* (1988). Passive immunoneutralisation of HIV in patients with advanced AIDS. *Lancet,* **ii**, 647–51.

Kahn, J. O., Lagakos, S. W., Richman, D. D., *et al.* (1992). A controlled trial comparing continued zidovudine with didanosine in human immunodeficiency virus infection. *New England Journal of Medicine,* **327**, 581–7.

Larder, B. A., Darby, G. & Richman, D. D. (1989). HIV with reduced sensitivity to zidovudine (AZT) isolated during prolonged therapy. *Science,* **243**, 1731–4.

McKinney, R. E., Maha, M. A., Connor, E. M., *et al.* (1991). A multicenter trial of oral zidovudine in children with advanced human immunodeficiency virus disease. *New England Journal of Medicine,* **324**, 1018–25.

McKinney, R. E., Pizzo, P. A., Scott, G. B., *et al.* (1990). Safety and tolerance of intermittent intravenous and oral zidovudine therapy in human immunodeficiency virus-infected pediatric patients. *Journal of Pediatrics,* **116**, 640–7.

Merrigan, T. C., Skowron, G., Bozzette, S. A., *et al.* (1989). Circulating p24 antigen levels and responses to dideoxycytidine in human immunodeficiency virus infections: phase I and II study. *Annals of Internal Medicine,* **110**, 189–194.

Mitsuya, H., Broder, S. (1986) Inhibition of the *in vitro* infectivity and cytopathic effect of human T-lymphocyte virus type III/lymphadenopathy associated virus (HTLV-III/LAV) by 2,3'-dideoxynucleosides. *Proceedings of the National Academy of Sciences, USA,* **83**: 1911–15.

Nunberg, J. H., Schleif, W. A., Boots, E. J., *et al.* (1991). Viral resistance to human immunodeficiency virus type I-specific pyridinone reverse transcriptase inhibitors. *Journal of Virology,* **65**, 4887–92.

Pizzo, P. A., Butler, K., Balis, F., *et al.* (1990) Dideoxycytidine alone and in an alternating schedule with zidovudine (ZDV) in children with symptomatic human immunodeficiency virus infection. *Journal of Pediatrics,* **117**, 799–808.

Pizzo, P. A., Eddy, I., Falloon, J., *et al.* (1988). Effect of continuous intravenous infusion of zidovudine (AZT) in children with symptomatic HIV infection. *New England Journal of Medicine,* **319**, 889–96.

Pizzo, P. A., Wilfert, C. M. & Working Group on Antiretroviral Therapy: National Pediatric HIV Resource Centre (1993). Perspectives on pediatric immunodeficiency virus infection. Antiretroviral therapy and medical management of the human immunodeficiency virus-infected child. *Pediatric Infectious Disease Journal*, **12**, 513–22.

Redfield, R. R., Birx, D. L., Ketter, N. *et al.* (1991). Phase I evaluation of the immunogenicity of vaccination with recombinant gp160 in patients with early human immunodeficiency virus infection. *New England Journal of Medicine*, **324**, 1677–84.

Richman, D. D., Fischl, M. A., Grieco, M. H., *et al.* (1987). The toxicity of azidothymidine (AZT) in the treatment of patients with AIDS and AIDS-related complex: a double-blind, placebo-controlled trial. *New England Journal of Medicine*, **317**, 1927–32.

St Clair, M. H., Martin, J. L., Tudor-Williams, G., *et al.* (1991). Resistance to ddI and sensitivity to AZT induced by a mutation in HIV-1 reverse transcriptase. *Science*, **253**, 1557–9.

Tudor-Williams, G., St Clair, M. H. & McKinney, R. E. (1992). HIV-1 sensitivity to zidovudine and clinical outcome in children. *Lancet*, **i**, 15–19.

van Leeuwen, R., Lange, J. M. A., Hussey, E. K., *et al.* (1992). The safety and pharmacokinetics of a reverse transcriptase inhibitor, 3TC, in patients with HIV infection: a phase I study. *AIDS*, **6**, 1471–5.

Volberding, P. A., Lagakos, S. W., Koch, M. A., *et al.* (1990). Zidovudine in asymptomatic human immunodeficiency virus infection: a controlled trial in persons with fewer than 500 CD4-positive cells per cubic millimeter. *New England Journal of Medicine* **322**, 941–9.

Yarchoan, R., Lietzau, J. A., Brawley, O., *et al.* (1992) Therapy of AIDS or symptomatic HIV infection with simultaneous or alternating regimens of AZT and DDI (abstract MOB0054). Amsterdam: VIII International Conference on AIDS.

Yarchoan, R., Mitsuya, H., Meyers, Cs, C. E. & Broder, S. (1989) Clinical pharmacology of 3-azido-2 3-dideoxythymidine (zidovudine) and related dideoxynucleosides. *New England Journal of Medicine*, **321**, 726–38.

Addenda

Concorde Coordinating Committee (1994). Concorde MRC/ANRS randomised double-blind controlled trial of immediate and deferred zidovudine in symptom-free HIV infection. *Lancet*, **343**, 871–81.

In ACTG 128, comparing 720 with 360 mg/m²/day ZDV in children with moderately symptomatic HIV infection, there were no significant differences in progression to AIDS, survival, neurodevelopment or toxicity between the two groups. The full report is awaited.

Combination therapies may hold promise over monotherapy, and trials are planned or ongoing with 2-, 3- or 4-drug combinations. The results of ACTG 175 and DELTA trials are expected in 1995 and early 1996.

13

An overview of American paediatric treatment trials

GEORGE D. McSHERRY and EDWARD M. CONNOR

Introduction

Since the first cases of paediatric AIDS were described in the early 1980s more than 4900 children with AIDS have been reported to the United States Centers for Disease Control and Prevention (Centers for Disease Control and Prevention, 1993). It is conservatively estimated that an additional 15 000 children are now infected with HIV and that an additional 1500–2000 infected infants are born annually. By 1990 HIV/ AIDS was the seventh leading cause of death among children 1–4 years old in the USA (Chu et al. 1991; Oxtoby, 1994). AIDS has become the leading cause of death among young women and men in many US cities. In Newark, New Jersey, AIDS was the cause of death of 43% of women between 25 and 44 years of age (Selik et al., 1993).

Virtually all children now being diagnosed as infected with HIV acquired it vertically from their mothers (Centers for Disease Control and Prevention, 1993). Diagnosis and monitoring of these HIV-exposed infants is a complex process. While many questions remain about both diagnostic testing and immune monitoring of these children still more are raised with regard to treatment and, more importantly, prevention of infection.

Despite these difficulties, the work of groups such as the European Collaborative Study, Institut National de la Santé et de la Recherche Médicale (INSERM), Agence Nationale de Recherches sur le SIDA (ANRS), the Paediatric European Network for Treatment of AIDS (PENTA) and the AIDS Clinical Trials Group (ACTG) of the National Institute of Allergy and Infectious Diseases (NIAID) in the USA means that paediatric HIV infection, while still an incurable disease, is no longer an untreatable one (Connor, 1991; Working Group on Antiretroviral Therapy: National Pediatric HIV Resource Center, 1993). In the USA all large-scale intervention trials aimed at HIV infection in children are conducted through the Pediatric ACTG. Reviewed here are the structure, accomplishments and current research agenda of that organisation.

History of the AIDS Clinical Trials Group

The AIDS Clinical Trials Group (ACTG) is a cooperative network of institutions that designs and conducts collaborative clinical trials and other studies of HIV infection in the USA. These include, but are not limited to, studies in antiretroviral chemotherapy, prophylaxis and treatment of opportunistic infections and vaccine trials (Agenda of the Pediatric Committee of the AIDS Clinical Trials Group, 1993). The ACTG is sponsored by the National Institute of Allergy and Infectious Diseases (NIAID). It is directed by NIAID's Division of AIDS (DAIDS) (Cotton *et al.*, 1993). The ACTG was established in 1986 and is now divided into adult and paediatric sections. The Pediatric ACTG was established in 1987 with the funding of four paediatric units. By 1988 13 paediatric units had been established. There are currently 22 NIAID-funded sites and an additional 28 sites sponsored by the National Institute of Child Health and Development (NICHD) (Agenda of the Pediatric Committee of the AIDS Clinical Trials Group, 1993). A specific paediatric laboratory infrastructure involving clinical and developmental virology, pharmacology, immunology and neuropsychology was established in 1993.

Current scientific agenda

Since its inception in 1987 more than 3200 HIV-infected children and 750 pregnant women have been enrolled into clinical trials sponsored by the Pediatric ACTG. Accomplishments during that time include the reduction in the age of diagnosis of perinatal HIV infection from 18 months to 3–6 months of age (Borkowsky *et al.*, 1992; Report of a Consensus Workshop, 1992); the definition of age-adjusted normal CD4+lymphocyte counts (Denny *et al.*, 1992); the completion of phase I/II trials of zidovudine (ZDV) and didanosine (ddI) in children allowing for paediatric licensing indications (McKinney *et al.*, 1990, 1991; Balis *et al.*, 1992); promotion of the parallel development of drugs in children and adults; definition of the role of intravenous immunoglobulin (IVIG) in the prevention of serious bacterial infections in HIV-infected infants and children (National Institute of Child Health and Human Development Intravenous Immunoglobulin Study Group, 1991; Spector *et al.*, 1993); definition of the safety and tolerance of ZDV in pregnant women and newborns (O'Sullivan *et al.*, 1993; Boucher *et al.*, 1993); delineation of clinical endpoints unique to the paediatric population, i.e. neuropsychological functioning and failure to grow (Working Group on Antiretroviral Therapy: National Pediatric HIV Resource Center, 1993); development of an infrastructure to facilitate the development of a perinatal vaccine; and the establishment of guidelines for the use of ZDV in clinical practice (Agenda of the Pediatric Committee of the AIDS Clinical Trials Group, 1993).

Research priorities and organisation of the Pediatric ACTG

Research priorities of the Pediatric ACTG include the prevention of transmission of HIV from mother to infant, the development of effective antiretroviral and immunomodulator therapy for children who are already infected, and the development of effective prophylactic regimens against opportunistic infections for children at risk.

The Pediatric ACTG is organised into five Scientific Core Committees and five Working Groups. The Scientific Core Committees are: Perinatal, Primary Therapy, Vaccine, Opportunistic Infections and Adolescents. Their responsibilities include the establishment of scientific priorities (or agendas) that address the most important scientific questions in a manner consistent with available resources. Review and revision of these priorities occur on a regular basis. Working Groups provide scientific support and quality assurance needed by the scientific committees for the development of investigational protocols (Agenda of the Pediatric Committee of the AIDS Clinical Trials Group, 1993). They work scientifically with Adult Working Groups so that important advances from each section are recognised and efforts are not duplicated, thereby avoiding the waste of limited resources. The Pediatric Working Groups are: Virology, Immunology, Pharmacology, Supportive Care/Quality of Life, and Neurology/Neuropsychology.

Perinatal trials

Since almost every new case of paediatric HIV infection results from perinatal transmission of the virus, the mission of the Perinatal Scientific Core Committee and the highest priority of the Pediatric ACTG is the development of effective measures to interrupt transmission of HIV from mother to infant (Centers for Disease Control and Prevention, 1993; Agenda of the Pediatric Committee of the AIDS Clinical Trials Group, 1993). Although the exact timing and events associated with transmission are not fully understood, available evidence suggests that > 50% of transmission occurs at the time of delivery. Lower percentages occur during gestation (as early as the first trimester) and in the postpartum period as a result of breastfeeding (Devash *et al.*, 1990; Dunn *et al.*, 1992). On the basis of these assumptions a number of methods are under study that may interrupt perinatal transmission, including the treatment of maternal infection to reduce viral burden, the reduction of the amount of virus to which an infant is exposed at birth and primary prophylaxis of the fetus/ infant (see also Chapter 1).

Trials that are currently in progress or planned involve the use of ZDV and newer antiretroviral agents, passive and active immunisation with HIV envelope vaccines, and studies of the influence of obstetric practices on perinatal transmission.

Antiretroviral trials

Zidovudine (ZDV)

Initial trials established the pharmacokinetics, safety and tolerance of ZDV in pregnant women and newborns (O'Sullivan *et al.*, 1993; Boucher *et al.*, 1993). Protocol ACTG 082 was the first formal study of ZDV in pregnant women and provided data that supported a larger efficacy trial (O'Sullivan *et al.*, 1993). In addition to this a survey conducted by the Perinatal Scientific Committee about the use of ZDV in pregnancy provided further safety information and supportive data for larger clinical trials (Sperling *et al.*, 1992).

The initial large-scale perinatal trial was protocol ACTG 076. This was a phase II/III double-masked, placebo-controlled trial to evaluate the efficacy of ZDV in decreasing transmission of HIV from mother to infant. Women were eligible for the trial if they did not have medical indications to receive ZDV. A standard adult dose of ZDV was used, supplemented by an intravenous infusion of ZDV during labour. For the first 6 weeks of life infants received the same study medication that their mother received. In February 1994, after just over one-half of the projected number of mother–infant pairs had been enrolled, the study underwent an interim efficacy analysis by the Data Safety Monitoring Board. This analysis found that the use of ZDV reduced transmission by 70% in the group that received the drug. As a result the study was stopped. At this time further data analysis is in progress. Toxicities among mothers and infants were approximately equal in the drug group and the placebo group (National Institute of Allergy and Infectious Diseases, 1994).

While the short-term toxicities appear to be negligible, there is a need for follow-up of non-infected children who have been exposed to ZDV to evaluate them for long-term effects. Children who participated in ACTG 076 are therefore encouraged to be enrolled into the long-term outcomes protocol (ACTG 219) which will follow them until their twenty-first birthday. One of the major aims of this protocol is to detect untoward effects of the receipt of ZDV during gestation and the newborn period.

Nevirapine (NVP)

Nevirapine is a non-nucleoside reverse transcriptase inhibitor that causes a rapid and significant but transient decline in HIV activity when administered to HIV-infected patients (Cheeseman *et al.*, 1993). It is safe and well-tolerated in both adults and children. Its use in monotherapy is limited by the development of high-level HIV resistance after only a few weeks (Richman, 1992; Sullivan & Luzuriaga, 1993). However, because of its safety profile and high level of initial activity against HIV a trial involving intrapartum dosing of nevirapine to prevent transmission is currently being developed. This protocol will study the ability of NVP to prevent transmission occurring at the time of delivery (Sullivan & Luzuriaga, 1993). The drug may be especially useful for women who receive no prenatal care and among women whose HIV infection is not diagnosed until late in the course of their pregnancies (Agenda of the Pediatric Committee of the AIDS Clinical Trials Groups, 1993).

Didanosine (ddI)

Didanosine is frequently used for second-line therapy in HIV-infected adults. It is certain that ddI will soon be used for maternal indications during pregnancy. In anticipation of this a phase I study of ddI to evaluate safety, tolerance and pharmacokinetics during pregnancy (ACTG 249) is currently being developed (Agenda of the Pediatric Committee of the AIDS Clinical Trials Group, 1993).

It is anticipated that as other antiretrovirals become available additional similar studies will be needed.

Immune-based interventions

Studies of active and passive immunisation for the treatment of HIV infection in women and the prevention of transmission of HIV to their infants recently began in the ACTG. The eventual model that is envisaged for these therapies is a combination of an active/passive approach similar to that used successfully for the prevention of vertical hepatitis B infection. Separate trials are designed to evaluate the individual safety and efficacy of active and passive immunobiologics prior to their use in a combination trial (McElrath & Corey, 1994).

Active immunisation

Active immunisation with HIV envelope vaccines is being evaluated in both pregnant women and HIV-exposed infants. Active immunisation carries the potential advantage of eliciting both cellular and humoral responses, which are felt to be optimally necessary to control or prevent viral infection (Weinhold et al., 1988). Immunisation of pregnant women may enhance immune response to the virus, improving the mother's overall disease status and reducing the amount of virus to which the fetus/infant is exposed (Letvin, 1993; Agenda of the Pediatric Committee of the AIDS Clinical Trials Group, 1993). A phase I vaccine programme has been developed with the goal of establishing active or active/passive immunisation strategies for the interruption of perinatal transmission (McElrath & Corey, 1994). Such strategies might involve administration of vaccine to a mother followed by active/passive immunisation of the infant at the time of delivery. At present three separate phase I studies are evaluating the safety of different gp120 and gp160 HIV envelope vaccines (Biocine/Chiron, MicroGeneSys and Genentech products) in HIV-infected pregnant women (ACTG 233, 234 and 235). A phase I study to evaluate the safety and immunogenicity of the Genentech and Biocine/Chiron vaccines in the newborn infants of HIV women (ACTG 230) is also under way.

Passive immunisation

Humoral immune responses play a significant role in initial control of the virus after infection (Letvin, 1993). Early, and somewhat controversial studies of perinatal HIV infection suggested that the presence of neutralising antibody was associated with a decreased risk of transmission (Goedert et al., 1989; Devash et al., 1990). Preliminary studies of an HIV hyperimmune immunoglobulin (HIVIG) derived from the plasma of healthy HIV-infected patients has been associated with a decrease in p24 antigen levels and viraemia when administered to adults with HIV infection (Jackson et al., 1988; Karpas et al., 1988; Jacobson et al., 1993). The preparation is treated with alcohol and solvent/detergent to remove viral particles and has been well tolerated (Connor & McSherry, 1994).

The initial perinatal study involving passive immunisation (ACTG 185) is a phase III randomised, double-masked, controlled study of the use of HIVIG versus intravenous immunoglobulin (IVIG) in prevention of maternal–fetal transmission of HIV in women receiving ZDV. Infants receive ZDV for 6 weeks postpartum and receive one infusion of the same study drug their mother received (i.e. HIVIG or IVIG).

Paediatric antiretroviral trials

In the USA drug development and licensing for use in children have historically lagged significantly behind that for adults. As a result of this the Pediatric Primary Therapy Core Committee attempts to identify the most promising new drugs as early as possible in their clinical development. Clinical trials to evaluate pharmacokinetics, safety, tolerance and preliminary efficacy in children are then begun almost simultaneously with adult trials. Data obtained from these paediatric trials when combined with data from adult efficacy trials, which can often be extrapolated to children due to similarities in disease and drug effects, help to facilitate earlier approval of antiretroviral therapies for use in children (Working Group on Antiretroviral Therapy: National Pediatric HIV Resource Center, 1993; Agenda of the Pediatric Committee of the AIDS Clinical Trials Group, 1993). In addition, there are certain clinical manifestations of HIV that are either unique to paediatrics or are more easily studied in children. Consequently, the Committee has emphasised development of paediatric trials prior to adult studies in these areas. An example of this is protocol ACTG 239, which studies the effect of antiretroviral therapy on the early onset and rapidly progressive HIV disease seen in certain perinatally infected infants.

A number of treatment trials have been completed in children. Other trials evaluating various monotherapy and combination therapy strategies in children naive to antiretroviral agents are now under way. In addition, treatment trials for children with advancing disease despite therapy are currently being conducted.

Monotherapy

Zidovudine

Use of ZDV in children with HIV infection has been associated with improvement in clinical and virological markers (McKinney *et al.*, 1991). It is currently recommended as the drug of choice for initial therapy in children with symptomatic infection or significant immunodeficiency. The recommended dose is 180 mg/m^2 given every 6 hours (Working Group on Antiretroviral Therapy: National Pediatric HIV Resource Center, 1993). A trial comparing the effectiveness of this dose with a lower dose (90 mg/m^2) (ACTG 128) recently ended. Data from that trial are now being analysed.

Didanosine (ddI)

ddI is approved for use in children who are intolerant to ZDV or who develop disease progression while receiving it (Working Group on Antiretroviral Therapy: National Pediatric HIV Resource Center, 1993.)

ddI for these indications is currently being studied more extensively, at two different doses (ACTG 144).

Zalcitabine (ddC)

Two different doses of ddC are being studied for safety and efficacy in patients intolerant of ZDV or who have developed disease progression while receiving it (ACTG 138).

Nevirapine (NVP)

The non-nucleoside reverse transcriptase inhibitor NVP is being evaluated in a phase I trial both as a single agent and in combination with ZDV (ACTG 180).

Stavudine (D4T)

A phase II (safety, tolerance and preliminary efficacy) randomised comparative trial of the nucleoside analogue D4T with ZDV for the initial treatment of HIV in children has recently opened (ACTG 240).

Combination therapy

Three trials comparing ZDV monotherapy with combination therapy are currently in progress. One is a phase III trial that compares initial therapy with ZDV with combination therapy with ZDV+ddI with monotherapy with ddI (ACTG 152). It has completed enrolment of 800 children and is continuing. The second is a phase II trial comparing continued monotherapy with ZDV in patients who have received at least 6 weeks of ZDV with continued ZDV+ddC (ACTG 190). The third combination therapy trial is directed at the subset of HIV-infected infants that develop rapidly progressive disease in the first few months of life (Byers et al., 1993). Infants will be randomised to receive either ZDV or ZDV+ddI.

An additional trial aimed at children with very advanced disease is in the final stages of development (ACTG 245). The phase I/II trial utilises the concept of triple or convergent therapy and will evaluate the virological efficacy, safety, tolerance and pharmacokinetics of combination therapy (Chow et al., 1993). Patients will be randomised to receive either ZDV+ddI, ZDV+ddI+NVP or ddI+NVP.

Paediatric opportunistic infections

Research efforts of the Pediatric Opportunistic Infections Scientific Committee have been directed at the prevention of the most frequent and serious opportunistic infections seen in HIV-infected children. Those efforts to date have had two major targets: bacterial infections and *Pneumocystis carinii* pneumonia (PCP).

The results of two studies of IVIG for the prevention of bacterial infections have been published. One (ACTG 045), carried out in collaboration with the NICHD, showed that IVIG prolonged the time to serious bacterial infection in children with CD4 counts > 200 cells/mm^3 (National Institute of Child Health and Human Development Intravenous Immunoglobulin Study Group, 1991). The other (ACTG 051), in which children also receive ZDV, showed that only when patients were not receiving prophylaxis with trimethoprim-sulfamethoxazole was an effect on serious bacterial infections seen (Spector *et al.*, 1993).

PCP prophylaxis

PCP is the most frequent opportunistic infection seen in children with HIV infection and is associated with severe morbidity and high rates of mortality (Connor *et al.*, 1991; Kovacs *et al.*, 1991; Simmonds *et al.*, 1993). In collaboration with the National Pediatric HIV Resource Center and the Centers for Disease Control and Prevention, the Pediatric AIDS Clinical Trial Group helped to develop guidelines for prevention of PCP in 1990 (Centers for Disease Control and Prevention, 1991). Trimethoprim-sulfamethoxazole was recommended as the drug of choice for prophylaxis. A phase I/II trial to evaluate a dapsone regimen (ACTG 179) and a phase I trial to evaluate atovaquone (ACTG 227) as alternatives to trimethoprim-sulfamethoxazole are currently being conducted.

The highest priority is this area, however, is the development of a Multiple Opportunistic Pathogens Prevention Study (MOPPS) comparing trimethoprim-sulfamethoxazole with azithromycin-atovaquone for the prevention of bacterial infection, *Mycobacterium avium intracellulare* and *Pneumocystis* prophylaxis (Agenda of the Pediatric Committee of the AIDS Clinical Trials Group, 1993).

Finally, a phase I study of oral ganciclovir for the prevention of serious cytomegalovirus (CMV) disease is being developed, as is a phase I trial of early administration of measles vaccine to infected infants.

HIV vaccine trials

The major goal of the Pediatric Vaccine Scientific Committee is the development of an active/passive immunisation schedule for the prevention of intrapartum transmission of HIV (Agenda of the Pediatric Committee of the AIDS Clinical Trials Group, 1993). Concepts currently in development include active immunisation of pregnant women in a parallel

attempt to influence favourably the course of disease in the mother, followed by active/passive immunisation of the infant or active/passive
immunisation of the infant alone. Active immunisation of pregnant
women may improve their disease status, thereby reducing the amount
of virus to which the fetus/infant is exposed. Theoretically, it may also
increase the amount of protective antibody crossing the placenta. Active/
passive immunisation of the infant may enhance the immune response
to HIV and prevent infection (Connor & McSherry, 1994).

Three HIV vaccines are currently undergoing placebo-controlled, safety
and immunogenicity trials in different patient groups. ACTG 218 is evaluating the envelope protein vaccines HIV gp160 (MicroGeneSys gp160) and
gp120 (Biocine/Chiron and Genentech) in asymptomatic infected children
older than 1 month of age.

Another concept currently under development involves the use of HIV
vaccines for immune-based therapy. An effective vaccine could, theoretically, stimulate neutralising antibody and the cytotoxic T lymphocyte
response, thereby prolonging immune vigilance and HIV suppression in
infected patients (Connor & McSherry, 1994).

In the summer of 1993 a phase I trial of the Genentech and Biocine/
Chiron vaccines (ACTG 230) was begun in infants born to infected
mothers.

Adolescent trials

Adults, 20–29 years of age, account for more than 18% of the cases of
AIDS reported to the Centers for Disease Control up to September 1993.
Although adolescents (13–19 years of age) account for less than 1% of all
cases of AIDS reported in the USA many of the 20- to 29-year-old adults
with AIDS may have been infected as adolescents, given the prolonged
incubation period seen in adults (Centers for Disease Control and Prevention, 1993).

In the light of this the Adolescent Scientific Core Committee has developed a protocol (ACTG 220) to identify, characterise and co-enrol HIV-
infected adolescents into ACTG interventional trials. The protocol also
assesses adolescent abilities to adhere to study-required treatment regimens. The Adolescent Scientific Core Committee is developing trials that
will identify possible pharmacokinetic and pharmacodynamic differences
between adolescents and adults. Uncomplicated trials that provide effective therapy while promoting compliance with treatment regimens are also
being developed (Agenda of the Pediatric Committee of the AIDS Clinical
Trials Group, 1993).

Summary

Paediatric HIV treatment trials are now offered at over 50 sites in the USA. More than 3200 HIV-infected children and 750 perinatal patients have been enrolled in these trials. Work of the Pediatric ACTG has led to the approval of various antiretrovirals for use in children and development of an effective strategy for the prevention of *Pneumocystis carinii* pneumonia. Of major importance are the results of a recent trial (ACTG 076) demonstrating that transmission of HIV from mother to infant could be prevented by the use of zidovudine (National Institute of Allergy and Infectious Diseases, 1994). The goals of the Pediatric ACTG research programme continue to be the prevention of perinatal infection, rapid development and approval of antiretroviral and immune-based therapy for infected children, development of new prophylactic strategies for opportunistic infections, and strategies to increase adolescent participation in clinical trials. Only through cooperative national and international efforts will steady progress continue to be made against this devastating disease.

Acknowledgements

This work was supported by grants 2-UO1-AI25883–06 from the National Institute of Allergy and Infectious Diseases and U64/CCU202219–07 from the Centers for Disease Control and Prevention.

References

Agenda of the Pediatric Committee of the AIDS Clinical Trials Group (1993). Bethesda, MD. 15–18 August 1993.

Balis, F. M., Pizzo, P. A., Butler, K. M. *et al.* (1992). Clinical pharmacology of 2′,3′-dideoxyinosine in human immunodeficiency virus-infected children. *Journal of Infectious Diseases*, **165**, 99–104.

Borkowsky, W., Krasinski, K., Pollack, H., Hoover W., Kaul A. & Ilmet-Moore, T. (1992). Early diagnosis of human immunodeficiency virus infection in children <6 months of age: comparison of polymerase chain reaction, culture, and plasma antigen capture techniques. *Journal of Infectious Diseases*, **166**, 616–19.

Boucher, F. D., Modlin, J. F., Weller, S. *et al.* (1993). Phase I evaluation of zidovudine administered to infants exposed at birth to the human immunodeficiency virus. *Journal of Pediatrics*, **122**, 137–44.

Byers, B., Caldwell, B., Oxtoby, M. (1993). Survival of children with perinatal HIV-infection: evidence for two distinct populations (abstract no. WS-C10–6). Berlin: IXth International Conference on AIDS.

Centers for Disease Control and Prevention (1991). Guidelines for prophylaxis against *Pneumocystis carinii* pneumonia for children infected with human immunodeficiency virus. *Morbidity and Mortality Weekly Report* **40**(RR-2), 1–13.

Centers for Disease Control and Prevention (1993). HIV/AIDS Surveillance Report, 5(no. 3), 1–19.

Cheeseman, S. H., Hattox, S. E., McLaughlin, M. M., et al. (1993). Pharmacokinetics of nevirapine: initial single-rising-dose study in humans. *Antimicrobial Agents and Chemotherapy*, 37, 178–82.

Chow, Y. K., Hirsch, M. S., Merrill, D. P., et al. (1993). Use of evolutionary limitations of HIV-1 multidrug resistance to optimize therapy. *Nature*, 361, 650–4.

Chu, S. Y., Buehler, J. W., Oxtoby, M. J., & Kibourne, B. W. (1991). Impact of the human immunodefiency virus epidemic on mortality in children in the United States. *Pediatrics*, 87, 806–10.

Connor, E. (1991). Antiretroviral treatment for children with human immunodeficiency virus infection (editorial). *Pediatrics*, 88, 390–2.

Connor, E., Bagarazzi, M., McSherry, G. et al. (1991). Clinical and laboratory correlates of *Pneumocystis carinii* pneumonia in children infected with HIV. *Journal of the American Medical Association*, 265, 1693–7.

Connor, E. & McSherry, G. (1994) Immune-based interventions in perinatal human immunodeficiency virus infection. *Pediatric Infectious Disease Journal*, 13, 440–8.

Cotton, D. J., Powderly, W. G., Feinberg, J., et al. (1993). Guidelines for the design and conduct of AIDS clinical trials. *Clinical Infectious Disease*, 16, 816–22.

Denny, T., Yogev, R., Gelman, R., et al. (1992). Lymphocyte subsets in healthy children during the first 5 years of life. *Journal of the American Medical Association*, 267, 1484–8.

Devash, Y., Calvelli, T., Wood, D. G., Reagan, K. J. & Rubinstein, A. (1990). Vertical transmission of HIV is correlated with the absence of high affinity/avidity maternal antibodies to the gp160 principal neutralizing domain. *Proceedings of the National Academy of Sciences, USA*, 87, 3445–9.

Dunn, D. T., Newell, M. L., Ades, A. E., & Peckham, C. S. (1992). Risk of human immunodeficiency virus type 1 transmission through breastfeeding. *Lancet*, 340, 585–8.

Goedert, J. J., Mendez, H., Drummond, J. E., et al. (1989). Mother-to-infant transmission of human immunodeficiency virus type 1: association with prematurity or low anti-gp 120. *Lancet*, 334, 1351–4.

Jacobson, J. M., Colman, N., Ostrow, N. A. et al. (1993). Passive immunotherapy in the treatment of advanced human immunodeficiency virus infection. *Journal of Infectious Diseases*, 168, 298–305.

Jackson, G. G., Perkins, J. T., Rubenis, M., et al. (1988). Passive immunoneutralisation of human immunodeficiency virus in patients with advanced AIDS. *Lancet*, ii, 647–54.

Karpas, A., Hill, F., Youle, M., et al. (1988). Effects of passive immunization in patients with the acquired immunodeficiency syndrome-related complex and acquired immunodeficiency syndrome. *Proceedings of the National Academy of Sciences, USA*, 85, 9234–7.

Kovacs, A., Frederick, T., Church, J., Eller, A., Oxtoby, M. & Mascola, L. (1991). CD4 T-lymphocyte counts and *Pneumocystis carinii* pneumonia in pediatric HIV infection. *Journal of the American Medical Association*, 265, 1698–703.

Letvin, N. L. (1993). Vaccines against human immunodeficiency virus, progress and prospects. *New England Journal of Medicine*, 329, 1400–5.

McElrath, M. J. & Corey, L. (1994). Current status of vaccines for HIV. In: *Pediatric AIDS: The Challenge of HIV Infection in Infants, Children, and Adolescents*, 2nd edn, ed. P. A. Pizzo & C. M. Wilfert, pp. 869–88. Baltimore: Williams & Wilkins.

McKinney, R. E., Maha, M. A., Connor, E. M., and the Protocol 043 Study Group (1991). A multicenter trial of oral zidovudine in children with advanced human immunodeficiency disease. *New England Journal of Medicine*, **324**, 1018–25.

McKinney, R. E., Pizzo, P. A., Scott, G. B. and the Pediatric Zidovudine Phase I Study Group (1990). Safety and tolerance of intermittent intravenous and oral zidovudine therapy in human immunodeficiency virus-infected patients. *Journal of Pediatrics*, **116**, 640–7.

National Institute of Allergy and Infectious Diseases (1994). Clinical alert: important therapeutic information on the benefit of zidovudine for the prevention of the transmission of HIV from mother to infant. Washington, DC: NIAID.

National Institute of Child Health and Human Development Intravenous Immunoglobulin Study Group (1991). Intravenous immune globulin for the prevention of bacterial infections in children with symptomatic human immundeficiency virus infection. *New England Journal of Medicine*, **325**, 73–80.

O'Sullivan, M. J., Boyer, P. J. J., Scott, G. B. and the Zidovudine Collaborative Working Group (1993). The pharmacokinetics and safety of zidovudine in the third trimester of pregnancy for women infected with human immunodeficiency virus and their infants: Phase I Acquired Immunodeficiency Syndrome Clinical Trials Group study (protocol 082). *American Journal of Obstetrics and Gynecology*, **168**, 1510–16.

Oxtoby, M. J. (1994). Vertically acquired HIV infection in the United States. In *Pediatric AIDS: The Challenge of HIV Infection in Infants, Children, and Adolescents*, 2nd edn, ed. P. A. Pizzo & C. M. Wilfert, pp. 3–20. Baltimore: Williams & Wilkins.

Report of a consensus workshop, Siena, Italy, 17–18 January 1992. Early diagnosis of HIV infection in infants. *Journal of Acquired Immunodeficiency Syndromes*, **5**, 1169–78.

Richman, D. D. (1992). Loss of nevirapine activity associated with the emergence of resistance in clinical trials. The ACTG 164/168 Study Team (abstract POB3576). Amsterdam: VIIIth International Conference on AIDS.

Selik, R. M., Chu, S. Y. & Buehler, J. W. (1993). HIV infection as leading cause of death among young adults in US cities and states. *Journal of the American Medical Association*, **269**, 2991–4.

Simonds, R. J., Oxtoby, M. J., Caldwell, M. B., Gwinn, M. L., & Rogers, M. F. (1993). *Pneumocystis carinii* pneumonia among children with perinataly acquired HIV infection. *Journal of the American Medical Association*, **270**, 470–3.

Spector, S. A., Gelber, R., McGrath, N. The Pediatric AIDS Clinical Trials Group and The NICHD Pediatric HIV Centers (1993). Results of a double-blind, placebo controlled trial to evaluate intravenous gammaglobulin (IVIG) in children with symptomatic HIV infection (ACTG 051) (abstract WS-B-05-6). Berlin: IXth International Conference on AIDS.

Sperling, R. S., Stratton, P., O'Sullivan, M. J. *et al.* (1992). A survey of zidovudine use in pregnant women with human immunodeficiency virus infection. The *New England Journal of Medicine*, **326**, 857–61.

Sullivan, J. & Luzuriaga K. (1993). Nevirapine activity and emergence of resistant virus in pediatric trials. The ACTG 180 Study Team (abstract PO-B26–2042) Berlin: IXth International Conference on AIDS.

Weinhold, K. J., Matthews, T. J., Ahearne, P. M., *et al.* (1988). Cellular anti-GP120 cytolytic reactivities in HIV-1 seropositive individuals. *Lancet*, **i**, 902–5.

Working Group on Antiviral Therapy: National Pediatric HIV Resource Center (1993). Antiretroviral therapy and medical management of the human immunodeficiency virus-infected child. *Pediatric Infectious Disease Journal*, **12**, 513–22.

Addenda

The results of the American/French Zidovudine trial (ACTG 076) have now been published as:

Connor, E. M., Sperling, R. S., Gelber, R., *et al.* (1994). Reduction of maternal–infant transmission of human immunodeficiency virus type 1 with zidovudine treatment. *New England Journal of Medicine*, **331**, 1173–80.

14

The role of the nurse

CANDY DUGGAN and FIONA MITCHELL

Introduction

'The lack of a biomedical response to AIDS offers nursing the opportunity – probably for the first time – to prove what nursing is worth and
to demonstrate that although the eventual outcome cannot be changed,
the path to the outcome can be made less rigorous and more tolerable
through nursing's interventions' (Wells, 1988).

This chapter does not tell nurses *how* to nurse children with HIV and
AIDS, but discusses some of the dilemmas posed by HIV infection in
children and encourages nurses to build on the skills and knowledge they
already have.

Nurses by virtue of their education and training are in a unique position
within the multidisciplinary team regarding the care and treatment of children with HIV infection. Because of their understanding of the medical,
social, developmental and psychological aspects of chronic illness they function as the pivotal point in providing, coordinating and directing the care of
the child with HIV infection and the involved caretakers (Eddy & Whittle-
Seiden, 1991). Different models of nursing care have been described, many
of which are appropriate to children with HIV infection. Examples of traditional nursing concerns are the child's skin integrity, nutrition, respiratory functioning and psychosocial comfort. Henderson's definition (1969) of
eleven basic needs as nursing's focus is a more complete list.

However, nursing can also be viewed as helping patients to solve, allevi-
ate, cope with or prevent problems related to activities of living rather
than as treating patients with specific disease conditions (Roper *et al.*,
1980). This fits very well with the notion of living with HIV and a holistic
approach.

Peplau (1991) saw illness as a practical learning experience through
interlocking or overlapping phases of interaction. For this relationship to
be achieved the nurse needs to have a clear understanding of what is communicated to the patient and how this is achieved.

In addition, nurses need to think carefully about their nursing knowledge, and their own beliefs about caring and attitudes towards care. Peplau (1991) identified several roles for the nurse and their long-term and short-term consequences. Nurses choose which role is appropriate at any one time. A nurse's relationship with a patient has to be dynamic and flexible.

The nurse as a stranger. Nurses must have basic respect for patients as for any stranger, and strangers must not be stereotyped or labelled. Each patient will have a different perception of how to be treated. Nurses should respect people with HIV infection and AIDS and not make assumptions.

The nurse as a resource person, and as a teacher. Children may be the first members of their family to present with illness due to HIV infection. Parents are often unaware of their own HIV status. As AIDS is a multi-system disease, its presentation is varied and often complex. Nurses should be able to give information about HIV, treatment options, and support agencies both locally and nationally. They should also offer families knowledge of the condition itself – its expected course, prognosis and treatment choices, and information about supportive interventions. They must provide the time and skill to share knowledge and counsel families. The family will bring information about the child's health, previous experiences with the health care system, the effectiveness of various previously tried regimens and intimate knowledge of the child's environment and daily pattern of behaviour. Families of children with chronic conditions quickly become expert in the care of their child.

The nurse as a leader and a counsellor. An important goal is for patients to be permitted and encouraged to organise and control some or all of their care. The role of a counsellor is a difficult one and requires confidence. It can be a realistic and positive role if education and practice for the nurse are provided and if the nurse is supported.

To be effective as a resource person, the nurse must be effective as a communicator. Hayes & Knox (1984) showed that, without exception, parents emphasised the importance of clear, honest, open communication of information, endlessly repeated if necessary.

Roles in nursing can be readily identified through the process of care. One of the strengths of nursing lies in the willingness and ability of a nurse to join with families in a partnership approach. Casey (1988) describes an active partnership between the nurse, child and family which allows for a very flexible approach to the delivery of care. This is especially important where the family is affected by HIV and AIDS. The partnership of care model aims for minimal intervention by health professionals whilst providing support and resources to parents to enable them to continue caring for their child. However, it also allows for extensive intervention and delivery of care by the nurse when this is indicated and appropriate.

This is not a new role for nurses, but a change in emphasis from the primary role of doing to that of educating and supporting parents and their families – particularly parents who undertake their children's care to varying degrees. To be successful, any partnership must be adaptable, flexible and supportive, and good communication is crucial.

In summary, the nurse's role within the patient–nurse partnership is to care, to teach, to support and to refer. Above all, nurses should be able to use a model that supports their practice and in doing so helps direct their thinking, feeling and doing.

HIV as a chronic illness

A chronic condition is any continuing anatomical or psychological impairment that interferes with the individual's ability to function fully in the environment. This definition of a chronic illness by Thomas (1983) reflects the course of HIV disease as we know it today.

Chronic conditions are characterised by relatively stable periods that may be interrupted by acute episodes requiring hospitalisation or medical attention. The individual's prognosis varies between a normal life span and an unpredictable early death. Chronic conditions are rarely cured but are managed through individual family effort and diligence. This rather broad definition reflects a concern not with the medical diagnosis, but with the consequences for the child. Nurses should consider:

How much does HIV or AIDS limit the child's ordinary behaviour?
What ranges of ordinary activities are available to the child and family?
How can we support the family to maximise the particular child's ability to play and learn?

Mutually negotiated goals are more likely to be realistic for the child and family and therefore more likely to be achieved.

Assessment

Assessment is the initial and essential step in the nursing process and creates a foundation upon which all interventions with a child and family rest. This should focus on three areas of the child's condition:

The pattern of actual or potential physical or psychological impairments the individual child has sustained as a result of the chronic condition
The extent to which the impairment interferes with the expected functioning for the child
The invisibility of the child's condition

Table 14.1 *Living with HIV as a chronic illness*

Repeated visits to doctors, clinics, wards or hospital departments for monitoring and treatment
Long-term drug regimens, perhaps with unpleasant side-effects
Chronic or continual episodes of pain or other discomfort, due to either the disease and/or interventions
Repeated separations from family, friends and school
Restrictions in activities, perhaps leading to isolation
Rigid or closely monitored diets
Constantly changing faces among caregivers
The threat of death

Each of these elements of the illness produces an impact on the child and family. Additional factors that appear to have the strongest impact on the child's experience are the characteristics of the disease and its treatment, the age and developmental level of the child, characteristics of the family and the supportive environment of the community.

The child with HIV, and his or her family, typically has many kinds of experiences which their uninfected peers do not, as listed in Table 14.1. In addition, the child may experience changes in the response of others to them, due to the stigma of HIV and AIDS (see Chapter 9). Parents may be unable to avoid feelings of grief and distress, and to pretend that life goes on as normal (Anderson, 1981). Alternatively they may be overprotective, or may think that education is not necessary since the child has no future. Friends may be lost through lack of contact.

Krulik (1980) stressed the importance of recognising the difference chronic illness can make to a child's life. He recommended that 'assisting the child and his family in reducing this feeling of being different and achieving as normal a life as possible, is one of the goals in nursing children with chronic illness'.

Caring for the family

If about 15 of every 100 children born to HIV-positive women in Europe will be infected with HIV, then the remaining 85 children will be affected as they will be born into a family where one or more of the family members will become sick and may die.

'There is a direct role for the nurse in treating the child, but there is an equally supportive role for the nurse with the family' (Kodadek, 1979). This is even more important when a child has HIV as he or she may have a parent and siblings who also require care and support.

A child with HIV inevitably tests a family's emotional, financial, organisational and adaptive resources. The unrelenting demands of medical

Table 14.2. *Dimensions of illness*

Onset:	Acute
	Gradual
Course:	Progressive
	Constant
	Relapsing
Outcome:	Fatal
	Non-fatal
Degree of incapacity	

From Rolland (1984).

treatment and adaptation to special needs and constant change take their toll on many families with HIV. Yet many families with similar circumstances and hardships manage to meet the challenges of illness successfully, as well as the needs of their ill children and other family members, despite the continuing problems of pain, disruption, uncertainty, family reorganisation and possibly life-threatening changes as the days go by. Rolland (1984) has established a useful categorisation of illness dimensions to help assess the likely impact of a particular condition on a family. These are listed in Table 14.2. Each of these illness dimensions and the many potential combinations of dimensions puts differing kinds, intensities and patterns of demands on the patient and family.

Another source of stress to parents is losing control of their child's care. Parents see themselves as ultimately responsible for this and need to be able to trust that the health professional is competent and cares for them as a family as well as for their child. Children and their parents are individuals with individual and constantly changing needs.

Nursing at home and in the community

Given that approximately 26% of children infected with HIV will become sick in their first year of life and that 17% of those children may die (European Collaborative Study, 1991), it is obvious that the majority of children will be well and cared for in the community.

As long ago as 1959, the Platt report stated that children should only be admitted to hospital if their care could not be provided at home. The Court report (1976) identified children as a priority group for whom community care and prevention should be the main focus for provision of care. This was reinforced by the United Kingdom Department of Health's 'Welfare of Children and Young People in Hospital' (1993).

In the UK there is now a recognition that community services, including nursing, have a valuable role to play in the discharge planning process.

Nurses should be involved in the planning of post-discharge care packages, in consultation with carers and the child. Parents must know who is managing their child's clinical care and where to go for help. Successful discharge depends on effective communication and liaison between agencies which, with adequate assessment of the family's needs, ensure that necessary services, appliances and equipment are in place ready for the child's discharge from hospital. Many hospitals have a discharge planning sheet that is completed with the family on, or soon after, admission. Inadequate notice of discharge causes difficulties for community nurses in trying to organise services at short notice and sometimes necessitates the re-admission of a child to hospital. More children could be discharged from hospital earlier with follow-up from the primary health care team or with continuing care from specialised secondary care teams.

Professionals caring for families within the community face a complex challenge. The major impact of HIV/AIDS on families in which more than one generation is affected will require health care workers to develop unique and flexible strategies to ensure the needs of this client group are met. It must be remembered, however, that for many families HIV will not be their most pressing concern, and for many the more pertinent issues of unemployment, poverty, discordant relationships, poor housing and child care problems will take precedence.

Parents who are drug users can present a special challenge to health care workers. The adverse social circumstances and chaotic lifestyle which can accompany drug misuse may make monitoring of children difficult. Fear of hostile attitudes can result in some women being reluctant to divulge their drug use and previous experience of judgmental attitudes from health care workers and other agencies may also serve to discourage women from attending for care.

Traditionally women have accepted the role as provider of child care and care of the sick. HIV brings this whole issue into question as the impact of a life-threatening illness on families begins to evolve. It may be that women have reduced access to services because they find them off-putting and not understanding of their needs, or because of difficulty in finding someone to look after their children (see Chapter 7).

Long-term follow-up of children

It is important that at the outset parents have an understanding of the value of regular surveillance (see Chapter 9). This knowledge is best reinforced by easily understood literature which is culturally sensitive. Parents should also have the opportunity to voice their fears or reservations regarding prolonged follow-up for their children, and their views should be taken into account when negotiating intervals between routine checks.

The stress and anxiety expressed by HIV-positive parents about the uncertainty of their child's diagnosis is immense. Parents become overwhelmed by guilt and can be excessively anxious whenever their child displays clinical signs or symptoms which they suspect may be HIV related. This is particularly so during the indeterminate stage when maternal HIV antibodies are still present. Improved technology has meant that specialist centres are able to diagnose HIV infection in children as early as 3 months of age. This information, though devastating for the parents, can be an immense relief as an early knowledge of the child's HIV infection will enable decisions to be made regarding intervention with prophylactic treatments.

As little is known about intrauterine exposure to HIV and its effects on the developing immune system, children born to HIV-positive mothers ideally should continue to be followed up even after they have cleared maternal antibody and are presumed uninfected. In practice follow-up of these children can be problematic. Many parents, satisfied that their children are not infected, no longer wish the continued involvement of the paediatric team, who serve as a distressing reminder of potential illness. The primary care team's involvement can be invaluable. Parents may still be in a state of denial regarding their own HIV infection and dread being questioned by their children. With growing awareness that, unlike their peers, they are the subject of investigations and procedures, children may raise unwelcome issues.

At times of great stress within families the presence of the paediatric team and what they represent can aggravate an already tense situation. Parents may therefore present as aggressive and intolerant of intervention. Some ex-injecting drug users have shown aversion to injecting equipment and can become agitated by its use on or near their child. In contrast to the situation described above, many parents do value the continued follow-up of their child and the regular reassurance that they remain apparently uninfected by HIV.

As children become older it is important to avoid disruption to their daily routine. The need to provide a flexible service may therefore require appointments being offered outwith school or nursery hours or during school holidays. This will ensure that children are not readily identifiable and subsequent breaches of confidentiality can be avoided.

Venue for follow-up

In order to ensure a user-friendly service, parents should be able to choose the venue where their children can be seen. By far the most popular venue

Table 14.3. *Strategies to encourage follow-up*

Respect for confidentiality
Appropriate choice of venue
Flexibility of appointment system
Multidisciplinary approach
Non-judgemental attitudes
Use of easily understood parent information literature
Respectful treatment of parents and children
Care for the family as a whole

is the child's own home, since a familiar environment is generally less distressing for both parent and child. Visits to hospital for follow-up can pose transport problems as well as being a difficult experience for families, since they serve as reminders of the potential threat of illness. Despite the convenience of the child being followed up at home, many parents prefer their home to be a sanctuary of normality, safe from medicalisation in order that their child feels safe and secure in accustomed surroundings. Other options for follow-up include the general practitioner's surgery, health visitor clinic or the home of a friend or relative.

Continuity of care

Frequent changes of health care workers can result in a lack of continuity of care for families. Health care workers who are unfamiliar with the family dynamics may feel intimidated and could be resistant to offering a flexible, non-judgemental service. This highlights the great need to coordinate services to ensure that resources are neither duplicated nor overlooked, and close liaison with generic staff is therefore essential. The strategies for ensuring continued follow-up are summarised in Table 14.3.

Uptake of services

It must be appreciated that due to chronic tiredness and/or effects of drugs, certain families may be unable to attend for appointments at designated times. This can result in them being labelled as unreliable, poor attenders. Health care workers must therefore be aware of the need to tailor services to ensure that health care is not denied to this group. A flexible and realistic attitude towards provision and expected uptake of health care resources will enable staff to plan a far more user-friendly service.

It must be acknowledged that providing a unique service such as this will undoubtedly be expensive. However, without such adaptability certain clients would not avail themselves of any health care.

Confidentiality

Following up children born to HIV-positive mothers can be particularly complex in situations where partners or other family members are unaware of the mother's HIV status. Because of the immense stigma associated with HIV, one of the greatest fears for families is a breach of confidentiality. Such an infringement can result in disastrous social repercussions for the parents and children. Disclosure in some instances can put personal, family and social relationships at risk.

School children can be taunted and ridiculed in the playground by their peers if it is known that one or both their parents are HIV infected. All establishments involved in caring for children, particularly schools and nurseries, should be following recognised guidelines for dealing appropriately with spillages of blood and other secretions. This avoids unnecessarily identifying children at-risk and also protects staff and children from exposure to blood-borne infections (see Chapters 9 and 16). When recommendations such as these are adhered to there is no need for parents to inform personnel that HIV is an issue for them. Consequently parents must take time to consider carefully who needs to know that their child may be infected or affected by HIV/AIDS (see Chapter 19).

Inter-agency referrals should be made only with a client's informed consent, as inadvertent breaches of confidentiality could occur where multiple agencies are involved with one family and the family's HIV status is wrongly assumed to be common knowledge. Identification of clients with HIV infection can also occur when workers are seen to be taking extreme and unnecessary hygiene precautions. For this reason some individuals may be reluctant to seek health care.

Specialist HIV services

Familiarity with specialist workers and confidence in those workers' understanding of their problems can encourage families with HIV to bypass generic services when seeking health care for themselves or their children. For patients who would not use resources other than those offered by specialist teams this is the only effective way of working. By endorsing the role of generic staff clients should be encouraged to use local services where their HIV infection should not prejudice their care. Liaison and a good working relationship can help to dispel any resentment or ill feeling between the specialist and generic member of staff.

With the client's consent early liaison, ideally in the antenatal period, with the generic health visitor can pave the way for a good working relationship. Sharing of information between generic and specialist staff will allow a greater understanding of each other's roles and joint visits may be indicated in certain situations. Demonstrating that staff do not work in isolation can help to avoid potential manipulation by problematic clients. Maintaining open channels of communication will also enable the specialist team member to act as a resource and consultant for community colleagues, thereby assisting them to provide the optimum service for the clients.

The infected child in the community

On learning of their child's HIV infection, parents may be unable to think rationally and may have difficulty taking in information. It is important, therefore, to provide a reliable supportive contact whom they can reach quickly and easily for information and advice.

Once a definite diagnosis has been reached, intervals between follow-up will depend on the stage of the disease, the need for prophylactic treatment, the child's age and the cooperation of the parents.

A large percentage of children with HIV infection will remain physically well for most of the time. However, during episodes of acute illness it is most likely that they will be nursed in hospital. Parents will require a great deal of support to come to terms with their child's HIV diagnosis and some may find it useful to visit the paediatric ward where the child is likely to be nursed during an acute illness and to meet ward staff who will be responsible for caring for their child during these episodes. Children receiving prophylactic treatment over long periods of time can establish very close relationships with ward staff, thus allowing them to talk over fears and anxieties surrounding their illness and its treatment. A familiar, friendly environment will be much less frightening to the child during times of acute ill health.

Child protection

While every effort is made to keep children with their natural parents, the safety of the child is paramount. There will be occasions when it is in the child's best interest that he or she is removed from the family home to a place of safety. Inevitably for some children long-term care will be necessary and this may involve children being placed for adoption. Before this major decision is reached a variety of child care options will have been explored with the child's best interests in mind. Every effort will have to be made by a variety of support services to keep children with their natural parents (see Chapter 15).

For some families a system of flexible foster care has enabled them to remain together in the secure knowledge that a known and trusted carer is available to look after their children at times of crisis (Mok & O'Hara, 1990). Some parents may have had their own experience of being in care, and have negative memories of this episode. They are therefore fearful of their own child experiencing a similar trauma. Social work intervention can be viewed with suspicion and fear, particularly by those already antagonistic to authority figures, and it is therefore essential that the multidisciplinary team works with the family to ensure optimum support and care.

Grandparents as carers

Due to the ill health, chaotic lifestyle or death of a parent, some grandparents have voluntarily taken on the role of carer for their grandchildren. In certain situations this arrangement has been mutually acceptable to all concerned. Difficulties may arise, however, where the relationship between grandparents and parent is fraught as a result of some unresolved childhood difficulty. This situation can be further exacerbated where grandparents have custody of their grandchildren as part of a statutory social work requirement.

The question will also arise of the ability and/or willingness of ageing grandparents to take on a parental role, particularly when they themselves may not be physically capable of coping with the rigours of child rearing for a second time. Grandparents will also be faced with acknowledging the potential death of their children and possibly grandchildren before their own.

Supporting families living with HIV in the community

Support from the statutory sector for families living with HIV includes counselling, welfare rights and benefits advice together with practical and emotional support (see Chapter 15). Ideally these services should be available from locally based generic sources which are also available to the wider community. Many clients, however, view voluntary agencies as being more sympathetic and understanding of their situation. The voluntary sector is able to offer support such as self-help groups, social functions, complementary therapies and counselling, as well as specific events for children.

Some people may resist using certain services which appear to be targeted towards particular groups. Health care workers need, therefore, to be sensitive when making referrals in order to avoid possible offence. In certain instances it may be appropriate to suggest peer support on either a one-to-one or a small-group basis.

There is a growing need to acknowledge the issue of supporting children infected and affected by HIV and consequently many of the statutory and voluntary services are endeavouring to help parents tackle the sensitive issue of talking with their children about HIV and plan for the future care of their children. Introducing these delicate issues requires immense skill and expertise. It may be appropriate to utilise colleagues who have particular experience in this field (see Chapter 17). For some families the intrusion of well-meaning professionals can serve to inhibit normal family life and for this reason it is important that families are enabled to maintain control over their lives and are not forced to lose their independence.

Terminal care

The unique function of the nurse is to assist the individual, sick or well, in the performance of those activities, contributing to health or its recovery (or to a peaceful death) that he or she would perform unaided given the necessary strength, will and knowledge (Henderson, 1969). In the face of uncertainty as well as the psychological and spiritual stresses caused by HIV infection, it is crucial that families continue to foster their child's growth and development despite the temptation to protect and nurture the children as though death was imminent. Van Eys (1974) stated 'we should not suspend the child's development until a cure is proven or a certainty'. Experienced paediatric nurses become aware of the dying process in children, and can be reasonably certain that a child in the terminal phase of the illness will die in the next few hours or days. Children with end-stage HIV disease may have an acute infection which if aggressively treated may resolve, leaving the child well for weeks or months before they get another infection. This roller-coaster may go on for months, if not years, and nurses may feel de-skilled and unable to offer the family help or information on which to make a decision.

There may be conflict between parents and health care professionals about when to stop active treatment, when experience has shown that a child has recovered from an acute infection and has had weeks, months, if not years of life. There is always the feeling that there may be a cure just around the corner, or that if the symptoms were investigated more aggressively a curable condition might be found and that it would not be in the child's best interests to do nothing. Sometimes, extremely difficult discussions between doctors and nurses acting as the child's advocate and the family have been helpful in planning short- and long-term care.

It is essential that the carers are encouraged to continue to be a member of the caring team if they wish, provided they are not in need of respite themselves.

Professional development

Information about HIV infection is changing so rapidly that it is important for nurses to remain aware of new developments. Close attention to AIDS and HIV-related research, conferences and information in the popular media can help nurses keep up with issues and information about HIV disease.

After the immediate and extended family, the hospital or specialised clinic is often the system most intimately involved with the child and family. The children and parents who spend a significant amount of time hospitalised or making repeated clinic visits develop long-term relationships with a large number of health care staff. Nurses often forget the fact that parents of chronically ill children are heavily dependent on them for continuing emotional support and approval. Parents often feel that friends and family (if available) cannot possibly understand their concerns and daily dilemmas in the way that health care staff can. Indeed the health care staff may be the only people who know the real diagnosis of the child and therefore the only people who can share the parents' fears. The attitudes and practices of hospital care givers affect the parents' feelings about their child's illness and about themselves as competent caretakers.

Hospital personnel have definite, if often unspoken, beliefs about appropriate family visiting behaviour, treatment practices and family relationships. When parents do not live up to staff expectations due to real inadequacies or family cultural differences, insecure or sensitive parents may find it difficult to respond to the subtle disapproval they sense from nursing or medical staff, particularly when the criticism is not directly discussed with them. Sick parents may be physically unable to visit and may be being cared for themselves in an adult ward far away from their children. At the other extreme, supportive and enthusiastic hospital staff members can successfully draw a parent more actively into the care of the child, through sensitive attention to the areas of success and competence exhibited by even the least skilled parental care taker (Libow, 1989).

Health care workers must examine their own prejudices, fears and attitudes if they are to support people with HIV compassionately, particularly if they are to be effective in educating others. The general public often consider health care workers to be an authority on the disease process. This places nurses in a unique position to discuss health education issues not only with colleagues and patients but with their own peer group.

Experience has shown that encountering judgemental attitudes can lead to lack of uptake of services by individuals with HIV infection. People who may already have a low self-esteem are particularly sensitive to perceived discrimination and may as a result be deterred from seeking health care. Education can help to dispel the damaging myths surrounding HIV and so prevent the terrible isolation and stigmatisation experienced by families living with HIV.

Ensuring that all health care workers have at least a basic awareness of the modes of transmission of HIV should be integrated into in-service and student programmes. Specialist members of staff can act as consultants for generic community and hospital personnel, enabling informal one-to-one discussion relevant to a particular workplace and/or caseload. Experience has shown that the general public and health care workers continue to be misinformed on many aspects of HIV and its transmission.

Personal safety

For the many children at-risk of HIV who are followed up in the community, the same principles of infection control should be applied as those followed in the clinical setting. The need to undertake universal precautions when dealing with body fluids is essential, as is ensuring the safe disposal of sharp and contaminated equipment. Discretion is required when carrying identifiable equipment such as sharps boxes into a client's home, as inadvertent breaches of confidentiality can occur.

For the personal safety of health care workers it is important to avoid where possible, potentially dangerous situations, and when working with families where there may be drug use, health care workers should avoid confrontational situations by emphasising their non-involvement in the carrying or prescribing of drugs. Sensitivity to the heightened emotions of parents and the ability to be alert to the danger signs in tense situations can help health care workers to diffuse potentially volatile situations, thus avoiding conflict.

Research

To meet the needs of existing clients and to improve future services it is essential that research is undertaken. Any such project must, however, be tackled in a sensitive, non-intrusive manner in order to avoid the feeling amongst individuals with HIV/AIDS that they are the subject of endless, non-essential analyses.

Health care workers asked to provide information or to participate in research projects should investigate the motives and integrity of those involved before taking part. Similarly health care workers approached by the media seeking information on 'the plight of HIV sufferers' need to balance protecting the privacy of clients against denying them an opportunity to air their views.

Conclusion

As the emotional and physical impact of the HIV epidemic unfolds, nurses and others have to work together to deal with the specific needs of children and families affected by this disease, particularly as parents are becoming ill and are dying. Undoubtedly many more children in the community will be profoundly affected by HIV/AIDS. The important message for all concerned is to work to a standard of care that meets the individual needs of the child and to ensure that the child's family has the appropriate support needed to provide it.

References

Anderson, J. M. (1981). The social constructing of illness experience: families with a chronically ill child. *Journal of Advanced Nursing*, **6**, 427–434.

Casey, A. (1988). A partnership with child and family. *Senior Nurse*, **8**, 8–9.

Court, S. D. M. (1976). *Fit for the Future: Report of the Committee on Child Health Services*, vols. 1 & 2. HMSO: London.

Department of Health (1993). *Welfare of Children and Young People in Hospital*. London: HMSO.

Eddy, J. & Whittle-Seiden, S. (1991). Nursing issues in the care of HIV infected children. In: *Paediatric AIDS*, ed. P. Pizzo & C. Wilfert, pp. 561–8. Baltimore: Williams & Wilkins.

European Collaborative Study (1991). Children born to women with HIV-1 infection: natural history and risk of transmission. *Lancet*, **337**, 253–60.

Hayes, V. E. & Knox, J. E. (1984). The experience of stress in parents of children hospitalised with long-term disabilities. *Journal of Advanced Nursing*, **9**, 333–41.

Henderson, V. (1969). *The Basic Principles of Nursing*. Geneva: International council of Nurses.

Kodadek, S. (1979). Family centre care of the chronically ill child. *Association of Operating Room Nurses Journal*, **30**, 635–8.

Krulik, T. (1980). Successful 'normalising' tactics of parents of chronically ill children. *Journal of Advanced Nursing*, **5**, 573–8.

Libow, J. (1989). Chronic illness and family coping. In *Children in Family Contexts. Perspectives on Treatment*, ed. L. Combrink-Graham. The Guilford Press.

Mok, J. & O'Hara, G. (1990). Placement of children from HIV-affected families: The Edinburgh experience. *Pediatric AIDS and HIV Infection: Fetus to Adolescent*, **1**, 20–2.

Peplau, H. E. (1991). Peplau's model in action. Howard Simpson, Macmillan.

Platt, H. (1959). *The Welfare of Children in Hospital*. Report of the Committee on Child Health Services. London: HMSO.

Rolland, J. (1984). A psychosocial typology of chronic illness. *Family Systems Medicine*, **2**, 2–25.

Roper, N., Logan, W. W. & Tierney, A. J. (1980). *The Elements of Nursing*. London: Churchill Livingstone.

Thomas, R. B. (1983). Family response to the birth of a child with a chronic condition. Unpublished manuscript, Seattle, WA: University of Washington School of Sociology.

Van Eys, J. (1974). The truly cured child. In: *Living with Childhood Cancer*, ed. J. Spinetta & P. Deasy-Spinetta P. St Louis: C. V. Mosby.

Wells, R. (1988). Foreword. In: *AIDS A Strategy for Nursing Care*, R. Pratt. London: Edward Arnold.

Suggestions for further reading

Batty, D. (ed.) (1993). *HIV Infection and Children in Need*. BAAF.

Claxton, R. & Harrison, T. (eds.) (1991). *Caring for Children with HIV and AIDS*. London: Edward Arnold.

Douglas, J. (1993). *Psychology and Nursing Children*. London: Macmillan.

Flaskerud, J. & Ungvarski, P. (1992). HIV/AIDS: a guide to nursing care. In: *Nursing Care of the Child*, 2nd edn. Philadelphia: W. B. Saunders.

Lwin, R., Duggan, C. & Gibb, D. (1992). *HIV and AIDS in Children: A Guide for the Family*. The Hospital for Sick Children, Great Ormond Street, London. Department of Medical Illustration.

Rose, M. H. & Thomas R. B. (eds.) (1987). *Children with Chronic Conditions*. New York: Grune & Stratton.

15

Supporting families affected by HIV infection

NAOMI HONIGSBAUM

Introduction

Increasing recognition that HIV infection is a disease of the family will inevitably raise questions as to how best the needs of all family members can be addressed within the context of the social changes that are profoundly altering family size, role and relationships, and traditional patterns of child rearing, socialisation and education. How will these changes in family structures, demographic trends and socio-economic factors impinge on the needs of families affected by HIV, and should these factors be taken into account when considering how different European countries might respond to the increased demand for services and support for families as HIV infection rates in women of childbearing age and in children continue to rise (European Observatory on National Family Policies, 1990)?

Social and demographic trends

A declining birth-rate and an ageing population is changing the age structure of most western European countries. This has coincided with a decline in marriage and an increase in divorce rates and cohabitation. The number of births outside marriage has increased in some countries and there is a significant rise in single parents and one-parent families (Kiernan & Estaugh, 1993). Although marriage is still popular the trend is towards shorter duration of marriages and post-marital cohabitation, where reconstructed families from previous marriages are established with new partners.

Whilst there are still marked variations of family structure between northern and southern European countries, with the more traditional family pattern of lower divorce rates and cohabitation in the South, the overall trend is remarkably similar, although the rate of change differs. In all countries family size has declined, and more women are taking up full-time or part-time employment outside the home (Eurostat, 1992).

However, migrant families who have settled in Europe from countries outside western Europe, including previous colonies in Africa, present a different population profile and age structure. Nearly half of all migrants come from other European countries such as Turkey and the former Yugoslavia, and about a quarter come from Africa (Eurostat, 1992). East European migration to the West is a more recent phenomenon following the break-up of the former communist states. Historically migrant families have settled in countries which needed a cheap unskilled labour workforce, and migrant families are usually found in menial and poorly paid occupations. But there is a significant and increasing number of migrant refugee families who are seeking asylum, often as a result of civil wars, famine or political persecution for religious, racial or cultural beliefs in their own countries. These migrant families tend to be made up of a younger population, with larger numbers of children; they may often have extended family networks in their country of origin, but may now be living in temporary housing and social isolation with few local support systems.

These demographic changes have produced a more pluralistic society with greater diversification of family models and patterns, and a reduced role for the family as the mainstay of social care and support for vulnerable members such as the sick, the young and the elderly. The traditional role of women as carers is changing as more women join the labour market and thus are unavailable to undertake these tasks. The level of social welfare benefits and services is becoming even more important in supplementing family roles, and needs to take account of the greater flexibility and duality of family relationships in the organisation and development of services for families under stress (Anon., 1989). These changing family needs have been recognised by the European Commission, which issued its first statement on European Community childcare policy in March 1992 (EC Network on Childcare, 1992). This policy refers to the need for action in four areas: services for children, improving leave arrangements for parents, ensuring that employers respond to the needs of workers with children, and promoting the sharing of responsibilities for children between men and women.

HIV infection in the family

Changing patterns of family life and socioeconomic factors are of crucial importance when considering the likely future needs of families in Europe in the second decade of the HIV/AIDS pandemic. HIV transmission rates from mother to child vary from 1 in 5 in Europe to 1 in 3 in parts of

Africa (see Chapter 1). Any headcount of HIV-infected children underestimates the full impact of HIV disease in children and their families, and in so doing may unduly influence the pattern and provision of services. It would be more appropriate in describing the social impact of HIV infection on the family to say that for every child infected, four uninfected children will be living in a family with HIV disease. In the European Collaborative Study, at age 5 years half the children born to HIV-infected mothers were still living with their mothers (M. L. Newell, personal communication 1994). In some families there may be inter-generational HIV infection which will affect siblings, grandparents and other relatives.

Whilst there is no cure for HIV at present, medical therapies have increased survival time, and HIV disease may well become more associated with issues relating to chronic illness and disabilities. In the USA some children with vertically acquired HIV infection have now reached 15 years and many adults remain reasonably well or asymptomatic for more than 10 years.

However, stigma, prejudice and fear of discrimination when HIV infection is diagnosed in the family are still the main barriers preventing families from seeking early intervention and support, and severely hinder the normalisation and integration of services. Disadvantaged families from ethnic minority communities or drug-using families may be more reluctant to ask for services for fear of discrimination, and families seeking political asylum may fear reprisals or repatriation if their HIV status is known. Some families may be illegal residents.

These families may be coping with multiple illness, death, loss and bereavement. Guilt, blame, poverty, lack of self-esteem and powerlessness will have an effect on family functioning and will influence the emotional and physical well-being of children. Problems of behaviour and psychosocial disturbance or educational difficulties may be manifest. Fear of losing control and anxieties about the long-term welfare and care of dependent children or vulnerable adults will interact with family dynamics and may lead to family breakdown and crisis. Coming to terms with terminal illness is painful, but fear of disclosure about a stigmatised disease often forces families to become secretive, isolated and withdrawn from normal social intercourse with friends and family. Children themselves are often bewildered by the secrecy and are uncertain and anxious about the nature of their illness or that of their parent or sibling. Children need opportunities to explore their own feelings and be allowed to participate in issues affecting them such as consent to treatment, undergoing HIV tests or planning their future care when parents can no longer look after them. These are all-important rights of children, which need to be acknowledged by adults whether they are professionals, parents or carers. Individual

counselling and family group work will be needed in supporting families
to resolve many of these painful experiences (Honigsbaum, 1991).

In the UK recent legislation in the National Health Service, the Community Care Act 1990 and the Children Act 1989 (Department of Health,
1989, 1990) support and provide increased opportunities for developing a
more needs-led assessment, which acknowledges parents' and children's
rights and encourages sharing power and responsibilities with parents.
This approach is mirrored in European Community child care policy
developments, where there is an increasing tendency to direct services
which focus on needs analysis for vulnerable children and families with
disabilities (Dumon, 1990, 1991).

Models of care

The organisation and provision of social care and support for HIV-affected
families varies depending on HIV infection prevalence, the range and
availability of social welfare provision in different countries, and family
preferences and attitudes.

In countries with a high prevalence of paediatric AIDS, such as Italy
and Spain, where injecting drug use is a major route of transmission in
HIV-affected families, the extended family still plays an important role in
providing care for its members. In these countries locally based social service provision outside hospital settings is less well developed, and varies
in the range of support offered. Some of this provision is supplemented by
charitable religious organisations and more recently some HIV specialist
non-governmental organisations have been established – but many of
these smaller organisations focus on giving intensive support to a few
families.

In France (which also has a high prevalence of paediatric HIV infection)
and the UK, HIV transmission is associated more with heterosexual contact as well as drug use, but with a more comprehensive array of social
welfare provision there is less expectation on the family as the provider
of all aspects of social care. The role of the voluntary sector in the UK is
also well developed and historically has played a pioneering role in providing a wide range of child and family services.

In northern European countries alternative care for children unable to
stay with their parents has moved away from institutional residential care
towards substitute family care programmes of fostering, adoption and day
care, such as child minders and nurseries. In some areas of Spain and
Portugal where support outside the family is variable, foster care and day
care is generally less well developed, and young orphaned children who
are not placed for adoption remain in institutional residential care. How-

ever, in all these countries (including Italy) there has been a growth in fostering schemes, in particular for children with special needs (Colton & Hellinckx, 1993).

The higher incidence of social deprivation, poverty, social isolation, illness, family fragmentation and breakdown in HIV-affected families has been well documented in studies undertaken in paediatric centres and social services in Europe and the USA (Oletto *et al.*, 1993; Levine, 1993). Stigma and fear of discrimination or disclosure of HIV status are still given as the main inhibiting factors preventing families from seeking early intervention and help with social problems. Denial of HIV disease and the lack of counselling and support prevents parents from making long-term alternative care plans for children in the event of their death, from helping children to acknowledge their own anxieties and fears about their future, or from seeking support for children in the school environment (Boland, 1987; Levine, 1993).

A recent multidisciplinary symposium of leading experts in Europe reached a unanimous consensus on the need to develop a family model of care which takes into account all family members whether they are HIV infected or HIV affected. This model of care should be based on a shared set of principles. These include developing multidisciplinary integrated and coordinated health and social service provision, providing family-based services which are child-centred, and acknowledging the individual needs of the child within the family to express his or her own views and rights in relation to care and treatment (Honigsbaum, 1994).

Similar conclusions have been reached in the USA, where paediatric HIV infection is now seen as a chronic disease and where models of care are family-focused, community-based and comprehensive. This model respects cultural and family diversity and recognises that HIV infection is a multi-generational disease which requires a holistic model of care to meet complex needs (Oleske, 1993).

Planning and coordinating care: an integrated approach

Services for HIV-affected families are at present fragmented and uncoordinated. There is a need to integrate health and social care programmes which shift the focus away from a 'medicalised' model of care to a more family-based multidisciplinary model of care located in the community.

Effective coordination of care can only be planned within a framework of an integrated approach which offers continuity of care and follow-up. Closer liaison between health and social services would assist family members, by providing a more seamless service. There is also a need to develop more effective working relationships with teachers, parents and pupils in the school environment, where knowledge and understanding about the needs of children with HIV infection or their parents is not well developed. Issues of caring for the school child and offering HIV awareness training and prevention in school communities is still largely absent (see Chapters 9 and 16).

A planned approach which spans all services including non-governmental agencies can also take account of age-related services. Planning provision for young families and children needs to integrate health, education and social care provision, so that a child and family perspective is incorporated. Young families are likely to need a range of day and respite care provision.

Services for school-age children are more likely to concentrate on aspects of schooling and on supporting children and parents in the school environment. Education services will need to liaise more effectively with health and social services in order to understand about HIV infection prevention, but also to develop school programmes for training teachers, parents and pupils on HIV infection as well as support in schools for the infected child which is non-stigmatising and confidential (see Chapter 16). Planning of services for older children and adolescents needs to focus more on community-based HIV prevention programmes. Such services for young people should also take account of the changing patterns of disease, where infected children will survive into adolescence and will need counselling and support services which recognise the particular stress and trauma of adolescence, within the context of HIV infection in families.

Family models of care

One-stop clinics

Discussion with HIV-affected families on their needs has provided a consistent response. Families want services which are flexible, accessible and are child and family centred. They prefer 'one-stop' clinics, where the needs of children and parents can be met within the framework of family concerns. This is practical, saves time and money, and prevents families with HIV infection from becoming too exhausted. This approach is also more likely to encourage the integration, continuity and co-ordination of care plans between health and social services provision. A 'one stop' centre should provide multidisciplinary care drawing on professional knowledge from different services (Duggan, 1993).

This model of care already works well in HIV specialist paediatric family clinics where general health and family problems are resolved, with the support of a multidisciplinary team of paediatricians, dietitians, health advisors, social workers, psychologists and liaison health visitors. These family clinics offer psycho-therapeutic work with children, counselling and support for parents, and follow-up and advice with locally based services and hospitals (Melvin & Sherr, 1993).

Pre-school provision and respite care

Many of those affected by HIV infection are single parents or one-parent families, and even where they have support from other family members there is a need to provide flexible day care for pre-school children. Parents prefer their children to attend local day nurseries or play groups which incorporate health, education and social care, and where children are integrated within normal provision. However, because parents may from time to time be too ill to care for children (or because the children have special health care needs), there is also a need to develop a range of flexible, respite care. This would include providing trained child minders, home helps, baby-sitters or foster parents who would care for children but offer flexible care for parents at times of family crisis and illness. In some social service organisations long-term respite and foster care programmes have been developed which offer opportunities to work closely with affected families, providing continuity of care for children. Children may be less traumatised by the illness or death of parents or siblings if an alternative family support system is available to help them cope. Such programmes aim to provide short-term respite care and fostering, but with the knowledge that permanent long-term fostering may develop from such arrangements. This allows time for both parents and children to anticipate separation and loss as well as to assess whether fostering or possibly adoption is appropriate.

Development of substitute care programmes

The majority of HIV-affected families in which parents are infected will, at some point, have to make plans for alternative care when the parents are no longer able to look after the children, or in the event of parental death. The preferred option is to seek alternative care which keeps the child within a family network of relatives or neighbours. But many parents will continue to care for children even in the late stage of their own illness if sufficient help is available in the form of domiciliary care, baby-sitting and respite care.

Long-term planning for children can be difficult. Social service organisations will need to recruit and train carers able to work in open-ended relationships with HIV-affected families which can ideally engender mutual trust. Foster carers will need to recognise that parents are reluctant to relinquish their parental rights and responsibilities, and the aim of good practice is to enable families to retain their independence for as long as possible.

Social service departments need to develop appropriate training and recruitment programmes for carers who can work flexibly. These carers will need training on HIV prevention, stigma, discrimination, health and safety, child care practice, confidentiality procedures, counselling children and understanding HIV disease in children.

Some local authorities in the UK have developed coherent HIV policies for children and families. Experience has shown that where departments have established and made explicit HIV child care policies there are greater opportunities to develop good child care practices and to recruit experienced foster parents who work closely with health, social services and community-based organisations (O'Hara, 1993). In the UK, policy guidance has been issued to all local authority social service departments on child care practice and HIV (Department of Health, 1992).

An important element in developing effective foster care programmes is to recruit experienced, older foster parents who are more mature and can cope with uncertainty and stress. Foster families themselves also need to be well supervised and offered counselling and support services, in order that they in turn can offer a professional service to parents.

Developing appropriate substitute care programmes can be problematic. In France, parts of the UK and Belgium there is a higher proportion of HIV-affected families from ethnic minority communities, many of whom are from sub-Saharan countries. These families are more likely to be socially isolated, have fewer local social support systems, and be reluctant to seek out services for fear of jeopardising their refugee status, racial discrimination, or more simply because they are unaware of how to gain access to services. However, additional problems can be encountered because of a family's possible fear of political persecution if they are put in touch with organisations from their country of origin. These families are more likely to have suffered traumas associated with separation, exile and possibly torture, and therefore need skilled counselling and support.

To develop culturally sensitive alternative care programmes it is necessary to take account of these issues, and the different perceptions of family cultures and beliefs on child rearing. Planning for children can be further complicated when parents may have left children in the country of origin and may be anxious to re-unite family members before they die. Specific recruitment programmes are currently being developed in the UK and France which take account of these concerns, and it is hoped that appropriate alternative family models of care for these families can be offered over time (Working Group on AIDS, 1990).

Providing social support and substitute care remains one of the key areas for further developmental work. Alternative ways of helping families and children to retain control of their own lives and remain at home wherever possible is the preferred option. Unnecessary hospitalisation and residential care should be avoided when possible. This will require a wide range of services including family support at home, respite and substitute parental care. More research is needed on the elements that contribute to developing good models of care.

HIV infection and schooling

A neglected area of service provision is related to the need to focus on the school environment. Developing links with education authorities appear to be more difficult than establishing liaison between health and social services. Yet it is essential to encourage effective collaboration between education services and the wider communities of health and social care.

Establishing mechanisms for a dialogue is important in developing collaborative projects. In Italy, the Government has launched an ambitious programme to train all head teachers in HIV prevention. In one Italian district collaborative work is being undertaken between health services and local schools to develop an HIV training programme for teachers and parents.

In the UK there have also been some imaginative programmes of HIV infection prevention and curriculum development on sexual health for older children. However, in general schools have not addressed the challenge of providing more comprehensive HIV policies which cover issues of care, counselling and support for HIV-infected children at school, discrimination and confidentiality policies and liaison with school communities (Young & Phillips, 1993).

In Europe, the main challenge for the education services and school communities is to combat the discrimination, social isolation and marginalisation of affected children. Integrating the HIV-infected child is still a major problem. Families have been victimised and forced to move following local protests from parents and teachers. Education authorities have often been slow to react until faced with a crisis of confidence (see Chapter 16).

Whilst many infected children are still below school age, they will soon be entering the school system. Schools need to draw up effective policies and guidance covering teacher training, confidentiality procedures, health and safety, sexual health and health education curriculum. Schools need to provide a safe and supportive environment for affected children, offering appropriate psycho-social help and counselling for children and their families (see Chapter 9).

Teachers need to be aware of HIV disease in children and to understand individual children's clinical care, as sometimes they may have to supervise a child's medication. Many schools are unskilled in working with drug-using families and tend to be rejecting; they will need guidance and support. Knowledge about drug use, and access to help, should be part of a teacher's armoury in offering support to children and their families.

HIV training and preparation for all school staff is an essential prerequisite for school-based strategies to offer confidential and supportive services for HIV-infected children, parents or uninfected siblings. Some families may wish to share information of their HIV status with school staff, not only to ensure the physical well-being of vulnerable children, but also to allow children to express fears, anxieties and worries, or be supported in coping with loss and bereavement. This can only occur if parents are reassured that confidentiality will be maintained, and teachers are well informed and have undertaken training which addresses their own attitudes and fears about HIV transmission.

Training

Access to HIV training programmes provides an important foundation on which to build good practice and to underpin policy and service developments. Systematic training programmes should be available for all staff who work in HIV services. Staff supervision and development are important aspects of training programmes. Professional staff need opportunities to up-date knowledge and explore their own training needs (Department of Health, 1992).

In general, whilst HIV prevention and awareness programmes have often been developed there has been little emphasis on developing communication skills in direct work with children. In particular, many adult-based organisations do not understand child care needs, and training should encourage all professionals to develop and identify elements of good child care policies and practice as part of their professional skills.

If services are to become more child centred then training needs to address child care needs, including topics such as sexual health, HIV prevention, drug use, working with terminal illness, loss and bereavement, living with stress and counselling children and families.

Support for older children

A recent study in Spain revealed the need for HIV prevention strategies aimed at all teenagers but especially those who were more at-risk of HIV transmission because of their lifestyle, such as run-away street children, the homeless and unemployed, young prostitutes and drug users. Many of these young people were ignorant about HIV transmission, but also lacked access to good information on HIV prevention, and did not know where to seek advice on health or social support when they became HIV infected.

Young people need advice which is non-judgemental and not patronising on issues such as HIV pre- and post-test counselling, safe sex and drug use and reproductive issues for young women. More effective outreach programmes should be developed with staff trained and experienced in communicating with young people. These programmes need to be well resourced and funded and located in informal social settings where 'hard-to-reach' young people at most risk are likely to congregate. HIV prevention strategies need to link the role of the school in providing a solid foundation of information and support with community services which can reach the older age group of teenagers who may respond more positively to peer-group education in a less structured environment.

Young people with HIV infection may also lack support from their families, and may have come from broken homes. There is a need to provide adolescent services which can offer a range of social and medical support including counselling services, housing and job creation schemes and rehabilitation services for young people with drug using problems (Echevarria, 1994).

Conclusion

The need to offer integrated and community-based services which maintain family strength and well-being for as long as possible is paramount. Problems of discrimination and stigma are still major obstacles in promoting integrated services. In developing services which support families more attention will need to be paid to the needs of migrant families and those from ethnic minority communities. Increased migration in Europe between countries has not necessarily led to greater understanding or tolerance, and migrant families are more likely to experience racial harassment, social rejection and discrimination in jobs and housing. Similarly health and social services have not developed culturally specific services which address issues related to language, culture and beliefs. Staff from ethnic minority backgrounds should be recruited to provide more sensitive services, and effective strategies for the recruitment, training and support of respite care staff should be discussed, so that children in need of substitute family placements are looked after within their own communities.

Families where drug use is associated with HIV infection also require strategies which acknowledge the difficulties presented in working and supporting them. The families may have a history of a disrupted family

life, chaotic behaviour, and estranged relationships with grandparents or
siblings or partners. Many are single parents, on low income and living in
poor housing (Gurbindo, 1994). Some HIV-infected women who are drug
users in the prison population are allowed to keep their young children
under the age of 6 years with them. Health and social care in the prison
services is poor and although some young children can attend nurseries
and day care services outside prison, many women want to keep their
children with them. However, policies which incarcerate children with
their parents fail to address the long-term developmental impact this may
have on the health and social well-being of children. Drug rehabilitation
services need to be developed, especially in areas of high drug use and
HIV prevalence. These services should offer supported accommodation for
parents and children, housing and harm reduction drug use programmes
as well as better primary health care facilities for child health surveillance.
Provision of family centres could offer training in parenting skills to those
parents who are often under considerable stress, and assist them in caring
for children by better provision of day nurseries, play and leisure activities.

References and further reading

Anon. (1989). Families in a Frontier-free Europe. Brussels: Coface.
Bradshaw, J., Dithc, J., Holmes, H. & Whiteford, P. (1993). A comparative study
    of child support in fifteen countries. *Journal of European Social Policy*, **3**,
    255–71.
Boland, M. G. (1987). *Helping Children with AIDS. The Role of the Child
    Welfare Worker*. Washington: American Welfare Association.
British Children in Need (1993). *Children and Disability*. London: National
    Children's Home.
Colton, M. J. & Hellinckx, W. (1993). *Child Care in the EC: Country-specific
    Guide to Foster and Residential Care*. Aldershot: Arena.
Department of Health. Children Act 1989. London: HMSO.
Department of Health. NHS & Community Care Act 1990. London: HMSO.
Department of Health. Health Publications Unit (1992). *Children and HIV*:
    Guidance for Local Authorities. London: HMSO.
Duggan, C. (1993). A family affair. *Child Health*, June/July 1993.
Dumon, W. (1990). *Family Policy in EEC Countries*. Luxembourg: Commission
    of the European Communities.
Dumon, W. (1991). *National Family Policies in EC-countries in 1991: European
    Observatory of National Family Policies*. Brussels: Commission of the
    European Communities.
Echevarria, J. (1994). Problemas en la adolescencia. Caceres: Paper delivered at
    2nd National Conference on AIDS.
EC Network on Childcare (1992). *Employment Equality and Caring for Children*.
    Commission of the European Communities.
European Observatory on National Family Policies (1990). *Families and Policies:
    Evolution and Trends in 1988–89*. Commission of the European
    Communities.

Eurostat (1992). *Europe in Figures*. Commission of the European Communities.

Gurbindo, M. (1994). Problemas Sociales Asociados a la transmision del VIH. Caceres: Paper delivered at 2nd National Conference on AIDS.

Honigsbaum, N. (1991). *HIV/AIDS and Children: A Cause for Concern*. London: National Children's Bureau.

Honigsbaum, N. (1994). *Children and Families Affected by HIV in Europe: The Way Forward*. Report of a Symposium in Torgiano, Italy. London: National Children's Bureau.

Kiernan, K. E. & Estaugh, V. (1993). *Cohabitation: Extra-marital Childbearing and Social Policy*. London: Family Policy Studies Centre.

Levine, C. (1993). *Orphans of the HIV Epidemic*. New York: United Hospital Fund of New York.

Melvin, D. & Sherr, L. (1993). The Child in the family: responding to AIDS and HIV. *AIDS Care*, **15**, 35–42.

O'Hara, G. (1993). Looking after children (abstract). Edinburgh: 2nd International Conference on HIV in Children and Mothers.

Oleske, J. M. (1993). When paediatric HIV infection becomes a chronic disease; caring for the late stages of HIV infection (abstract). Edinburgh: 2nd International Conference on HIV in Children and Mothers.

Oletto, S., Giaquinto, C., Ruga, E., Cozzani, S., Giacomelli, A. & Mazza, A. (1993). Foster care in HIV-positive children (abstract PO D22.4088). Berlin: IXth International Conference on AIDS.

Working Group on AIDS (1990). *HIV Infection and the Black Communities*. London: Local Authority Association Offices.

Young, J. H. & Phillips, K. (1993). HIV/AIDS: sharing the voice of young people. *Education and Health*, **11**, no.5.

16

HIV infection in schools

A PRIMARY SCHOOL HEADTEACHER

Introduction

When HIV infection first became an issue in education there was naturally uncertainty about the effect this would have in schools. Due to lack of research and minimal knowledge of HIV infection the whole subject was approached with understandable concern by all staff. We were entering an unknown area, and no one was sure what having HIV-infected children in the school would imply. There were obvious doubts and some apprehension. It was we felt important to learn as much as we could, as quickly as we could, as to the nature of this new disease.

Meeting the challenge

There were several key questions that needed answers:

Would HIV-infected children be mentally or physically impaired in terms of their education?
Could the infection be passed easily from one person to another?
What were the necessary precautions staff and children should take?
Would HIV-infected children be likely to die while at school?
Did parents have to inform the school if their children were infected?
How confidential was the matter supposed to be?

In quite a short time all these issues were addressed both by information packs from the UK Education Department and by in-service sessions in which teachers could discuss any concerns or questions they had with an expert in the field.

Effect on the child's education

It was clear that HIV infection would have no effect on the educational abilities of a child other than the fact that he or she might be absent from school more frequently than most other children. Certainly in our experience HIV-infected children have shown no difficulties, developing at a normal pace, participating in all school activities both mental and physical, and contributing as much to the life of the school as other children. Of course this is now obvious. Our own ignorance was the problem, and not that of any possibly infected children. Staff were understandably concerned about the educational development of HIV-infected children but they now know that the disease does not limit educational progress. If children are absent from school they are always given the opportunity to catch up on work they have missed. This is not an insurmountable problem.

We have learnt that it is possible but extremely rare for the AIDS virus to have some effect on the brain. Certainly in the school's experience this has never been an issue. We were quickly satisfied that in terms of their education HIV-infected children would have only the same problems as any other child when it came to progressing through an increasingly complex curriculum.

Taking care at school

A greater concern was how easily the disease could be passed from one person to another. Again there were the usual exaggerations and distortions. This was in the early days before we had knowingly enrolled any HIV-infected children. We knew that transmission of the disease had something to do with bodily fluids but noone was quite sure what this meant. Obviously in a primary school there are many incidents when blood is spilt, children vomit on a classroom floor, in the corridor or the playground, or urine accidentally ends up where it should not; there is also phlegm, which some children have a habit of discharging to make some gesture to their peers.

The immediate response was to worry about all these 'bodily fluids' as though all of them might be a danger. We now know that the emphasis is on blood, not the emission of blood but the chance of a member of staff or another child coming into contact with infected blood through a cut on their own body. A child with a cut is not likely to have that wound come in to direct contact with another child's open wound, and even then it is probable that at least one of these wounds will be dry and therefore not be so exposed to any mixing of blood. Saliva, vomit or urine are no longer seen as a problem. We now understand that it is only through blood that HIV infection can be passed on. This, we realise, may not be completely understood or accepted by certain sections of the general public. We know that many of the parents of our schoolchildren still have the old fears about HIV, and through lack of information see it as being a highly contagious infection. It is a problem that only more publicity and education can redress. Too many people still do not accept that HIV is basically a sexually transmitted or drug-related infection caused by the mixing of blood through either unsafe sex or the sharing of contaminated needles.

In our experience the most common causes of blood spillage are nose bleeds and cuts on hands or legs from a fall in the playground. These are usually one-off incidents involving individual children, so the likelihood of one child's blood contaminating another's is extremely slight. Our playground is a very busy place and accidents do happen, but because the entire staff is more knowledgeable in dealing with these, the situation is no longer as problematic as it was. With the right responses and the correct hygiene procedures it is unimaginable that a child could be infected by another child.

The emphasis is obviously on the necessary precautions. Again this has been clearly spelt out in the guidelines from the Education Authority. The approach is based on the possibility that every child in the school is HIV infected, so that every child is dealt with in the same way. Every teacher, playground supervisor, dinner supervisor, janitor, secretary and auxiliary responds to a situation in exactly the same manner and everyone follows similar procedures. These are based on a thorough, consistently implemented policy. All staff are clearly briefed on the correct procedures for dealing with any bodily spillage, and there are regular updates to remind everyone. These updates are essential, especially as HIV infection no longer has the high profile it once had. In a crisis it is easy to forget what actions are appropriate. The staff are reminded always to wear medical gloves before treating any cut or when cleaning up any other kind of spillage. In every classroom, in the auxiliary's room, in the janitor's and secretary's room, and in the hall, there are distinctly marked medical boxes in which there are gloves, cotton wool and plasters. Also in every room is a specially designed waste bin for used tissues, cotton wool and other soiled dressings only. This bin has its own waste bag inside so the school cleaners can tie it up at the end of each day and easily dispose of it separately from the rest of the classroom waste.

A child who has an accident in the playground will usually be brought into the school to be dealt with. When this is not possible the playground supervisors always have a pack of medical gloves with them. The precautions with the right kind of emphasis should become automatic. They are now standard procedures. The staff obviously realise their importance.

The children are continually advised on their own safeguards, such as always to tell an adult if they have an accident or to tell a member of staff if someone else has one, and never to try and deal with it themselves. They are warned of the dangers of picking up anything sharp, such as needles, in the street or in the school area. This is important as we know of several occasions when children have come across hypodermic needles and syringes in their local area. One child accidentally pricked himself with a needle he found on the pavement on his way to school one morning.

The continuing process of education about HIV infection for both children and staff is essential. Simple awareness of hygiene and necessary precautions reduces the risks involved to the extent that if the procedures are followed, everyone working in the environment of the school should be safe from any possibility of being infected.

Confidentiality

Another key issue as regards HIV-infected children is that of confidentiality. A parent does not have to inform a school concerning their child's infection – that is why a school's hygiene policy is based on the possibility that any of its children could be HIV infected. It is entirely up to the parents whether they inform the school or not. If they wish to do so it is essential that they realise such information will remain totally confidential. The day-to-day success of any school depends on its parents feeling confident that whatever is discussed with a member of staff will go no further than the person they have spoken to unless they wish it. Obviously there are many delicate matters discussed within the privacy of the headteacher's office. Parents have to feel they are in a situation which they control. Their trust in the professionalism of school staff is the basis of a school working for the benefit of the children in that school's care. Without that trust a school cannot function properly. This is not just an issue with parents of HIV-infected children; it is something that is crucial to the whole ethos of a school. It is completely up to the parents who they want to share that information with. They may wish to discuss something with a headteacher and nobody else. If that is the case that information goes no further. We have failed as professionals if the parents do not feel confident that anything they say remains totally confidential. It is the same with any teacher. They realise the utter importance of being trusted by a parent. So much essential information that might help in dealing with a child would be sacrificed if any parent felt unsure as to how confidential such information would be. The only qualification to this would be my expectation as a headteacher that a member of my teaching staff would discuss with me anything relevant about a pupil that had been mentioned by a parent so long as the teacher informed the parent that they were going to do this. As the person finally responsible for the well-being of all the pupils in the school a headteacher has to know anything significant that might affect the development of one of them. A discussion between a member of staff and headteacher is just as confidential as that between a parent and the headteacher or other member of staff.

Certainly if a parent came to enrol a child and at the same time informed me that their child was HIV infected it would have no effect whatsoever on the enrolment of that child. There are basically no reasons for refusing the enrolment of a child other than the capacity of the school. No parent has any grounds for concern on that point and the information given would not have to be registered on an enrolment form unless the parent wished it. Of course some parents might wish that anyone dealing with their child is told of the diagnosis. That is their decision. In our experience the information given to the headteacher or class teacher has gone no further. We have HIV-infected children in the school whom noone else knows about because that is what the parents wanted. We have enough evidence to know that confidentiality in a school does work. Professionally that has to be the case or the school would not work for the full benefit of all its pupils.

A chronic illness

A few years ago we were prepared for the fact that HIV-infected children might not survive through their primary school years. Of course at the time this was an extremely difficult issue. But with more research and monitoring of infected children it now seems that their life expectancy is much greater than was at first thought. The problem is now open ended, and only in the fullness of time will we know more about the longevity of these children.

At some time it may be that a school will have to deal with a bereavement. Teachers need support in how to deal with such a situation, whether or not it is related to HIV infection. If the death is related to HIV infection it might involve helping the parents or classmates of an HIV-infected pupil, or dealing with an uninfected child who has lost an HIV-infected parent. Whatever the situation it will be difficult and complicated. In some cases the family may wish the whole thing to remain private; alternatively it may be that the bereavement and its causes are openly discussed. Whatever the circumstances it is something that a school sadly has to prepare itself for as we may be required to help and counsel those involved (see Chapter 18).

Conclusion

Many of the myths about HIV infection have been destroyed, and for teachers the problem has been given a proper perspective. That is not to say that HIV infection is not still of huge concern. It is of fundamental significance to the whole of society, and schools by their very nature have to deal with many of society's problems. We are not naive in thinking that HIV-infected children are no longer seen by everyone as an uncomfortable issue. Unfortunately we realise that some of our parents are still sensitive to the idea that their children might be sharing a school with HIV-infected pupils. Only more education will help lessen the worries they have. That is why confidentiality and the proper hygiene procedures are crucial. No child should be tainted with a label, and it is the job of teachers to ensure this does not happen. Our school welcomes any child. Thanks to our Education Department's own educational policy on HIV infection we are now more confident in dealing with any problem that might arise. This is more important for parents to realise than their children. As teachers our concern is for the safety and well-being of our pupils. They are placed in our care, and whether they are HIV infected or not makes no difference to how we manage that care.

17

Talking with the dying child

REBEKAH LWIN

Time is not gentle with a last goodbye –
the body changes while the mind
remembers and forgets the things
that yesterday were consciousness –
Ralph Wright 1983

Joe is 6 years old. He has AIDS and is dying. He was first admitted to hospital 12 months ago, 1 month after his arrival in Britain. Since then he has been discharged and readmitted several times for increasingly longer stays. The latest has lasted 3 months; two attempts to allow him home for the weekend have failed because of his oxygen requirements. During the last year he has had blood tests, transfusions, intravenous antibiotics, immunoglobulin, naso-gastric tubes, pleural taps, biopsies, CT scans, oxygen and constant medication. His mother also has AIDS and recently her health has deteriorated; she is frequently too sick to visit; there have been times when Joe has been well enough to go home but his mother has been hospitalised. There is no one else at home to look after him. Fear, culture and personal belief prevent Joe's mother from talking to him, not only about their HIV diagnosis, but also about being ill and the fact that he is dying. She would like staff to respect her wishes and to maintain the silence about illness and death. This, she strongly believes, is in Joe's best interests. She fears that to talk about such things would frighten Joe and may lead him to ask questions of her that she would be unable to answer.

On the ward Joe has been cheerful, friendly, cheeky and very engaging. He has also been sad, angry, disappointed, frightened and silent. He asks no questions and talks little of how he feels or what sense he makes of all that is happening in his world. The hospital staff feel increasingly uncomfortable about his silence and ignorance of his and his mother's condition.

The above case illustrates the dilemmas common to families facing terminal illness in their child. In cases of children suffering from HIV infection and AIDS, the stigma of the disease and the multiple illnesses and losses within the family contribute additional burdens which reinforce the barriers to communication with the dying child.

Why talk with children?

It is now widely acknowledged within the health care professions that it is important for dying children to have the opportunity to talk, to understand, to communicate their feelings and put life and death in perspective (Anthony & Koupernick, 1973; Burton, 1974; Spinetta, 1982; Baum, 1990). However, it is not uncommon for the parents of these children to fear that knowledge of the seriousness of the illness will frighten their child and perhaps prevent possible recovery or even accelerate death. The agony of accepting that a child is going to die can inhibit communication with the child about death. It can also deter parents from discussing any aspect of the illness for fear that the conversation and their emotions may escalate out of their control. Parents sometimes take refuge in the protective adage: 'What children do not know, cannot harm them'. But, for children who are ill, hospitalised, facing frequent and sometimes painful medical procedures, ignorance is not bliss.

Children, even very young ones, are skilful at picking up the cues of worry, concern and tension within their family. It does not take much for a child to realise that what is happening to them does not happen to most other children. If questions are evaded or explanations denied, then sooner or later they formulate their own answers. They pick up fragments of details, listen to the whispered speculations of others, hear talk about other children and think it is about them. They will interpret what they can and create the rest to complete the picture, colluding with the secrecy by not asking questions.

Normality and predictability decrease and the child may begin to distrust the world about him.* 'If children are aware of the serious nature of their illness and this is then hidden under a veil of secrecy or even hypocrisy, their curiosity can become inhibited, they distrust their own senses, and tend to find everything unreal. All this can lead to a chronic distrust of others' (Judd, 1989). Silence does not eliminate worry and fear and often reinforces a belief that what is happening is too appalling to talk about. The child may lose all previous sense of mastery and may become psychologically very vulnerable. Responses such as withdrawal, regression and aggression are not uncommon.

Although children who are made aware of the seriousness of their condition are also psychologically vulnerable, if allowed to explore and question their perceptions, they can anticipate events and make predictions and choices based on their knowledge. This will reduce anxiety and leave them with a sense of control.

The aim of talking is therefore to reassure, build trust and maintain a sense of effectiveness and self-confidence. It is not a one-way action nor a fast solution, but more a continuous circular process of giving,

* Throughout this chapter the use of the male pronoun implies the female also.

receiving, interpreting and seeking knowledge. Understanding the perspective of those involved is fundamental. For example, in the case of
the child dying from AIDS, the deteriorating health and imminent
death of the child may be uppermost in the thoughts of a parent. For
the child, however, particularly if not yet aware of the seriousness of
their condition, foremost thoughts may be of separation or pain, or
equally what friends are doing at school or whether a favourite pet is
okay. A starting point to communication is therefore often not 'telling'
anything but understanding where the child is in an interpretation of
what is happening and what meaning the illness holds for him or her.
It is perhaps helpful at this stage to consider the development of the
concepts of illness and death in young children before addressing the
more specific issues of how, when and who should talk with dying
children about these subjects.

Development of the concept of illness and death in young children

Understanding the nature of illness and the concept of death is a learning
process and such knowledge develops gradually over time and with experience (see also Chapter 18). From the moment a child is diagnosed as
HIV infected a new routine of hospital visits, blood tests and medications
commences. A child may later start to link these experiences with pain,
feeling unwell, or being separated from family. If there has been previous
illness in the family or close experiences with other children in hospital
then these associations may occur earlier. Bluebond-Langer (1978) and
Lansdown (1987) both discuss the child's growing awareness of his illness
as proceeding through distinct stages from 'I am ill' through 'I am seriously ill but will get better' to 'I am seriously ill and will not get better'
and finally 'I am dying'. Parents, on hearing the diagnosis of their child,
may pass through similar stages of awareness. Their perceptions, for
example that their child has a fatal illness which may kill others but will
not claim the life of their child, may have profound influence on the
child's beliefs about himself.

The development of a child's view of death is not necessarily linked to
his awareness of illness and may be influenced by previous experience of
death as well as cultural and religious factors. Initially death may be con-
fused with sleep but, generally, by the age of 6 years most children will
understand that death means separation, immobility and is irreversible
(Kane, 1979). By this age many children will also be aware of how
the body changes after death and of death's universality (Lansdown &

Benjamin, 1985). Certainly by the age of 9 or 10 years most children will have a fully formed concept of death similar to that of adults. Beliefs in God, heaven, ghosts and life after death vary considerably from child to child and culture to culture. Such beliefs may often provide comfort for the child but not necessarily so, and it is important when exploring these issues to understand according to the child's interpretation and not to make assumptions.

How children react psychologically to the knowledge of their own illness and impending death depends on many factors and will reflect the individual nature of the child's inner world. Judd (1989) describes a distinct psychological process taking place 'that bears much similarity with the stages of bereavement'. Anger, fear, disbelief, fantasy and profound sadness may all, at various stages, be features of a child's response to this knowledge.

How do children communicate?

Children communicate their fears and worries in many different ways. Even at a very young age, before speech develops, they may express through their behaviour and their temperament that they are not feeling well, or that they are frightened or unhappy. Correct interpretation of non-verbal as well as verbal cues will encourage further communication and, where possible, conversation. When children do talk, they may seek answers to many questions about the practical aspects of their current experiences, or perhaps more searching questions about others. It is rare for the 'dreaded' direct questions such as 'Am I going to die?' or 'Have I got AIDS?' to be asked before any other general awareness of illness or death has been explored.

Emotions may be expressed not only in words but also through play, drawing, writing and through changes in mood and behaviour. How to respond depends on the method of expression that the child is adopting, and on his age and level of development. Children should not be made to feel pressurised into talking but should be given the opportunity to express their feelings and concerns, in a way that is flexible and feels comfortable and secure for them. Talking directly is often difficult for many children, but the use of dolls, puppets, drawings, symbolism, games, books and stories can all be used to help children express themselves. Positive as well as negative feelings should be explored and emphasis should be placed on what is good and works well in their lives and bodies as well as on the converse. Wherever possible, children should be left with a sense of balance and competence.

Children under 5 years of age*

Very young children may view their illness in terms of separation and pain. There will be a preoccupation with their immediate experiences as a more long-term understanding of what might happen to them will probably not yet be fully developed. They may also be particularly vulnerable to the fact that their parents, far from protecting them from painful and uncomfortable procedures, seem to be partners in this treatment. Parents may be equally distressed at having to put their child through anything that is painful or frightening.

Children of this age may talk about how they feel but expressive language may not be fully mature. The listener should therefore be careful of semantic errors and not place adult interpretations on what the child has said but rather ensure that they have understood the child's perspective. The latter point is important for all ages, particularly where the main language of the child differs from that of the listener.

Young children may indicate anxiety and discomfort through their behaviour. Inability to verbalise or otherwise adequately explain their feelings may lead to behaviour or moods not normally seen in that child, such as a fear of going to sleep, or to regressive behaviours such as over-attachment or bed wetting.

Children between 5 and 9 years of age

By this age, children may begin to link their illness with a long-term understanding that they may not get better. However, they may continue to speak in terms of dreams and ambitions, and make references to 'when I grow up'. A more realistic view of death begins to develop. As with the younger child, fears of separation and pain will still be prominent, but the school age child may begin to verbalise his feelings more. He may become increasingly aware of how his life differs from that of other children of his age, and he may become more inquisitive and more angry at insufficient explanations. Concepts of 'good' and 'bad' may form dominant images and it is important to ensure that children do not attribute 'being ill' with 'being bad'.

Most children, but especially this age group, are susceptible to the beliefs of others and are significantly influenced by what they see in the world around them. It may still be difficult to separate fantasy from reality, and understanding of the moment of death may be coloured by the often violent and bloody deaths seen from fairy stories through to

---

* All ages given here are approximate. A child's needs and level of understanding will depend on many factors, not age alone.

modern films. Such images can be frightening and frequent reassurance that their death will not be like this may be necessary.

Children over 10 years of age

By the age of 9 or 10 years most children will begin to suspect they are seriously ill if they have not already been told. This is especially true if the diagnosis of HIV infection has been made at an early age and if other family members have also been ill. They may collude with the secrecy and silence within the family, but may also actively seek 'proof' they are not well. A child who does know the seriousness of his condition may begin to ask more searching questions, be more specific about whom he chooses to talk to and begin to show more independence in coping with it.

Adolescence is a particularly difficult time as conflicts can arise between dependence on parents and desire for autonomy. The inability to live life to the full and the loss of control over life may lead to rebellion and depression. In these cases one-to-one professional help may be valuable. Peer groups, as a source of learning, confiding and support, become increasingly important. If the adolescent is aware of his diagnosis, the need for continued secrecy and the inability to discuss feelings around HIV with close friends may be frustrating and restricting. Similarly certain symptoms such as changes in body image can be distressing. Being able to identify purpose and achievement in their lives may be important. Children from this age, or even younger, will often benefit from being able to take an active role in their treatment, thereby feeling they have some element of control. Whatever the age of the child, caregivers and staff may need to be supported in receiving what the child has to 'say', in encouraging further openness and in acknowledging that this is a stressful and difficult time for themselves too.

What should be talked about?

For most children now infected with the HIV, the time between diagnosis and death is increasing. Ideally, therefore, by the time the child reaches the terminal stages of illness much preparatory talking can and should have taken place. As early as possible after diagnosis of HIV infection, parents should try to create an environment that encourages open and honest discussion about all aspects of life that may be relevant to the child at that time. Communicating in an unforced, general way about emotive, sensitive and potentially embarrassing subjects such as separation and loss, the 'facts of life' or prejudice, will give the parent practice at talking about such issues with their child and will give the child confidence to trust and confide in the parents. This will help prepare the way for both parent and child if and when a more frank discussion about the child or the parents' health becomes appropriate. Such discussion can and should start at any age and the child will learn from it to trust that his parents will listen, understand and respond to his questions. Knowing what to say at each stage depends, in part, on what the child already knows and it is important, therefore, to start from wherever the child is. Giving information about his condition does not mean that the child understands it. Care should be taken to check how the child interprets what he has been told and to correct any misunderstanding.

Wherever possible, questions should be answered truthfully. It is best not to lie or be obviously evasive. It is not helpful, for example, to claim a painful procedure will not be painful, or indeed to deny any reality, as the child will soon discover the deception. It is far better to admit the truth and offer the child strategies for coping with it. However, if it is the express wish of the prime caregiver to conceal certain facts then this should be respected. If this concealment is considered not to be in the best interests of the child, efforts should be made to help the child's carers understand the effects of their secrecy while at the same time trying also to understand their motives. This may be particularly crucial when parents or caregivers disagree on how much their child should know or where the parents are having difficulty containing and coping with their own feelings. Parents, however, should not feel pressurised into taking a course of action that they feel would be detrimental to their family and child.

This is an extremely sensitive area with HIV infection where communication about a child's condition risks four separate but related disclosures to the child.

1. You are seriously ill
2. You are seriously ill and will die
3. You have AIDS
4. Other family members also have AIDS or will develop AIDS or have already died from AIDS

The latter two disclosures are highly significant and require careful consideration. A child who knows anything of HIV infection will understand that AIDS is a family disease and may make the leap from 3 to 4 without the need for its explicit disclosure. Knowledge of 4 will raise questions unique to the field of HIV infection, such as 'Who will look after me if my mother is also ill?' or 'Will I get sick in the same way as my mother?'

Deciding how much information to give is difficult. Providing new information is an irreversible process and parents are often understandably cautious about disclosing the diagnosis, particularly if the child is in a terminal condition. HIV is not an easy illness to explain. Disclosing the diagnosis to children usually means that parents are bringing children into the secret, not that they are exploding the secret. To do this would therefore be giving the child information and then saying that it must not be discussed this with anyone else. It is hard to see the benefits of this disclosure at such a late stage in the child's life but at the same time continued secrecy may foster the continued 'mutual pretence' that develops as a way of parent and child shielding each other from emotional pain (Bluebond-Langer, 1978). There is no rule of thumb that provides a solution to this dilemma; each family and each child is different and the cues of how to proceed and how far to go should be taken from them.

Talking about death

The realities of death carry so many personal emotions that it may be difficult for some people to dissociate these and work objectively with the dying child. It is important, before any discussion of death with a terminally ill child, that the cultural and familial beliefs on death and dying are understood. A child's personal beliefs will be influenced by these and his experiences both present and past. Professionals must take care not to impose their own attitudes which may conflict with those of the family. A difference in belief should not, however, preclude any discussions with the child on death in general or his own death in particular. As with other issues, books, drawings and stories can all be employed, according to the maturity of the child, to help explore feelings around death and dying as well as related areas such as change, fear and memories. Frankness about real life events, such as the death of a child on the ward, may also be encouraging for the child.

Care should be taken not to patronise or underestimate a child's ability to cope. Whilst children can feel afraid and sad when considering their own death there can also be great courage and maturity of attitude. It is not unusual for parents to report that it is the way their child has coped that has been their own greatest source of strength.

In acknowledging their imminent death, children are freed to explore and appraise their life. Completing a scrap book or facilitating discussions and memories about their life, though often poignant, can be very therapeutic for children who are dying. In this way they can attribute meaning and value to their lives and reaffirm that they will always be loved and remembered.

To what extent children should be involved in the decision making about their own treatment and exercise control over how they die is a matter for the individual child and his family. Children who know they are dying may want to state a preference for where and how they die. They may also benefit, as adults do, from being able to prepare for this event by making some final wishes along the lines of a will which may bequeath personal things to special people. This may be as important for the bereaved person as for the child who is dying.

Talking about HIV and AIDS

HIV is usually a very closely guarded secret and the fears around disclosure frequently mean that children are unaware of their diagnosis. If disclosure of HIV infection has been made, it does not mean that the process of understanding and coping with this knowledge is necessarily complete. Children may still have many questions, and they deserve answers, not only with respect to their own illness but that of other family members as well. Many myths surround people's understanding of HIV and AIDS and much fear is often based upon inaccuracies. Health care workers should therefore be cognisant with the facts and realities of HIV infection. A child's fears that he may have already, or might still, transmit the virus to others, concern about a parent or parents who might also be infected, and concern for siblings who will be left behind are common and will require repeated reassurance.

The secrecy surrounding the diagnosis may contribute to feelings of shame or worthlessness which can overwhelm the child who is dying. The ease with which others who know the diagnosis relate to the child and discuss issues of HIV infection can greatly influence the child's acceptance of himself.

It is possible that children dying from AIDS have also experienced the death of parents or siblings from the same disease. Parents may be ill or dying at the same time as their children. The practical and emotional effects of this increase fear and anxiety. Ill parents, for example, may not be able to visit their children in hospital or provide the care they had wished or planned for. Great sensitivity is required to help the child understand his parents' absence and perceived unreliability. If HIV has been discussed openly in the family, it may still have been kept secret from the outside world. Not everyone, even close family members, who visits the child, in hospital or at home, may know the diagnosis and the continued need for confidentiality is vital.

Who should talk with the child?

Anyone who is involved with a terminally ill child may be drawn into communicating with him about illness and perhaps death. Often, when the child is in hospital where there are other people around, the child will choose the person or people he feels he can most comfortably talk to. Specialists trained in helping children discuss their feelings may not necessarily be the best people if only because such conversations are not always easy to time. Sometimes the greatest worries emerge through play, or after a chance remark or in the quiet moments before sleep. The person who is most frequently available when the child needs to talk and who can be trusted to listen and give honest responses is probably the person most likely to be taken into the child's confidence. In this case the role of the specialist should be to support and provide back-up for that person. Likewise, where the child is being cared for at home, support for the care-givers is vital. There will, however, be some children and some situations that require more intensive specialist help. It is important that signs of distress and poor coping are recognised early and appropriate referral is made.

Ideally, though not always appropriate, the child's family should be involved as much as possible in all aspects of a child's treatment, and this includes discussions about death and dying. Clearly, there are times when a child may wish to speak confidentially to someone, but generally parents and health care workers should communicate with each other to ensure consistency. It is unwise to give 'new' information to a child without the parents' prior knowledge and consent. Indeed, it usually more desirable for such information to be given by the parents or in the parents' presence.

For the child with HIV infection and his family there may be much professional, social and volunteer help. Sometimes there may be, as in Joe's case, an assigned foster mother to 'parent' the child if the mother is unwell or otherwise unable to do so herself. The risk here is that with so many people involved, a child may easily be given conflicting messages. An identified person who can monitor and liaise with all those who are involved is essential. Such a person can also ensure that parents, even if unwell, can be kept informed and that their wishes are respected.

Special considerations

There are some children for whom talking may not be easy or may be impossible. Many children with HIV infection are babies; for others the working language may not be their first language. Every attempt should be made to find someone who can communicate in their language and to find working material in that language. However, it is important to remember that even though the words may not be meaningful, the tone of the voice and the touch of the hand can be.

Another special group of children are those who have developed neurological deficits which may inhibit their expressive and/or receptive speech abilities. Again, the importance of non-verbal communication and reassuring physical contact must not be underestimated. The continued need of these children to be allowed to express their feelings and be understood, despite their neurological condition, should not be ignored.

Finally, there are the children whose parents will not agree to any discussion of dying. Like Joe, they are to be told nothing. This can often give rise to great unspoken conflicts between staff and family and feelings of rage that the child's best interests are not being met. There is little the professional can do in this situation but work with the parents or caregivers around the child's needs and to work obliquely with the child about his feelings. This is highlighted by Goldman & Christie (1993) who comment that 'although the child's welfare is usually the first priority, this may be balanced by the needs of the family, who will live on and must maintain its integrity and ability to function. For some families this is only possible if their defences are intact.' For Joe, his mother in time accepted the need to talk to him about being ill though not about death. He died, calmly, having been able to talk just a little but perhaps just enough.

Conclusion

For the professional working with HIV-infected children it is important to remember that children are not isolated individuals but that they live within a social, influential environment, usually dominated by the adults who care for them. At its most fundamental level this is the family system, although this may be represented in different ways for different children. For children who are terminally ill, hospital wards and health care workers may represent another significant faction. Before discussing illness or death with a child it is imperative, therefore, to understand first the context and the culture in which the child lives. Most of these children, for example, have acquired their infection perinatally, so within the family there is a mother, perhaps others, who are also infected, who may be ill, or who may have already died. It is equally common also for no one, apart from the parents and immediate health care workers, to know of the diagnosis.

Another point of general consideration is that whilst children have a right to know about their illness they also have a right not to talk about it if this is their way of coping. The terminally ill child, whether hospitalised or being treated at home, has to endure so much that is beyond his control that he may choose to exercise his independence through silence.

If and when a child chooses to talk, what is discussed will depend on the child's needs, age and level of maturity, previous experiences of illness and death, and parental and cultural beliefs. How this is communicated will again vary according to the individual child. Some terminally ill children exhibit a wisdom and maturity about their condition which seems beyond their years. Others seem to grapple and struggle with events in silence. Adults need to respond appropriately to restore confidence and trust, always remembering that the child who is dying is also still living.

References and further reading

Anthony, E. & Koupernick, C. (1973). *The Child in his Family: The Impact of Disease and Death*. New York: Wiley.

Baum, J. D. (ed.) (1990). *Listen. My Child has a Lot of Living to Do: Caring for Children with Life threatening Conditions*. Oxford: Oxford University Press.

Bluebond-Langer, M. (1978). *The Private Worlds of Dying Children*. New Jersey: Princeton University Press.

Burton, L. (1974). *Care of the Child Facing Death*. London: Routledge & Kegan Paul.

Goldman, A. & Christie, D. (1993). Children with cancer talk about their own death with their families. *Paediatric Hematology and Oncology*, **10**, 223–31.

Gyulay, J. (1978). *The Dying Child*. New York: McGraw-Hill.

Judd, D. (1989). *Give Sorrow Words: Working with a Dying Child*. London: Free Association Books.

Kane, B. (1979). Children's concepts of death. *The Journal of Genetic Psychology*, **134**, 141–53.

Lansdown, R. (1987). The development of the concept of death and its relationship to communicating with dying children. In *Current Issues in Clinical Psychology*, ed. E. Karas. New York: Plenum Press.

Lansdown, R. & Benjamin, G. (1985). The development of the concept of death in children aged 5–9 years. *Child: Care, Health and Development*, **11**, 13–20.

Spinetta, J. (1982). Behavioural and psychological research in childhood cancer: an overview. *Cancer*, **50**, 1039–43.

Some suggested books for use with dying children and children who want to know more about HIV and AIDS

Aliki (1987). *Feelings*. London: Pan.

Baker, L. (1991). *You and HIV: One Day at a Time*. Philadelphia: Saunders.

Bryant-Mole, K. (1994). *We're Talking About AIDS*. Hove, UK: Wayland Press.

Good Grief 1 (1988). *Talking about Loss and Death*. London: Good Grief.

Good Grief 2 (1989). *Exploring Feelings of Loss and Death*. London: Good Grief.

Grollman, E. (1990). *Talking about Death: A Dialogue Between Parent and Child*. Boston, Mass.: Beacon Press.

Heegaard, M. (1991). *When Someone Special has a Very Serious Illness*. Minneapolis, Minn.: Woodland Press.

Heegaard, M. (1991). *When Someone Very Special Dies*. Minneapolis, Minn.: Woodland Press.

Jordan, M. K. (1989). *Losing Uncle Tim*. Illinois: Albert Whitman & Company.

Mathias, B. & Spiers, D. (1992). *A Handbook on Death and Bereavement: Helping Children Understand*. National Library for the Handicapped Child, UK. (This is a reference list, with short summaries, of 113 books.)

Mellonie, B. & Ingpen, R. (1983). *Beginnings and Endings with Life Times in Between*. Paper Tiger.

Merrifield, M. (1990). *Come Sit By Me*. Toronto: Toronto Women's Press.

Sanders, P. (1990). *Let's Talk about Death and Dying*. London Aladdin.

Sanders, P. & Farquhar C. (1990). *Let's Talk about AIDS*. London: Aladdin.

Tasker, M. (1992). *How Can I Tell You?* Bethesda, Md.: Association for the Care of Childrens' Health.

Varley, S. (1984). *Badger's Parting Gifts*. London: Picture Lions.

18

The bereaved child

PETA HEMMINGS

Introduction

Childhood bereavement presents a threat to normal development but the threat does not necessarily lie in the experience of death. The significant factor that determines whether this experience is a challenge or a trauma is the quality of care afforded the child in the months and years that follow the loss (Furman, 1974; Sandler, 1980; Raphael, 1984; Cassidy, 1988; Silverman & Worden, 1992). It is argued that we need to be guided by the child's experience of his* bereavement and allow him a greater part in the family's shared experience of mourning.

Some of the common assumptions made about the appropriateness of involving children, the development of the concept of death, the issues surrounding explanations and the ways in which children mourn differently from adults will be discussed. The ways in which children respond to loss of this nature and how adults can help create a secure and supportive environment for them will be explored.

Although reference will be made to the bereaved child this does not do justice to each child's unique experience and is used with that understanding in mind.

Children, death and mourning

It is a paradox that loving parents often present problems for young bereaved children. Parents have two main roles: one is to nurture and care for the emotional and physical needs of their children and the other is to protect them from physical and emotional hurt and harm. A good parent will anticipate danger and protect a child from hurt or will comfort the upset child with reassuring words. These everyday situations are within the power of parents to manage and help resolve for their child.

* Throughout this chapter the use of the male pronoun implies the female also.

The emotional pain that is an intrinsic part of death and bereavement can not be assuaged in this way. When parents are bereaved and experience the intense and often overwhelming distress such loss generates it is understandable if their first response is to want to protect their child from that same hurt. It is only natural and, in other circumstances, the measure of a loving parent. However, when a parent or sibling dies, this protective behaviour is inappropriate and will come between the child and his ability to resolve his own loss.

It is neither desirable nor reasonable to expect a child who has experienced the protracted illness of a family member and then their death to be unaffected by this experience. It is unrealistic to think that avoidance of the topic will lessen the child's painful memories or his need to express his feelings, yet this 'protective' approach is not uncommon in the most caring families. Parents will often suppress their grief until the children are out of the house or in bed and then give vent to their feelings in the belief that they are sparing the children. What they are actually doing is silencing them. The implicit message is that it is not all right to cry or to express or share sadness and despair. Children quickly become isolated in their sadness and worried about the meaning of those feelings which are not allowed to be expressed within their family.

Michelle

Michelle was 9 when her mother, Jill, died. She and her father had cared for Jill at home throughout her long illness. Michelle had watched her mother slowly and painfully deteriorate. She knew she would die although nobody told her or talked to her about what that would mean. She just went on, day by day, helping around the house and doing little things for Jill as and when she needed them. She was an only child and very close to both her parents.

When Jill eventually died both Michelle and her father were stunned. They managed all the funeral arrangements in a state of suspended animation. When all the family and friends had gone and their lives had settled into some sort of routine, the meaning of the loss hit them hard. They began to realise that their days which had formerly been so full of caring for Jill and managing the home, were empty now. There was only the two of them left and their despair hung about them like a dark cloud.

Michelle's father felt fiercely protective of his little girl and vowed that he would make every effort to ensure that nothing would ever hurt her again. Although he felt absolutely distraught at the loss of his wife, he held on tightly to his feelings during the day. Only when he thought Michelle was asleep in bed would he allow himself to think about and cry for Jill. He smothered the sound of his sobbing in a cushion so that Michelle would not hear him and be upset. Unknown to him, Michelle was doing exactly the same in her bed, saving her sadness until she was safely private and able to cry into her pillow. She felt that because so many people had told her it was a blessed relief to her mother to be free of the pain which had been part of her illness, she should be pleased for her and that her sadness and tears were wrong in some way, especially as she thought her father was not feeling as she did.

This state of affairs persisted for many weeks until Michelle's teacher noticed that she was becoming increasingly withdrawn and suggested that she might benefit from some professional help. The situation was resolved by arranging a visit to Jill's grave where it was easier for Michelle and her father to share their sadness and talk about Jill and how important and loved she was. Once this door had been opened between them, they were able to continue supporting each other through their shared grief.

As well as being excluded through 'protection', children are frequently considered to be intellectually too immature to be able to appreciate the significance of events around them. All too often a 4-year-old will be assumed to be too young to understand what death means, or a 2-year-old thought too young to appreciate that daddy is not around any longer, and yet this is clearly not so. The 'immaturity' argument is more a reflection of the concern adults feel about the effects of experiencing the child's pain than a cogent and convincing argument for non-involvement of children. It becomes a collusive game played above the heads of children in which one adult may ask of the parent 'How are the children?', to which the parent will answer that they are fine and just as they have always been.

That adults are able to do this with a degree of sincerity is a reflection of the way in which children respond to bereavement, as well as a tendency in adults to apply the adult model of mourning to children. When they see a child who is able to play with their friends, go to school and do all the things they have always done, it is assumed that the child is untouched by the loss, but this is a false assumption based upon an inappropriate premise. The premise applied here has two elements. The first proposes that the child is too young to understand death and therefore unable to appreciate the personal implications of the event. The second is that the child's apparent lack of emotional response indicates that he is not affected by the loss and, therefore, does not have the need to mourn in the way that adults do. Both these need closer examination as they constitute a dangerously dismissive attitude and come between children and the help and support they need.

Development of the concept of death

The child's cognitive capacity to appreciate what death is underpins our appreciation of his potential in this situation. Children discover death quite naturally during their development through play and observation.

Table 18.1. *Factors that constitute a mature concept of death*

1.	Realisation	An awareness of death as an event which happens and results in the living dying
2.	Separation	A knowledge that death involves being physically apart from the dead person, that they are located elsewhere
3.	Immobility	An appreciation that the dead person can no longer move or initiate any activity
4.	Irrevocability	An acceptance of the degree of permanence and irreversibility connected with the status of death
5.	Causality	The beliefs about what brought about the death, especially the child's part in that
6.	Sensitivity	An awareness that the dead person has no sensory or mental function
7.	Dysfunctionality	The beliefs about the inability of the dead person to have any bodily functions
8.	Appearance	An acceptance that the dead person looks different from living people
9.	Universality	The ability to accept death as everyone's eventual fate

Their intrinsic interest in the subject is reflected in their fascination with fairy stories, nursery rhymes and games that focus on death. Research findings have demonstrated that children start to acquire an understanding of death at around 3 or 4 years of age (Anthony, 1940; Huang & Lee, 1945; Lansdown, 1991; Lansdown & Benjamin 1985: Nagy 1948). Subsequently, understanding is a protracted process which normally reaches maturity when the child is 9 or 10 years old. It is not a smoothly linear progression but one of progress and consolidation. Nagy's seminal Budapest study (1948) examined the maturation process among a group of 3- to 10-year-olds and concluded that the concept developed in three distinct phases culminating in a mature awareness at around 9 years. Her research findings have inspired many other studies which have extended and refined understanding in this area.

The concept of death is multi-faceted and there are nine main components which constitute a mature concept (see Table 18.1). Although most 10-year-olds will have grasped the implications of death, it should not be assumed that all children of this age have done so, or that only children of this age have the ability to do so. Indeed, further studies have demonstrated that, in certain circumstances, children as young as 4 years old can fully understand the implications of death (Bluebond-Langer, 1978; Kane, 1979; Lansdown, 1991).

The data from these studies help to dispel the myth that young children are protected from the impact of bereavement by their cognitive immaturity. In fact they demonstrate quite the reverse: that children who have experienced bereavement as the outcome of protracted illness acquire a precocious maturity in this respect (Lampl-de Groot, 1976; Koocher, 1986). First, they will have had relevant experiences which accelerate their awareness of this aspect of life and second, given the right quality of explanation, they are able to accept the information readily because it serves to reduce anxiety by helping make sense of a difficult and stressful situation. The child's ability to understand highlights the need for explanations to be carefully considered.

Explaining death to children

It is a measure of society's unease about the subject of death that there is a wealth of clichés and euphemisms about death. There are a host of acceptable phrases and established imagery that provide a comforting buffer against the harsh reality of that taboo word. Adults use them in conversation to reduce the stress of the subject matter, but when they are used in conversation with children they have a very different effect. It is worth considering some of the more popular ready-made phrases and images commonly used and explore their possible meanings for children.

(1) *'Grandma has fallen asleep; it's a special kind of sleep and she won't ever wake up again.'* The child develops fears that he too might not wake up the next time he goes to sleep and develops fears associated with bed, night-time and sleep.

(2) *'Daddy has gone on a long journey to be with God and he won't be coming back.'* There are two possible reactions to this statement. One is that almost all the separations the child has previously experienced, that resulted from a long journey, ended in reunion. It would be reasonable to hope for a reunion in this instance too, in spite of being told that it is not possible. The second reaction is that the child may well become afraid that anyone who goes on a long journey may not return.

(3) *'Mummy has gone to heaven to be with Jesus.'* Often this sort of religious explanation is given to children who have no established family belief system and yet suddenly are expected to develop a whole new way of thinking in order to incorporate this event. Young children think very concretely and if this explanation is given without any real exploration of what the child believes about heaven, it can lead to all sorts of problems.

Jenny

Jenny was 5 when her father died. She was told that he had gone to heaven and that heaven was somewhere way above the clouds in the sky. A few months later the family decided to go on holiday to Italy. Jenny was very excited and could hardly wait to get on the plane. She insisted on having a window seat and sat glued to the window from the moment she got on.

The plane took off and gained height quickly. Jenny got more and more excited and held her teddy to the window. After they had been flying for about 20 minutes she started to cry, saying that she couldn't see Daddy even though there weren't any clouds. Her mother was puzzled for a while and then realised that her little girl had thought they were high enough in the plane to see heaven and that her daddy would surely know that she would want to see him.

Jenny's mother then had to explain properly about the meaning of death. The whole holiday was ruined for all of them because Jenny was understandably furious with her mother for her lack of honesty, bitterly disappointed at not seeing her father and deeply saddened by the realisation that she would never see him again.

(4) *'Jesus needed another angel in heaven and that is why he took your baby brother because he was so good.'* This is a lovely image that comforts grief-stricken parents, but what does it say to the child who is left behind? Does it mean that they are not good enough to be an angel? Does it mean that if they don't want to become an angel and lose mum and dad they ought to be naughtier in the future? Either interpretation leads to difficulties.

(5) *'I was sorry to hear about the loss of your husband.'* The child who hears death referred to as 'loss' will naturally think that his mother has been remarkably careless to lose such an important person as his father. It is logical for the child to ensure that they too are not lost and the only way they can reliably do this is to shadow their mother. This explanation feeds existing anxieties the child will inevitably have about other separations and losses, real or feared.

These are just some of the commoner explanations given to children to protect adults from having to explain honestly the meaning of death and their possible uncertainty about what happens to us after death.

If children are given the opportunity to explore their thinking around this subject they will often come up with some perfect images. Many children will choose those associated with light (e.g. stars, candles), some may prefer those associated with the natural world (e.g. the wind, sea, countryside). Through their efforts to construct personal pictures the child is helped to embark upon the process of mourning. They need guidance and support and not to have their thinking clouded by adults' need for self-protection. It is only when children know what death really means that they can start the work of mourning; therefore, all good explanations of death will use age-appropriate language for each child and incorporate the salient points contained within the mature concept of death (Grollman, 1964; Raphael, 1984).

Peter (7 years)

'When I think of my Daddy I see him on a rainbow. He climbs up one side of it and when he is on the top he waves to me. Then he sits down and slides down the other side, just like when we used to go to the park. I know he is happy.'

Susan (9 years)

'Grandpa is in a special place and he is a beautiful silver trout swimming in a pond. There is sunlight on the water, sparkling like diamonds, and he will be beautiful for ever.' (Her grandfather was a keen angler.)

Both these sets of images gave these children comfort and enabled them to think of the dead person realistically in terms of their new status and construct personally meaningful pictures of them now.

Patterns of mourning

The second premise is that children do not mourn. This is a common assumption based on the difference between children's and adults' responses to bereavement.

Adult grief is often described as an all-embracing state, a dull cloud of sadness and despair that surrounds the mourner every moment of the day. Inside there is a leaden weight of sadness and an empty feeling. Life has nothing to offer. It is impossible to concentrate for any length of time and all thoughts return to the one theme. Gradually the cloud develops patches of light and the weight becomes less heavy. This process may take several years and involves a lot of strenuous emotional and intellectual work. For children the experience of grief is very different and this causes many problems.

A bereaved child does not look like a bereaved adult and does not look different from any other child. He may not behave differently from any other child for a large part of the day. The difference lies in the internal state. These are children who have knowledge of the world beyond their years, knowledge which can not be shared with their peers, for which other 5-year-old would understand the profound longing they feel to be held once more by their mother, or to hear their father come through the front door at the end of his working day?

The bereaved child will seem to be as he has always been, but there will be times when he experiences deep pockets of sadness and these times are not within his control. He may be playing with friends when a memory of past times comes upon him and he is immersed in intense memories and the emotions associated with them. Children have described this experience in terms of it being like a film which suddenly starts to roll. They are powerless to turn it off. Sometimes the film makes them feel good and the memories are comforting, sometimes they are painful; whichever is the case, the child is totally committed to watching. Returning to the real world at the end is always difficult as the child is out of step with what is going on around them.

The other salient feature of childhood mourning is that it is not an experience contained within a matter of a few years. The child's ability to mourn is limited by his developmental ability, therefore it is an issue which will re-emerge at each new developmental phase. The bereaved child will always be aware of that aspect of himself to a lesser or greater extent, so his mourning is a life-long commitment to resolving the loss.

To use the adult model as a template for all mourning is to do the child a disservice as it diminishes his experience and dismisses his need for support. The intermittent nature and developmental features of childhood grief are the essential descriptive elements.

The bereaved child

It is perhaps helpful to highlight some of the commoner problems experienced by the bereaved child. The frequency with which these problems occur indicate the need for them to be included in any assessment of the child. The onset of each of these problems is associated with certain age ranges but, once a feature of childhood bereavement at a particular age, they are found in subsequent ages and in adult mourning. Three of the more common ones are searching behaviour, causal thinking and magical thinking.

Searching behaviour: 9 months onwards

During the last quarter of the first year the infant develops an awareness that when people disappear from sight they can be recalled. The baby achieves this very effectively through crying. When the parent returns and comforts the infant the crying stops. If the parent does not return the infant continues to cry, searching for the parent until, worn out and dejected, he becomes withdrawn and depressed by the inexplicable and intolerable absence. Repeated experiences of stressful separations create a sensitivity in the child to all situations which threaten their security and the child experiences both anticipatory and reactive separation anxiety.

The experience of protracted illness means that the child is primed for separation anxiety often long before the separation through death.

The parallels between this early experience and bereavement responses are clear. The bereaved person calls out for the dead person, imploring him to return and searches for him in other ways. The infant is not ambulant but older children will actively search for the dead person, looking in the rooms of the home, in places where he used to go regularly and in less expected places such as cupboards, drawers and behind furniture. It is a necessary process of confirmation that the separation is real and absolute.

James

James was 14 months old when his father died. James' mother, Mary, thought he was too young to appreciate the significance of the death and felt sure he was completely unaffected. Her husband had been ill and away from the family for most of the previous year, so she thought James would hardly notice his father's permanent absence. She was convinced of this in spite of James' need to go back to using a feeding-bottle and his reluctance to let her out of his sight, two changes in his behaviour which indicated an increased anxiety level.

One day James got up from where he was playing quietly on the floor, walked across the room and picked up the telephone. He then proceeded to dial some random numbers. Mary remarked that he did this several times a day. He lifted the handset to his ear and listened intently for a short while, then he said plaintively, 'Daddy. Daddy gone. Daddy where you?', and looked into the handset searching for some sight of his father inside it.

Mary had three other children, much older than James, all of whom were able to express themselves through words which could be more easily heard than James' expression of bewilderment and anxiety, and yet he was communicating exactly the same feelings as his older brothers and sister. When Mary considered other changes in his behaviour she was able to see that he too was mourning his father. She had taken comfort in the well-intentioned advice from family and friends who reassured her that James was too young to know and she thought he would be spared the pain the rest of the family were experiencing. By Mary adopting this attitude James was actually experiencing more distress because he was not being given the extra help he needed at that time.

Causal thinking: 3 years and onwards

The 2-year-old child starts to acquire several skills as part of normal development, such as feeding, washing and dressing, with varying degrees of success. He becomes more adept socially and manages separations from his mother at playgroup, nursery or friends' houses. As he becomes increasingly competent in these areas he develops a greater sense of self and power. This developmental phase is accompanied by a cognitive shift. It is during this time that the child starts to think in a linear fashion. The child observes the world and draws conclusions about the causes of events witnessed. In this way the child learns about expected outcomes and how to anticipate them. This is an essential part of learning development but it can lead to some bizarre conclusions being drawn in relation to death.

Gemma

Gemma was 4 when her baby sister, Alana, was born. Alana was a beautiful, healthy baby and Gemma proudly paraded her in the pram. Gemma was allowed to give Alana her first bottle of the day and would arrive in her parents' bedroom as soon as she heard her first cries, and sometimes even before the baby had a chance to cry. She would pick her carefully from the cot and cradle her, ready for her mother to give her the warmed bottle.

One morning she came into the bedroom, leant over the cot and went to pick Alana up when she realised something was very wrong. Alana looked different, she felt cold, she was not moving. Gemma stepped back from the cot and called for her mother. When her mother saw Alana she screamed, pushed Gemma to one side and yelled, 'My God! What has happened to the baby?' Pandemonium followed: the parents desperately tried to resuscitate the baby, the ambulance arrived and she was rushed to hospital. Gemma watched everything from the end of the bed where she was sitting.

Several weeks later, after the post-mortem and the funeral, Gemma hazarded the question about how it had happened. Her mother said that nobody knew, but Gemma thought she knew. She had been the last person to touch Alana, therefore it was obviously her fault. She thought she had some very bad naughtiness inside her which had somehow come out of her fingers when she went to pick Alana up and this had caused her to die. She dared not voice this but went on, over the following weeks and months to punish herself in a variety of ways.

After months of self-injury and increasing depression she was referred for therapeutic help. By this time she was a withdrawn, fearful child who was convinced of her responsibility for the death. Her conviction had become entrenched because nobody had taken the time to make sure she understood how the death had occurred.

Magical thinking: 5 years onwards

Magical thinking is a strong feature for children who are five or six years old. The term is descriptive of a cognitive process which is influenced by the emotional content those thoughts arouse. The emotions are so strong that they diminish the rational element and transform it beyond the realms of logic. Adults can recognise this way of thinking in themselves and superimpose higher logic in order to keep the fanciful thoughts within a more realistic framework. Children do not usually have the level of insight and can not control the influence of their magical thinking in the same way. Consequently, it becomes a dominant feature of their attempts to rationalise the irrational.

A child who tries, unassisted, to understand the meaning of events surrounding death and his part in them, will inevitably fall into the traps within magical thinking. The effects of this can be devastating as the resulting logic invariably has negative implications for the child.

Lucy

Lucy (9 years) and her father Jim were very close. They were both interested in music, wildlife and painting. During the 4 years of Jim's illness Lucy would happily spend time with him, whether he was at home or in the hospital. All her questions about his condition were answered honestly and she was kept informed of any changes as and when it was appropriate. When he was in bed but well enough, they would draw and paint together or she would lie next to him and he would play his guitar as they sang their favourite songs. She was with him a few hours before he died, saw him afterwards and went to the funeral. She had been willingly and appropriately involved throughout his illness and death.

Eight months later Lucy was a profoundly worried little girl. She was sure she had been responsible for Jim's death because she had not been a good enough daughter. During the later months of Jim's illness she had been told in school assembly by her head teacher, so it must be true, that if we pray hard enough miracles can happen. She only wanted a small miracle, for her father to get better.

She had searched in her prayer book for the right prayer and had made up several of her own. She prayed hard but, not only did he not get better, he died. She felt sure that there was some connection between the two. If she had searched harder and found the right prayer, the right magic formula, then she could have saved him. All the hard facts about the illness which she knew, all the experiences she had leading up to Jim's death counted for nothing as she reviewed the process and 'rationalised' it anew.

Magical thinking reflects the importance adults place upon the significance of the love felt for someone who dies. When someone who is ill recovers this is thought to be partly due to the effects of the medication and partly to the love given him. If someone dies then it is natural for adults to scrutinise their part in the process and examine the adequacy of their contribution.

Lucy had done just that. She concluded that the only reasonable explanation for this unreasonable experience was that her love for her father was lacking in some respect. All bereaved people experience some loss of self-esteem and torment themselves with the ways in which they could have been a better person in their relationship with the dead person or taken better care of them in some way. Children are no exception. Regardless of their experience of illness and death, this aspect of their understanding of the meaning of events needs to be checked rigorously to avoid misconceptions such as Lucy's.

Counselling bereaved children

Children living with serious illness are bereaved long before the actual death. Their loss of normal routines and hopes for a shared future constitute a bereavement. This is ideal time for intervention as it allows time for prevention. Post-death counselling has a different purpose; it aims to help each family member reconsider their experience and learn to live with the multitude of losses that one death contains. There is no template of perfect practice because of the uniqueness of each person's experience, but there are some useful guidelines for children.

Creating the secure mourning environment

For healthy development children need two primary conditions to prevail in their environment: security and love. Security refers to an ability to assume that people and situations can be relied upon to remain the same or change only gradually. Bereavement undermines security, shaking faith in this assumed world. It is understandable that the bereaved child may fear for his personal safety when a loved one can be snatched away by death. The child's realisation of this possibility poses a profound threat to his development, forcing him to concentrate his energy upon ensuring he is secure. His exploration of the world is inhibited and, consequently, there is less opportunity for him to acquire skills and insights through new experience (Matas *et al.*, 1978; Arend *et al.*, 1979; Hazen & Durrett, 1982; Belsky *et al.*, 1984).

The second condition essential for a child's healthy development is the need to know he is loved. At times of great stress children need extra affection, but on their terms. The bereaved parent may be so immersed in his own grief that he is less sensitive to his child and may be unaware of his increased need. This reduced sensitivity is often felt acutely by the child and the parent is perceived as emotionally and physically inaccessible and unavailable. Children bereaved of one parent often feel that they are effectively orphaned, losing one parent to death and the other to grief. Although this situation is tolerable for a short while, any prolonged experience of this quality of care places the child at considerable risk of developmental disturbance (Bowlby, 1969; Tracy & Ainsworth, 1981; Radke-Yarrow *et al.*, 1985; Pederson *et al.*, 1990).

The effect of bereavement upon these two critical factors indicates the need for the child to have predictability in his daily routine, to counteract the former, and extra demonstrations of his lovableness to meet the change in the latter. Predictability of routine can mean as little as the ability to expect that his parent will provide a meal, clean clothes and regular bedtimes, just basic boundaries to daily life. The provision of physical care inspires confidence in the child that the parent is competent and this quells the common fears that children have about their physical well-being.

Demonstrations of affection are not as simple. Each parent–child relationship develops its own ways of expressing affection so there are no universally applicable means of achieving this. However, most children like to sit close and have a cuddle with their parent while watching television or having a story. Many children like to share activities with their parents such as baking, playing games, jigsaws, walks or non-grocery shopping, and there is an implicit intimacy in these activities. Affection can be shown in a number of ways, according to personal preference, but it needs to be shown. The child needs to recognise that the parent's deep sadness does not mean that he is less lovable.

In the presence of these two factors the child will be able to explore his own grief and learn to express himself as part of the family's shared conversation about their loss. Ideally he will be supported in his struggle to resolve the emotional pain in that intimate milieu. If that is not possible, either because the parent is too overwhelmed by his own grief, or because the child is unable to share with them for whatever reasons, then professional counselling is advised. It is not necessary for most children to be referred for psychiatric help; their grief is not usually a mental illness but a manifestation of their intense sadness, bewilderment, anger at abandonment and reasonable fears for the safety of their remaining family.

More than anything else the bereaved child needs to have someone he can trust, someone who will listen to and treat with respect his expressed emotions and thoughts. As well as trust and respect he needs privacy, confidentiality and secure boundaries. The child needs to know that he is safe with the counsellor, physically and emotionally. Only when the child knows the counsellor is trustworthy and strong will he feel able to explore his feelings and thoughts and express the pain they generate, safe in the knowledge that this person will believe him and help him try to find some resolution of his distress.

The substance of the therapeutic work with bereaved children will vary for each child, but there are recurring themes within the work. Much has been written on the subject and there is a wealth of children's literature which focuses on death and bereavement. As awareness of the importance of this area of work has increased so specific play techniques and materials have been developed to assist in this work, as has groupwork with such children (Quarmby, 1990; Hemmings, 1991; Pennells & Smith, 1992).

Although there are many practical tools available nothing is more important to the child than the offer of a chance to share his experience with someone he knows he can trust, someone who will listen to what he has seen, heard, thought and felt, and help him to understand what it all means to him.

Conclusion

This chapter establishes the case for allowing the child to have his own experience of death and bereavement. The arguments for excluding the child on grounds of protection and/or immaturity have been shown to be fallacious and possibly reflective of adult needs for protection from the child's experience. It has also been argued that, given security and love, the child will be able to tolerate the vicissitudes of the parent's grief and pursue his developmental goals. Furthermore, given a person who is trustworthy and sensitive to his needs, the child will be able to explore his mourning and come to some resolution.

Resolution is not a matter of living untouched by the loss but of learning to adjust to the new order. The bereaved child will always be bereft of his parent or sibling – that is his status. Resolution is the ability the child has to be sensitive to the significance of that experience without that awareness overwhelming the joy of his childhood. The ability to be spontaneous, creative and to discover the world through experience is the true mark of healthy resolution and the aim of all therapeutic intervention.

References

Anthony, S. (1940). *The Discovery of Death in Childhood and After*. London: Penguin.

Arend, R., Gove, F. L. & Sroufe, L. A. (1979). Continuity of individual adaptation from infancy to kindergarten: a predictive study of ego-resiliency and curiosity in pre-schoolers. *Child Development*, **50**, 950–9.

Belsky, J., Garduque, L. & Hrncir, E. (1984). Assessing performance, competence and executive capacity in infant play: reactions to home environment and security of attachment. *Developmental Psychology*, **20**, 406–17.

Bluebond-Langer, M. (1978). *The Private Worlds of Dying Children*. New Jersey: Princeton University Press.

Bowlby, J. (1969). *Attachment and Loss*, vol. 1, *Attachment*. London: Penguin.

Cassidy, J. (1988). Child–mother attachments and the self in 6-year-olds. *Child Development*, **59**, 121–34.

Furman, E. (1974). *When a Child's Parent Dies*. New Haven: Yale University Press.

Furman, E. (1986). When is the death of a parent traumatic? *Psychoanalytic Study of the Child*, **41**, 191–208.

Grollman, E. (1964). *Explaining Death to Children*. Boston: Beacon Press.

Hazen, N. L. & Durrett, M. E. (1982). Relationship of security of attachment to exploration and cognitive mapping abilities in 2-year-olds. *Developmental Psychology*, **18**, 751–9.

Hemmings, P. (1991). Direct work techniques with bereaved children. *Journal of Child Psychology and Psychiatry*, Occasional Paper no. 7, 23–7.

Huang, I. & Lee, H. W. (1945). Experimental analysis of child animism. *Journal of Genetic Psychology*, **66**, 69–74.

Kane B. (1979). Children's concepts of death. *Journal of Genetic Psychology*, **134**, 141–53.

Koocher, G. (1986). Coping with death from cancer. *Journal of Consulting and Clinical Psychology*, **54**. 623–31.

Lampl-de Groot, J. (1976). Mourning in a 6-year-old girl. *Psychonalytic Study of the Child*, **31**, 273–81.

Lansdown, R. (1991). The child's concept of death. *Journal of Child Psychology and Psychiatry*, Occasional Paper no. 7, 2–6.

Lansdown, R. & Benjamin, G. (1985) The development of the concept of death in children aged 5–9 years. *Child Care, Health and Development*, **11**, 13–20.

Matas, L., Arend, R. & Sroufe, L. A. (1978). Continuity of adaptation in the second year: the relationship between quality of attachment and later competence. *Child Development*, **49**, 547–56.

Nagy, M. (1948). The child's theories concerning death. *Journal of Genetic Psychology*, **73**, 3–27.

Pederson, D. R., Moran, G., Sitko, C., Campbell, K., Ghesquire, K. & Acton, H. (1990). Maternal sensitivity and the security of the infant–mother attachment: a Q-sort study. *Child Development*, **6**, 1974–83.

Pennells, M. & Smith, S. (1992). Bereavement and adolescents: a groupwork approach. *Association of Child Psychology and Psychiatry Newsletter*, **14**, 173–8.

Quarmby, D. (1990). Coming to grief. *Times Educational Supplement*, 2 June.

Radke-Yarrow, M., Cummings, E. M., Kuczynski, L. & Chapman, M. (1985). Patterns of attachment in 2- and 3-year-olds in normal families and families with parental depression. *Child Development*, **56**, 884–93.

Raphael, B. (1984). *The Anatomy of Bereavement*. London: Unwin Hyman.

Sandler, I. N. (1980). Social support resources, stress and maladjustment of poor children. *American Journal of Community Psychology*, **8**, 41–52.

Silverman, P. & Worden, J. W., (1992). Children's reactions in the early months after the death of a parent. *American Journal of Orthopsychiatry*, **62**, 93–104.

Tracy, R. L. & Ainsworth, M. (1981). Maternal affectionate behaviour and infant–mother attachment patterns. *Child Development*, **52**, 1341–3.

19

Living with HIV

A PARENT

Introduction

Throughout our day to day routine HIV does not really affect us as a family. It is simply the name of a virus requiring nothing more than a few minor adjustments to our life and those so insignificant and familiar as to now be normal. And then, without warning, an apparently minor incident turns our lives upside down, has us holding our breath waiting for something to happen and discussing at length contingency plans for what might be.

This could perhaps be a description of living with the illness associated with HIV infection but it is not; I am referring to the social aspects of life with the virus.

Family life

My daughter Kate was infected with HIV at birth and has remained positive since. The effects of the virus have not touched her in any obvious sense yet; she is now a sturdy, healthy, cheerful 8-year-old, not in the least delicate or sickly, so I do not know what it is like to live with the illness, only the threat of it. But I do know very well what living with HIV today means to a family in other ways and I know how doing so has damaged my previous trust of 'professionals', and of agencies generally, although my respect for certain individuals within those agencies has grown.

Living with Kate is not a problem. She arrived at 22 months and any adjustment then was entirely due to the upheaval a small child causes in any family and not to the virus. Life is for us as it is for most other families. Kate does and has always done everything other children of her age do; she attends the local primary school, joined the Brownies, took dancing lessons. She has a wide group of friends who play at our house, stay for tea, sleep overnight and invite her to do the same. She fights with her brother, argues with her friends, behaves badly at times and like an angel at others. She swallows medicine three times a day with no more than a normal amount of resistance and her regular (though not frequent) visits to the hospital with their associated blood tests are treated in an offhand manner. If she falls and bleeds she returns home for sympathy and plasters, or reports the injury to her class teacher or the parent of a friend. For minor damage, 'do it yourself' first aid is the order of the day for Kate; we dampen the tissue or cotton wool and let her mop up the blood and apply the plaster. For more major events we use plastic gloves from one of the many sources around in the house, in the cars or in my bag. This is the same procedure we use whenever any adult or child bleeds. I believe most of the people faced with Kate bleeding do the same and I am also fairly certain they do not take these simple precautions routinely with anyone other than Kate. I do not know for sure and I try not to worry about it.

So life is normal and Kate is normal and we drift along in a complacent sort of way for most of the time as we have done for 6 years until something happens to force us to wake up to the reality of HIV and the fear it instills in others. Initially this was likely to be necessary contact with some agency; now it could be something Kate has said to someone who did not previously know of her HIV status and who is reacting with panic. Whatever the start of it we are quickly aware that our apparent acceptance and surface normality is just that: apparent and superficial. The process of education of the general public and its ensuing understanding is still far from complete and most contacts need information and reassurance at first. Acceptance of Kate and the rest of the family comes later. Sometimes it feels we are living in a particularly nasty track event where, just as the field seems clear, we start to congratulate ourselves on having survived and we can breath more easily, another series of obstacles appears from nowhere and we must start to negotiate them again. And sometimes we do not want to; argument is tiring, especially when it feels (as it does at times) that there is not likely to be an end to it.

Confidentiality and the right to know

When Kate arrived her HIV status was known only by a few people: our general practitioner, the social workers who had responsibility for her, our closest family and friends. Once we had lost our initial anxiety about her health we lived as any family does until eventually she was old enough for playgroup. Our village playgroup had not addressed the issue of HIV. I do not think many had at that time, and the staff were not using any sensible first aid procedures. After a great deal of anxious discussion we decided we had to be fair and advise them of the need to be more cautious. This was intended to be information for the benefit of the playleader, but it was soon public knowledge and the reactions from the villagers were very strong. The playgroup committee discussed the situation endlessly with a variety of professionals, experts and with the other parents. We were invited to some meetings though not to many others, and in time they accepted that there was no danger. Meanwhile Kate's entry into play-group was delayed and medical information about her was public. During that period we faced all the fear and prejudice surrounding this disease and we learned the pain of gossip, rejection and isolation. We had the added worry then of the effects of this on our son Iain, who was 11 at the time. Thankfully it seemed his friends did not equate the hostility with Iain's little sister, the child they had known for over a year. They carried on with nothing more than an occasional comment.

In time Kate joined the playgroup, familiarity relieved the anxiety and life became normal again. The village people became our supporters and advocates for Kate and we were grateful for their support. However, we knew then and I know now that it came because of the information they had been given; their expectation of their right to know had been satisfied so they were willing to work through their fears. I also know that even after a year with Kate among them, many would still expect that right to know; they would not accept Kate's or any other child's right to privacy. Nor would they accept they could or should provide the means to make 'needing to know' unnecessary.

Starting school

Later Kate went to nursery with some of the children from playgroup, a nursery in a nearby town run by the education authority. I was less anxi-ous here since the staff were professionals – colleagues of the same pro-fessional social workers, health board staff and educationalists who had advised us that Kate should have her privacy – and confidentiality was her right. They were also employed as childcare workers by the same local authority and would therefore be knowledgeable and safe. I was wrong to be less anxious. After a discussion with a senior education authority worker I decided I would inform the headteacher since it was his responsi-bility to ensure that first aid and hygiene standards in the school were adequate and in line with the authority standards, which were taken from the Education Department guidelines issued in 1987 on the subject of HIV in schools. So I went along to see him and I found that my contact, through whatever channel, had got there first. He already knew and I had been denied my right to control that information. This aspect is common throughout my experiences with Kate. Information which belongs to me, about Kate, is taken from me and controlled by others against all of the official lines. I wonder how I would have felt if I had changed my mind and decided I did not want him to know; if, after reconsidering, I had decided I would rather tell the class teacher; if I later decided to tell no one at all or even chose not to send Kate to nursery. None of that would have mattered because someone felt they had the right to manage confidential information in the way they chose without my consent. I was very angry that they dared to do this to us but there was little I could do. I could and I did complain but I could not take back the information, it was out of my control. I felt utterly powerless; I was denied the opportunity to look after my child's interests in the way I believed (and had been advised) was best for her.

Later came school – back in the village this time. I felt sure this would be straightforward since everyone in the village knew about Kate and she had already had a good year in an educational establishment. I was wrong and once again I had to accept that I did not know very much about what went on behind the scenes. It was purely by chance and by the sheer professionalism of a doctor that I even found out the school staff were holding meetings to discuss Kate and her entry into school. We were not told these were happening, much less invited to be present while our child was discussed; a child who was not at that time even enrolled at the school. I was angry at and frustrated by the system again.

In time, though, and with the support of our friends in the village, Kate went to school and spent a very successful and happy 2 years there. This time the field really looked flat and it was a comfortable time for us. Everyone accepted Kate, she could join in with whatever activities were going on and the school staff were exceptionally aware and caring. It would have been easy to sit back and enjoy life, but by then we were only too conscious that the situation we lived in was not mirrored throughout Britain, nor was it achieved in the right way. It had its price and that price was too high to expect most people to pay. We felt it was necessary to bring this issue to the top of the agenda for education authorities, for other childcare establishments or agencies and for the general public. We decided to speak out then, to describe our experiences and to call for changes in practice.

Shortly after this we became aware just how superficial our own comfort and acceptance were when a house move to another area became necessary. All the fear and concern returned with a new school, different families, no friends to support us and no real belief that there had been significant changes in practice or attitude. The decision to tell the headteacher this time was made partly in the belief that schools were still not using safe first aid measures, but also because I believed if I had not told the school someone else would. I cannot believe I would have been allowed to hold that information without someone, possibly from the education department again, exercising the right they claim to pass on such information. Anyway I preferred to do it myself so I spoke to the headteacher and I was relieved to find things had changed a little. At least this time no one questioned Kate's right to be in the school. Hurdle one was over, Kate went to school and she settled in well. The school staff inform me of any infectious diseases around and they supervise her lunchtime dose of medicine, so I am grateful.

Hurdle two came when two sets of parents arrived on my doorstep in a very anxious state because Kate had explained to their children why she had to visit the hospital. This, I have decided, is the inevitable result of refusing to allow my daughter to feel ashamed. She does not see the need for secrecy and that is her right. As her parent I do not feel I have the right to pass out information about her, however easy that makes it for everyone else, but she can if she chooses even at 8 years old. I was fortunate in my initial contact with those parents. They were prepared to listen and learn and in time they understood what I was saying, that there was no danger, and they accepted Kate. However, the information then spread about the village in a very haphazard way, unlike the original village where everyone learned about it in a few short days. I have heard the 'child with AIDS' discussed in the village shop by people who obviously do not know me, but I still do not know how wide the information has spread. Nor do I know who knows, so I operate on the basis that most do and if they do not it is not up to me to enlighten them. There has been sufficient media coverage of varying standards to ensure that every adult knows the risks and the way to protect themselves and their family. If they choose not to use that knowledge it is their decision.

This all sounds very controlled and considered and I suppose it is; it seems quite hard, but my attitude has grown through years of experience of the reactions of other people and from the need for self protection. Put bluntly, like this, it gives no indication of the pain and fear, the times when I have cried, when I have had to take a deep breath to walk into a shop with my head up, when I have flinched at an insensitive comment, when I have had to fight to overcome the urge to take Kate away somewhere safe so she will not be hurt by cruelty or thoughtlessness. It does not show the added stresses of moving house in these circumstances or the sleepless nights and anxious days as I wait to see if Kate has someone to play with after school.

Coping with illness

And this is just the social aspect. The medical side has been of a lesser priority for us so far. At the moment the knowledge that although Kate is well now she could become very ill soon just sits, underlying everything. It is not allowed to raise its head too much; it is as tightly controlled as the urge to ring the doctor with every cold or tummy pain. To give in to it would mean Kate's life would not be normal, she would be restricted by too much care. It is a balancing act between doing all we can to keep her well and yet allowing her the normal experiences of life. Some years ago I read an article which suggested people who were HIV infected could benefit from a macrobiotic diet because this had, in some circumstances, been shown to boost the immune system. It did not promise a cure but simply suggested a means to help the body fight for itself. Obviously I want to do all I can to help Kate stay well so I considered this at length, and with considerable pangs of conscience decided against it. My reasons for rejecting this diet were about Kate having a normal life. For my family a macrobiotic diet is not normal. It is time consuming, it would require a complete change for the entire family and it could well cause problems for outings, parties and school meals. I felt my time could be better spent playing and talking and living with the children rather than investing great chunks of it in the kitchen preparing food. I felt Kate would be better for that than with some extreme diet which again identified her as different. I do not know if I was right but it seemed the right decision for us as a family and for Kate, and I do not regret it now.

During all of this the hospital and its staff have been a major support in my life. I have heard other parents say they do not like the hospital visits because of the implications, the waiting for news, the anxiety surrounding any test results, etc. This has not been my experience. My contact with the hospital has been positive and comforting.

I found myself at the hospital almost by chance because I had discovered through my own research that doctors there were working with HIV-infected children. At that time I desperately needed to know if they or anyone could give me information, if they could offer a more optimistic prognosis than the ones I had been given elsewhere, and most of all if they could treat Kate. The paediatric clinic she attended until then had little experience of these children and seemed to me to be waiting for her to become ill; an approach I found difficult to accept. At each visit I reported on Kate's progress, she was weighed and measured and another appointment made. I was certainly not encouraged to ask questions, to discuss any information I had acquired or to expect advice. When I had to report some concerns about Kate they were duly noted and I was told it was only to be expected. I felt they were waiting for her to deteriorate physically, I had no confidence that there would be any intervention in an attempt to prevent this happening and I could not believe this was how it had to be, that we were all to sit back and wait. I was convinced the situation could not be that hopeless even if a cure was not available and I wanted her to have the very best treatment by doctors who had a particular interest in the subject and who were not giving up. I wanted to fight this disease for Kate. In my experience this need to believe your child is getting the best possible treatment is all-consuming and it concerns me that I only have that confidence because of my own efforts, my determination and the contacts I made. Also I was in a position financially to spend whole days on the telephone calling everyone I could and everywhere including America. Surely all families affected by HIV should have available the information I have, to be used as they choose?

The multidisciplinary team

The hospital ward and clinic are places I feel comfortable, supported, respected and accepted. When I am there I can ask questions and expect a straight answer, I can explain any worries without feeling foolish, I can moan without feeling a timewaster, I can lean without feeling inadequate and I am reassured after each visit. My need of the hospital is far more than just medical. It provides a social service for me too and without it I suspect I would be using a lot of other services for myself and Kate, including social workers, counsellors and perhaps psychotherapists. Maybe it is not right to use a hospital in this way but it is perfect for me and, I think, for Kate. We do not need several different agencies with a lot of different staff, all wanting information from us, all expecting an input to our life, all needing to refer to each other and maybe with conflicting views or opinions. We have the hospital; our centre point for all relevant agencies, our referral agency when necessary and a constant factor in the mass of medical, paramedical, social and educational threads of Kate's life. It seems important to me that all families have a similar contact point; someone who will provide all the hospital provides for us; who will work through the maze of services with the family and will protect them from unnecessary intrusion by agencies but can direct these same agencies if desired by the family or required by the child. And apart from all this, the hospital staff are my friends now and I need them.

Conclusion

Living with Kate and HIV has brought with it experiences I never thought I would face in my lifetime and it has taught me a lot about myself, about other people, about the society we live in and in particular about the things most of us take for granted such as our right to live as we choose, our right to privacy and confidentiality, an education, a job and a childminder if we need one. As a nurse I believed I had seen a lot of life. I thought I was politically and socially aware, but now I know I was naive in the extreme. I had more confidence in our establishments than they actually deserve, I was too trusting of other people and I had no real knowledge of life on the wrong side of acceptable. Now I think I am more tolerant and more understanding of individuals; in some ways I judge people less, and yet in other ways I expect more from them. I can accept ignorance from the general public but not unwillingness to learn. Yet I will not accept either of these from public agencies or employees. I have learned to speak out when I see things that are wrong. I have also learned how dangerous that can be and I have discovered you cannot use the normal measuring sticks of friendship, intelligence or education to gauge the response of people to HIV. This leaves a strange feeling of uncertainty about all aspects of life.

Most of all, I have learned that the family living with HIV and the child affected by it have the same physical, intellectual, emotional and social needs as anyone else and to deprive us is unkind and unnecessary. We do not need patronising assistance, decisions made for us or special conditions, we just need to be accepted. Every HIV-affected child can be provided with a normal life for as long as he or she is well enough to enjoy it if every agency and individual involved in the life of a family has the will and commitment to make it possible whatever the effort required.

Index